T0323940

UNDEREXPLORED MEDICINAL PLANTS FROM SUB-SAHARAN AFRICA

UNDEREXPLORED MEDICINAL PLANTS FROM SUB-SAHARAN AFRICA

PLANTS WITH THERAPEUTIC POTENTIAL FOR HUMAN HEALTH

Edited by

NAMRITA LALL

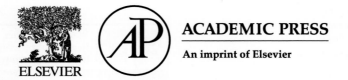

ELSEVIER

ACADEMIC PRESS
An imprint of Elsevier

Academic Press is an imprint of Elsevier
125 London Wall, London EC2Y 5AS, United Kingdom
525 B Street, Suite 1650, San Diego, CA 92101, United States
50 Hampshire Street, 5th Floor, Cambridge, MA 02139, United States
The Boulevard, Langford Lane, Kidlington, Oxford OX5 1GB, United Kingdom

Notices
Knowledge and best practice in this field are constantly changing. As new research and experience broaden our understanding, changes in research methods, professional practices, or medical treatment may become necessary.

Practitioners and researchers must always rely on their own experience and knowledge in evaluating and using any information, methods, compounds, or experiments described herein. In using such information or methods they should be mindful of their own safety and the safety of others, including parties for whom they have a professional responsibility.

To the fullest extent of the law, neither the Publisher nor the authors, contributors, or editors, assume any liability for any injury and/or damage to persons or property as a matter of products liability, negligence or otherwise, or from any use or operation of any methods, products, instructions, or ideas contained in the material herein.

Library of Congress Cataloging-in-Publication Data
A catalog record for this book is available from the Library of Congress

British Library Cataloguing-in-Publication Data
A catalogue record for this book is available from the British Library

ISBN: 978-0-12-816814-1

For information on all Academic Press publications visit our
website at https://www.elsevier.com/books-and-journals

Publisher: Andre Wolff
Acquisition Editor: Erin Hill-Parks
Editorial Project Manager: Timothy Bennett
Production Project Manager: Maria Bernard
Cover Designer: Christian J. Bilbow

Typeset by TNQ Technologies

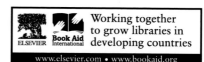

Disclaimer

This book provides a summary of different medicinal plants, their ethnobotanical usage, and scientific validation of usage. The information presented in its current form has been culled from scientific journals, book chapters, and online resources. The chapters have been peer reviewed by specialists in the field of medicinal plant sciences, phytomedicine, and ethnopharmacology. This book makes no claim with regard to the pharmacology and possible toxicity of the plants, and care should be taken when considering the plants' application. Many of you have already experienced herbal medicines and/or plant-derived compounds' positive effect on your health. We hope that through the content of this book, you gain tools to take an even greater role in your well-being. The information provided in this book is not intended to be a substitute for medical treatment. If you have any specific questions about any medicinal matter, you should consult your doctor or other professional healthcare providers. The authors take no responsibility for any wrongful or misuse of any plant mentioned in this book.

Contents

1. *Acalypha integrifolia* Willd

Nawraj Rummun, Cláudia Baider, Theeshan Bahorun, and Vidushi S. Neergheen-Bhujun

2. *Aloe lomatophylloides*

Joyce Govinden Soulange, Devina Lobine, Mala Ranghoo Sanmukhiya,
Melanie J.R. Howes, and Paul Chazot

3. *Aloe macra*

Joyce Govinden Soulange, Mala Ranghoo Sanmukhiya, Devina Lobine, Christophe Lavergne,
Melanie J.R. Howes, and Paul Chazot

4. *Aloe purpurea*

Mala Ranghoo Sanmukhiya, Joyce Govinden Soulange, Devina Lobine,
Melanie J.R. Howes, and Paul Chazot

5. *Aloe spicata*

Bianca Fibrich and Namrita Lall

6. *Aloe tormentorii*

Devina Lobine, Mala Ranghoo Sanmukhiya, Joyce Govinden Soulange, Kersley Pynee,
Melanie J.R. Howes, and Paul Chazot

7. Bauhinia galpinii
Joseph O. Erhabor and Lyndy Joy McGaw

8. Bruguiera gymnorhiza
Nabeelah Sadeer, Nadeem Nazurally, Rajesh Jeewon, and Mohamad Fawzi Mahomoodally

9. Buddleja saligna
Danielle Twilley and Namrita Lall

10. Combretum molle
Sunelle Rademan and Namrita Lall

11. *Commelina benghalensis*

Bianca Fibrich and Namrita Lall

12. *Elaeodendron transvaalense*

Thilivhali E. Tshikalange and Fatimah Lawal

13. *Equisetum ramosissimum*

Karina Szuman and Namrita Lall

14. *Eriosema kraussianum*
Riana Kleynhans, Ivy Masefako Makena, and Babalwa Matsiliza-Mlathi

15. *Erythrophleum lasianthum*
Sipho H. Chauke and Quenton Kritzinger

16. *Euclea natalensis*
Carel B. Oosthuizen and Namrita Lall

17. *Eugenia crassipetala*
Mala Ranghoo Sanmukhiya, Joyce Govinden Soulange, Jean-Claude Sevastian,
Avinash Budloo, Rachel Brunchault, and Srutee Ramprosand

18. *Eugenia tinifolia*

Nawraj Rummun, Cláudia Baider, Theeshan Bahorun, and Vidushi S. Neergheen-Bhujun

19. *Ficus glumosa*

Analike Blom van Staden and Namrita Lall

20. *Ficus lutea*

Analike Blom van Staden and Namrita Lall

21. *Ficus sur*
Analike Blom van Staden and Namrita Lall

22. *Greyia radlkoferi*
Marco Nuno De Canha and Namrita Lall

23. *Haemanthus albiflos*
Balungile Madikizela and Lyndy Joy McGaw

24. *Heteropyxis canescens*
Dikonketso Bodiba and Namrita Lall

28. *Lannea schweinfurthii*
Fatimah Lawal and Thilivhali E. Tshikalange

29. *Lippia scaberrima*
Anna-Mari Kok and Namrita Lall

30. *Newtonia buchananii*
Katlego Ellena Motlhatlego and Lyndy Joy McGaw

31. *Nymphaea caerulea*
Carel B. Oosthuizen, Matthew Fisher, and Namrita Lall

32. Ocimum labiatum

Isa A. Lambrechts and Namrita Lall

33. Phyllanthus phillyreifolius

Mohamad Fawzi Mahomoodally, Beebee Noushreen Kissoon, and Sameerchand Pudaruth

34. Plantago longissima

Bianca Fibrich and Namrita Lall

35. *Plectranthus ecklonii*
Isa A. Lambrechts and Namrita Lall

36. *Plectranthus neochilus*
Isa A. Lambrechts and Namrita Lall

37. *Rapanea melanophloeos*
Analike Blom van Staden and Namrita Lall

38. *Ravenala madagascariensis*
Shanoo Suroowan and Fawzi Mahomoodally

39. *Searsia lancea*
Murunwa Madzinga and Quenton Kritzinger

40. *Siphonochilus aethiopicus*
Anna-Mari Kok and Namrita Lall

41. *Stillingia lineata* subsp. lineata
Nawraj Rummun, Cláudia Baider, Theeshan Bahorun, and
Vidushi S. Neergheen-Bhujun

42. *Terminalia bentzoe* subsp. *bentzoe*

Nawraj Rummun, Cláudia Baider, Theeshan Bahorun, and Vidushi S. Neergheen-Bhujun

43. *Terminalia prunioides*

Fatimah Lawal and Thilivhali E. Tshikalange

44. *Vigna unguiculata*

Sipho H. Chauke and Quenton Kritzinger

45. *Wikstroemia indica*

Shanoo Suroowan and Fawzi Mahomoodally

46. *Zantedeschia aethiopica*

Karina Szuman and Namrita Lall

Contributors

Theeshan Bahorun ANDI Centre of Excellence for Biomedical and Biomaterials Research, University of Mauritius, Réduit, Republic of Mauritius

Cláudia Baider The Mauritius Herbarium, Agricultural Services, Ministry of Agro-Industry and Food Security, Réduit, Republic of Mauritius

Analike Blom van Staden Department of Plant and Soil Sciences, University of Pretoria, Pretoria, Gauteng, South Africa

Dikonketso Bodiba Department of Plant and Soil Sciences, University of Pretoria, Pretoria, Gauteng, South Africa

Rachel Brunchault Faculty of Agriculture, University of Mauritius, Réduit, Mauritius

Avinash Budloo Faculty of Agriculture, University of Mauritius, Réduit, Mauritius

Sipho H. Chauke Department of Plant and Soil Sciences, University of Pretoria, Pretoria, Gauteng, South Africa

Paul Chazot Department of Biosciences, Durham University, Durham, United Kingdom

Marco Nuno De Canha Department of Plant and Soil Sciences, University of Pretoria, Pretoria, Gauteng, South Africa

Joseph O. Erhabor Phytomedicine Programme, Department of Paraclinical Sciences, Faculty of Veterinary Sciences, University of Pretoria, Pretoria, Gauteng, South Africa; Phytomedicine Unit, Department of Plant Biology and Biotechnology, University of Benin, Benin City, Nigeria

Bianca Fibrich Department of Plant and Soil Sciences, University of Pretoria, Pretoria, Gauteng, South Africa

Matthew Fisher Department of Plant and Soil Sciences, University of Pretoria, Pretoria, Gauteng, South Africa

Melanie J.R. Howes Natural Capital and Plant Health Department, Jodrell Laboratory, Royal Botanic Gardens, Kew, United Kingdom

Rajesh Jeewon Department of Health Sciences, Faculty of Science, University of Mauritius, Réduit, Mauritius

Beebee Noushreen Kissoon Department of Health Sciences, Faculty of Science, University of Mauritius, Réduit, Mauritius

Riana Kleynhans Tshwane University of Technology, Pretoria, Gauteng, South Africa

Anna-Mari Kok   Department of Plant and Soil Sciences, University of Pretoria, Pretoria, Gauteng, South Africa

Quenton Kritzinger   Department of Plant and Soil Sciences, University of Pretoria, Pretoria, Gauteng, South Africa

Namrita Lall   Department of Plant and Soil Sciences, University of Pretoria, Pretoria, Gauteng, South Africa

Isa A. Lambrechts   Department of Plant and Soil Sciences, University of Pretoria, Pretoria, Gauteng, South Africa

Christophe Lavergne   Conservatoire Botanique National de Mascarin, La Reunion, France

Fatimah Lawal   Department of Plant and Soil Sciences, University of Pretoria, Pretoria, Gauteng, South Africa

Devina Lobine   Faculty of Agriculture, University of Mauritius, Réduit, Mauritius

Balungile Madikizela   Phytomedicine Programme, Department of Paraclinical Sciences, Faculty of Veterinary Sciences, University of Pretoria, Pretoria, Gauteng, South Africa;   University of KwaZulu-Natal, Durban, KwaZulu-Natal, South Africa

Murunwa Madzinga   Department of Plant and Soil Sciences, University of Pretoria, Pretoria, Gauteng, South Africa

Mohamad Fawzi Mahomoodally   Department of Health Sciences, Faculty of Science, University of Mauritius, Réduit, Mauritius

Ivy Masefako Makena   Tshwane University of Technology, Pretoria, Gauteng, South Africa

Babalwa Matsiliza-Mlathi   Tshwane University of Technology, Pretoria, Gauteng, South Africa

Lyndy Joy McGaw   Phytomedicine Programme, Department of Paraclinical Sciences, Faculty of Veterinary Sciences, University of Pretoria, Pretoria, Gauteng, South Africa

Katlego Ellena Motlhatlego   Phytomedicine Programme, Department of Paraclinical Sciences, Faculty of Veterinary Sciences, University of Pretoria, Pretoria, Gauteng, South Africa

Nadeem Nazurally   Department of Agricultural and Food Science, Faculty of Agriculture, University of Mauritius, Réduit, Mauritius

Vidushi S. Neergheen-Bhujun   ANDI Centre of Excellence for Biomedical and Biomaterials Research, University of Mauritius, Réduit, Republic of Mauritius; Department of Health Sciences, Faculty of Science, University of Mauritius, Réduit, Republic of Mauritius

Carel B. Oosthuizen   Department of Plant and Soil Sciences, University of Pretoria, Pretoria, Gauteng, South Africa

Sameerchand Pudaruth   Department of ICT, Faculty of Information, Communication and Digital Technologies

Kersley Pynee The Mauritius Herbarium, Ministry of Agro Industry and Food Security, Mauritius

Sunelle Rademan Department of Plant and Soil Sciences, University of Pretoria, Pretoria, Gauteng, South Africa

Srutee Ramprosand Faculty of Agriculture, University of Mauritius, Réduit, Mauritius

Nawraj Rummun ANDI Centre of Excellence for Biomedical and Biomaterials Research, University of Mauritius, Réduit, Republic of Mauritius; Department of Health Sciences, Faculty of Science, University of Mauritius, Réduit, Republic of Mauritius

Nabeelah Sadeer Department of Health Sciences, Faculty of Science, University of Mauritius, Réduit, Mauritius

Mala Ranghoo Sanmukhiya Faculty of Agriculture, University of Mauritius, Réduit, Mauritius

Jean-Claude Sevastian Faculty of Agriculture, University of Mauritius, Réduit, Mauritius

Joyce Govinden Soulange Faculty of Agriculture, University of Mauritius, Réduit, Mauritius

Shanoo Suroowan Department of Health Sciences, Faculty of Science, University of Mauritius, Réduit, Mauritius

Karina Szuman Department of Plant and Soil Sciences, University of Pretoria, Pretoria, Gauteng, South Africa

Thilivhali E. Tshikalange Department of Plant and Soil Sciences, University of Pretoria, Pretoria, Gauteng, South Africa

Danielle Twilley Department of Plant and Soil Sciences, University of Pretoria, Pretoria, Gauteng, South Africa

About the editor

Professor Namrita Lall is truly passionate about evaluating the wonders of medicinal plants and not only concludes her findings on collating information on ethnobotanical usage but takes it beyond proving their efficacy and eventually resulting in valuable pharmaceutical and cosmeceutical products. Professor Lall is a distinguished scientist in Medicinal Plant Science at the University of Pretoria. She has been placed in the Essential Science Indicators list of the top 1% of publication outputs (citations) in the discipline pharmacology and toxicology. She has international recognition for her research into the potential of medicinal plants for pharmaceutical and cosmeceutical purposes. She has made a significant contribution to the field of Medicinal Plant Science. Several medicinal plants with valuable biological activities have been discovered which led to several national and international patents. She has coauthored about 135 research articles in peer-reviewed journals and 24 book chapters. The book by Professor Lall, entitled "Medicinal Plants for Holistic Health and Well-being," was published by Elsevier in 2018.

Among several awards received in recognition for her work, a few are "The Order of Mapungubwe," South Africa's highest honor from the Honorable South African President Jacob Zuma (April 2014), Distinguished Young Women in Science Award by Naledi Pandor, Honorable Minister of the Science and Technology of South Africa (August 2011), prestigious United Kingdom Royal Society/National Research Foundation Award, South Africa (2005), "National Research Foundation/Center National de La Recherche Scientifique (CNRS) Award" (2004—05), University's "Young Exceptional Performers award (2002), S2A3-Gencor bronze medal by South African Association for the Advancement of Science (April 1997), Council Award of a Gold medal for BSc Honors (April 1994), Outstanding achievement award for PhD (March 2002), and UNESCO-L'Oreal Award for Women in Science (March 2002).

Professor Lall has presented numerous keynotes and plenary talks at international conferences. She has demonstrated commitment to community development by interacting positively with traditional health practitioners and engaging them in advancing traditional medicines toward conventional pharmaceutical products.

Readership

Professors, academics, graduate students, and amateur botanists in the areas of medicinal plant science, pharmacognosy, phytochemistry, phytomedicine, and herbal science courses, as well as the drug discovery and development scientists engaged in natural product research in the pharmaceutical and cosmeceutical industries.

Foreword

Who will doubt that medicinal plants are essential and an important resource for the future? Well, in fact, many do doubt it. Globally there is a drive to improve health care, to achieve the Global Development Goals. While these have been widely accepted as global public policy goals, there often has been a lack of recognition of the importance of medicinal plants and local/traditional medicines in this context. After considerable discussions, traditional medicine is now included in the "Declaration of Astana" (2018), which in assessing the future success of global primary health care (PHC) states: "We will apply knowledge, including scientific as well as traditional knowledge, to strengthen PHC, improve health outcomes and ensure access for all people to the right care at the right time and at the most appropriate level of care, respecting their rights, needs, dignity and autonomy." Traditional medicine is mentioned only twice, but it is included.

In this context, the book edited by Prof Namrita Lall "Underexplored Medicinal Plants from Sub-Saharan Africa" comes in as an exciting addition to our scientific and therapeutic resources. It provides an overview of such traditional uses (which is important in itself) and also includes an evaluation of the bioscientific data available on selected medicinal plants in Sub-Saharan Africa. It follows in the traditions of monographs, which are written to provide an evidence-base for their (medical) use. Prof. Lall is a distinguished scientist in medicinal plant sciences and has published extensively on the topic of ethno-pharmacology and phytomedicines. Her contribution has been recognized through various awards, including the "Order of Mapungubwe," the highest civilian honor granted by the president of South Africa for an individual's achievements internationally.

Southern Africa is a region with a unique biocultural diversity including the exceptional Cape Flora (Flora Capensis) and Africa's rich tropical flora. The entire continent is undergoing a fast and dramatic change, so summarizing and analyzing such data firstly offers an essential basis to document this richness and to ascertain that the regions of origin of these plants are fully known and recognized, and at the same time it may offer ideas for a sustainable and equitable use. Prof. Lall's effort can provide a knowledge-base, which will feed into future uses as a part of ecosystem services benefiting local people in Sub-Saharan Africa.

Compiling and assessing such data is a major undertaking, and in this volume, about 46 "underestimated and understudied" medicinal plants from Sub-Saharan Africa are included. With the numerous species present in this region, this is a tiny share, but also a very important one. Each monograph is carefully compiled covering all the ethnopharmacological aspects and very well referenced. They offer a concise and at the same time comprehensive overview of these medicinal plants. I found them fascinating to read, and the book will certainly be of interest to researchers and practitioners with an interest in medicinal plants and ethno-pharmacology, but also the "informed amateurs," i.e., the many people interested in medicinal plants.

So, for those of you who have doubts about herbal medicines, or who simply want to learn more about these fascinating plants, this book is an ideal starting point to learn about selected medicinal plants and their scientific study. And the same can be said for those who have worked in the field of ethnopharmacology and medicinal plant research. I really loved browsing through these great monographs.

Declaration of Astana (2018) World Health Organization and the United Nations Children's Fund (UNICEF), 2018. (CC BY-NC-SA 3.0 IGO licence).

Michael Heinrich
Research Group 'Pharmacognosy and Phytotherapy'
UCL School of Pharmacy, Univ. London
29 — 39 Brunswick Sq., London WC1N 1AX
Co-Chair of the UCL Research Ethics Committee (ethics@ucl.ac.uk)
https://ethics.grad.ucl.ac.uk/index.php.
Tel.: 0044-20-7753 5844/Email: m.heinrich@ucl.ac.uk.
https://scholar.google.co.uk/citations?user=jWHm_7oAAAAJ&hl=en.
https://iris.ucl.ac.uk/iris/browse/profile?upi=MHEIN39.

List of abbreviations

5637	Human primary bladder carcinoma
A431	Human vulva carcinoma cells
A549	Adenocarcinomic human alveolar basal epithelial cells
ABTS	2,2′-azinobis-3-ethylbenzothiazoline-6-sulfonic acid
AChE	Acetylcholinesterase
AGS	Human gastric epithelial adenocarcinoma cells
AIDS	Acquired immune deficiency syndrome
AlCl$_3$	Aluminum chloride
ANDI	African Network for Drugs and Diagnostic Initiative
AP	Activation protein
ARKP	Ampicillin-resistant *Klebsiella pneumoniae*
ATCC	American type culture collection
B16—F10	Murine melanoma cell line
BAE	Benzene/ethanol/ammonium hydroxide
βL$^+$EC	β-Lactamase isolated from *Escherichia coli*
BChE	Butyrylcholinesterase
BIA	Biofilm inhibition activity
CaCl$_2$	Calcium chloride
CAD	Cath.-a-differentiated
CAT	Catalase
CBA	Cytometric bead array
CBNM	Conservatoire Botanique National de Mascarin
CC$_{50}$	50% cytotoxic concentration
CCK5	Cholecystokinin 5
CEF	Chloroform/ethyl acetate/formic acid
CGMFC-21	Continuous Mangrove Forest Cover for the 21st century
CH$_2$Cl$_2$	Methylene chloride
CH$_2$OH	Hydroxymethyl
CHO	Chinese hamster ovarian cells
CITES	Convention on International Trade in Endangered Species
CNE2	Nasopharyngeal carcinoma cell line
Co115	Human colon carcinoma
CO$_2$	Carbon dioxide
COX	Cyclooxygenase
Cox B2	Coxsackie B2
CRCF	Chloramphenicol-resistant *Citrobacter freundii*
CRPA	Carbenicillin-resistant *Pseudomonas aeruginosa*
CUPRAC	Cupric reducing antioxidant capacity
DCFH-DA	2′,7′-dichlorofluorescein-diacetate
DCM	Dichloromethane
DNA	Deoxyribonucleic acid
DOPA	Dihydroxyphenylalanine
DPBAE	Diphenyl boric acid aminoethyl ester
DPPH	Diphenylpicrylhydrazyl

ED	Erectile dysfunction
ELISA	Enzyme-linked immunosorbent assay
EMW	Ethyl acetate/methanol/water
EtOAc	Ethyl acetate
EtOH	Ethanol
F254	Fluorescent indicator F254
FaDu	Hypopharyngeal carcinoma
FCBN	Fédération des Conservatoires botaniques nationaux
FCR	*Plasmodium falciparum* strain
FEC	Percentage fecal egg
FeCl$_3$	Ferric chloride
FRAP	Ferric-reducing ability of plasma
GABAA	Gamma-aminobutyric acid A
GBIF	Global Biodiversity Information Facility
GC	Gas chromatography
GCMS	Gas chromatography—mass spectrometry
GIT	Gastrointestinal tract
GOLD	Genetic optimization of ligand docking
GPx	Guaiacol peroxidase
GSH-Px	Glutathione peroxidase
H1N1	Influenza A virus subtype (swine flu)
H$_2$O	Water
H$_2$O$_2$	Hydrogen peroxide
H$_2$SO$_4$	Sulfuric acid
H37Rv	*Mycobacterium tuberculosis* strain
HaCaT	Cultured human keratinocyte cells
HeLa	Cervical carcinoma
Hep 3B	Human hepatoma
HEp-2	Human epithelial type 2
HepG2	Human liver cancer cell line
HIV	Human immunodeficiency virus
HOCl	Hypochlorous
HPLC	High-performance liquid chromatography
HPV	Human papillomavirus
Hs578T	Breast cancer cell line
HSV	Herpes simplex virus
IC$_{50}$	50% inhibitory concentration
IL	Interleukin
INF	Interferon
IRAP	Inter-retrotransposon amplified polymorphism
IRD	Institut de Recherche pour le Developpement
ISSR	Inter-simple sequence repeats
ITS	Internal transcribed spacer
IUCN	International Union for Conservation of Nature
K5625	Chronic myeloid leukemia
KB-HeLa	Subline of cervical carcinoma/cervical carcinoma derivative
Kr2	Kraussianone 2
LAB	Labdane diterpenoid
LC	Liquid chromatography
LCMS	Liquid chromatography—mass spectrometry
LC$_{50}$	50% lethal concentration
LD$_{50}$	50% lethal dose

L-DOPA	3,4-dihydroxy-L-phenylalanine
LMG 21263	*Listeria monocytogenes*
L-NAME	N_ω-Nitro-L-arginine methyl ester hydrochloride
LOX	Lipooxygenase
LPS	Lipopolysaccharide
LXFL529L	Lung tumor cells
MCF	Breast adenocarcinoma
MCF7	Human mammary adenocarcinoma
MDAMB	Breast cancer cell line
MDA-MB-231	Human mammary adenocarcinoma
MDA-MB-435S	Cancer/melanoma cell line
MED	Minimal erythema dose
MeOH	Methanol
MIC	Minimum inhibitory concentration
MMP	Mitochondrial membrane potential
MNHN	Muséum national d'Histoire Naturelle
MRC	Medical Research Council
MRSA	Methicillin-resistant *Staphylococcus aureus*
MS	Mass spectrometry
MS medium	Murashige and Skoog medium
MTS	3-(4,5-dimethylthiazol-2-yl)-5-(3-carboxymethoxyphenyl)-2-(4-sulfophenyl)-2H-tetrazolium
MTT	3-(4,5-dimethylthiazol-2-yl)-2,5-diphenyltetrazolium bromidefor
NCIB	National Center for Biotechnology Information
NF-kB	Nuclear factor kappa-light-chain-enhancer of activated B cells
NH_4OH	Ammonium hydroxide
NMR	Nuclear magnetic resonance
NO	Nitric oxide
NP/PEG	Natural products/polyethylene glycol reagent
NT	Nearly threatened
O_2^-	Superoxide anion
OH	Hydroxyl
ORAC	Oxygen radical absorbing capacity assay
ORR	Oxidation rate ratio
PBMC	Peripheral blood mononuclear cells
PC	Phosphocholine
PC-3	Human prostatic adenocarcinoma
PDA	Photodiode array
PEO	Peppermint essential oil
PHA	Phytohemagglutinin
PNE	Crude ethanol extract
PNH	Crude hexane extract
PR	Protease
Ps73	c-Jun (phospho)
PV	Poliovirus
qTOF	Quadrupole time of flight
RAPD	Relative afferent pupillary defect
RAW264.7	Mouse monocyte macrophage
RNA	Ribonucleic acid
RNase H	Ribonuclease H
ROS	Reactive oxygen species
RT	Reverse transcriptase

SANBI	South African National Biodiversity Institute
SCC-25	Squamous cell carcinoma
SCX	Si-propylsulfonic acid
SERT	Serotonin reuptake transport
SF A7	Semliki forest virus
SH-SY5Y	Neuroblastoma cells
SI	Selectivity index
SK-MEL-28	Human melanoma
SOD	Superoxide mutase
SPF	Sun protective factor
sPLA2	Secretory phospholipase A2
STZ	Streptozotocin
SVX	Shuttle vector
T24	Urinary bladder transitional cell carcinoma
TAC	Total antioxidant capacity
Tat	Trans-activator of transcription
TB	Tuberculosis
TBARS	Thiobarbituric acid reactive substances
TEAC	Trolox equivalent antioxidant capacity
TK10	Human renal cell carcinoma
TLC	Thin layer chromatography
TNF	Tumor necrosis factor
TWC	Total worm count
TZM	HeLa cell derivative
U1 cells	HIV-1 infected U937 Cells
UACC62	Human melanoma cell
UHPLC	Ultrahigh-performance liquid chromatography
UICN	L'Union internationale pour la conservation de la nature
UK	United Kingdom
UPLC	Ultra-performance liquid chromatography
UV	Ultraviolet
v/v	Volume/volume
VSV	Vesicular stomatitis virus
WCSP	World checklist of selected plant families
WI-38	Human caucasian fibroblast-like fetal lung cell
WS1	Normal fibroblast cells

Introduction

Throughout history, humankind has relied on plants for their survival. Not only does it serve as a primary food source and as building material and weapons due to its structural properties but also as a source of medicine. All cultures have their own indigenous knowledge systems that are transferred from generation to generation. Although for some cultures this knowledge has been well documented in scripts, books, databases, and online, for others this is not always the case.

Medicinal plants from Africa boast a wide variety of biological properties, which need to be discovered, documented, and explored. While other countries have extensive pharmacopoeias to use as a guideline when it comes to medicinal plants, Africa has only but a number of books which contain basic information. There have been some strides recently with the publishing of the African Herbal Pharmacopoeia, a truly valuable resource. While a second edition is in the pipeline, it focusses on the most prominent and well known and well-used medicinal plants from different countries in Africa.

There is an extreme abundance of potential drug candidates that can be discovered in the lesser known understudied medicinal plants from sub-Saharan Africa. This book attempts to showcase some of these understudied and underestimated medicinal plants. It combines the general description with traditional usage and phytochemistry. Additionally, an effort has been made to incorporate the scientific evaluation of these plants, not only to show what has been done but, more importantly, what still needs to be done.

This book presents up-to-date information on a total of 46 native and nonnative medicinal plants growing in sub-Saharan Africa. Comprehensive and useful information from published literature, including plant descriptions and origin, traditional medicinal uses, phytoconstituents, pharmacological activities, toxicity, and reported drug—herb interactions, is presented in an easy-to-read manner for easy and quick reference. There is no minimum level of knowledge required to read this book, and scientific and medical glossaries are also provided for the reader's convenience.

This book will be of great practical benefit to a wide-ranging audience. Educators and students in complementary medicine and health, pharmacognosy, medicinal chemistry, natural products, pharmacology, toxicology, pharmacovigilance, medicine, pharmacy, botany, biology, chemistry, and life sciences will find the information useful. This book is not only for scientists and advanced botanists but for any person interested in learning more about what this wonderful part of the world can offer with regard to medicinal plants, pharmacognosy, ethno-pharmacology, and botany.

Prof Namrita Lall
Editor
Dr Carel B. Oosthuizen
Editorial Assistant and Project Manager

CHAPTER

1

Acalypha integrifolia Willd

Nawraj Rummun[1,2], *Cláudia Baider*[3],
Theeshan Bahorun[1],
Vidushi S. Neergheen-Bhujun[1,2]

[1] ANDI Centre of Excellence for Biomedical and Biomaterials Research, University of Mauritius, Réduit, Republic of Mauritius; [2] Department of Health Sciences, Faculty of Science, University of Mauritius, Réduit, Republic of Mauritius; [3] The Mauritius Herbarium, Agricultural Services, Ministry of Agro-Industry and Food Security, Réduit, Republic of Mauritius

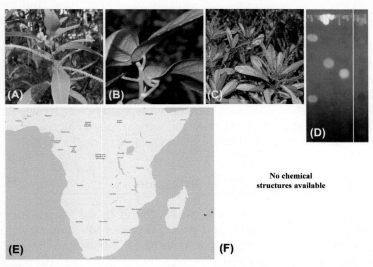

No chemical
structures available

FIGURE 1   Flowering specimen of *Acalypha integrifolia* Willd. with green leaves (Florens, V) (A), detail of a leaf with a red tinge in the abaxial side (The Mauritius Herbarium) (B), a flowering specimen with green leaves and red margin (Florens, V) (C), TLC chromatogram for flavonoid. Lane 1 bottom; rutin, top; quercitrin; Lane 2 bottom; hyperoside, top; quercetin; Lane 3; chlorogenic acid; Lane 4; *A. integrifolia* leaf extract (D), distribution of *A. integrifolia* in sub-Saharan Africa (GBIF, 2018) (E), no chemical compounds have been previously reported (F).

1. General description

1.1 Botanical nomenclature

Acalypha integrifolia Willd.

1.2 Botanical family

Euphorbiaceae

1.3 Vernacular names

Mauritius: Bois queue de rat
Réunion: Bois de crève coeur, Bois de Charles

2. Botanical description

Shrub up to 2 m tall. Branches erect; young branchlets usually glabrous, sometimes with tiny appressed hairs. Stipules 1—9 mm, triangular. Leaves variable, alternated or whorled, 4—13(−18) × 1—4.5(−6.5) cm; blade elliptical-ovate, elliptical, elliptical-obovate or oblong; base truncated or cordated; tip acute or rounded; glabrous, sometimes with hairs along the veins when young; coriaceous or papyraceous; secondary veins sometimes indistinguishable, green both sides, green with red margin or green above, red or purple below. Male inflorescence axillary, up to 20 cm long, many flowered, flowers in groups, axis hairy; female inflorescence axillary or at the base of male inflorescence, 2—5 cm long, 1—5 flowered. Flowers unisexual, more or less sessile; male flowers with small bracts; female flowers with large bract, styles 3, ovary covered with spines. Fruit 3—4 mm long. Seed, 2.5—3 mm long, pale brown. (Adapted from Coode, 1982).

3. Distribution

Acalypha integrifolia Willd is a species found in the Mascarenes only (Montero Muñoz et al., 2018) and do not occur in Madagascar as previously thought (WCSP, 2018; Tropicos, 2018). On Mauritius, the species is found at Le Pouce, Perrier and Magenta, among other sites (Coode 1982).

4. Ethnobotanical usage

The leaf is traditionally used for their astringent and purgative effect. The leaf decoction is ingested orally for their anthelmintic activity against intestinal worms. Moreover, the decoction is also applied topically to treat skin infections (Gurib-Fakim and Guého, 1996; Mahomoodally and Aumeeruddy, 2017; Rouillard and Guého, 1999; Seebaluck et al., 2015).

5. Phytochemical constituents

No isolated phytochemical has been reported from this species. The leaf, stem, and root have been reported to contain saponins, tannins, sterols, terpenes, and traces of alkaloids (Gurib-Fakim and Guého, 1996). The leaf decoction contained terpenes, tannins, coumarins, sesquiterpene lactones, and cardiac glycosides. In addition, the methanolic leaf extract also contained flavonoids (Seebaluck-Sandoram et al., 2018).

6. TLC fingerprinting of plant extracts

The air-dried leaves were exhaustively extracted with aqueous methanol (80%, v/v) and partitioned with dichloromethane. The aqueous phase was lyophilized and 5 mg of the powdered extract was dissolved in 1 mL of aqueous methanol (80%, v/v). For the reference standards, Quercitrin, quercetin, rutin, hyperoside, and chlorogenic acid were purchased from extrasynthèse (France), and 1 mg of each standard was dissolved in 1 mL methanol. For the chromatographic separation, 10 µL of extract and 5 µL of the reference standards were spotted on a silica gel 60 F254 thin layer chromatography (TLC) plate (20 cm × 20 cm). The samples were left to dry and placed in a TLC tank, presaturated with 100 mL mobile phase. The mobile phase comprised of ethyl acetate, formic acid, and water in a ratio of 8:1:1 (v/v). The samples were allowed to separate until the solvent front reached about 15 cm from the baseline. The plate was dried and sprayed with 1% methanolic diphenyl boric acid amino-ethyl ester (DPBAE) and examined in ultraviolet light at 365 nm to detect the bands on the TLC plate.

7. Pharmacological properties

Antibacterial and antifungal activity of a decoction prepared from the leaf of *Acalypha integrifolia* [=*Acalypha integrifolia* ssp. *integrifolia* var. *integrifolia*], as well as, organic extracts were reported recently (Seebaluck-Sandoram et al., 2018).

7.1 Antibacterial activity

The leaf decoction showed antibacterial activity against *Pseudomonas aeruginosa, Staphylococcus aureus, Acinetobacter* spp., *Proteus mirabilis*, and *Klebsiella* sp. The methanolic extract, however, showed more potent antibacterial activity against *S. aureus* compared to the decoction. On the other hand, the methanolic extract was equally potent against *Escherichia coli, Salmonella typhimurium, Vibrio parahaemolyticus, Propionibacterium acnes, Enterococcus faecalis*, and Methicillin-Resistant *S. aureus* (MRSA). The methanolic extract further potentiated the antibacterial activity of clinically used antibiotics such as ciprofloxacin, streptomycin, and chloramphenicol against *S. aureus*. Similarly, a synergistic effect of the methanolic extract combined with streptomycin was observed against *E. coli*.

7.2 Antifungal activity

The organic extracts including ethyl acetate extract, dichloromethane extract, and the methanolic extract of the leaves exhibited antifungal activity against *Candida albicans* and *C. tropicalis*. The methanolic extract being the most potent. On the contrary, the decoction was inactive against both *Candida* species.

8. Additional information

8.1 Therapeutic (proposed) usage

Antibacterial and antifungal

8.2 Safety data

Both the leaf decoction and methanolic extract showed low in vitro cytotoxicity against normal adult African green monkey kidney cells (Vero cells) (Seebaluck-Sandoram et al., 2018).

8.3 Trade information

The species would be classified under Least Concerned following the IUCN Red List category (IUCN, 2001).

8.4 Dosage

Not available

References

Coode, M.J.E., 1982. 160. Euphorbiacées. In: Bosser, J., Cadet, T., Guého, J., Marais, W. (Eds.), Flore des Mascareignes - La Reunion, Maurice, Rodrigues. MSIRI/ORSTOM/KEW. Imprimerie du Gouverment, Mauritius.

GBIF, 2018. *Acalypha integrifolia* Willd. In: GBIF Secretariat (2018). GBIF Backbone Taxonomy. Checklist Dataset. https://doi.org/10.15468/39omei.

Gurib-Fakim, A., Gueho, J., 1996. Plantes medicinales de Maurice, Tome 2. Editions de l'Ocean Indien, Mauritius.

IUCN, 2001. IUCN Red List Categories and Criteria, Version 3.1. IUCN Species Survival Commission, Gland, Switzerland and Cambridge, United Kingdom.

Mahomoodally, M.F., Aumeeruddy, M.Z., 2017. Promising indigenous and endemic medicinal plants from Mauritius. In: Máthé, Á. (Ed.), Medicinal and Aromatic Plants of the World - Africa. Springer Netherlands, Dordrecht, pp. 231—248. https://doi.org/10.1007/978-94-024-1120-1_9.

Montero Muñoz, I., Cardiel, J.M., Levin, G.A., 2018. Nomenclatural review of Acalypha (Euphorbiaceae) of the Western Indian Ocean Region (Madagascar, the Comoros Archipelago, the Mascarene Islands and the Seychelles Archipelago). PhytoKeys 108, 85—116. https://phytokeys.pensoft.net/articles.php?id=27284.

Rouillard, G., Guého, J., 1999. Les plantes et leur histoire à l'Ile Maurice. MSM, Mauritius.

Seebaluck-Sandoram, R., Lall, N., Fibrich, B., Van Staden, A.B., Mahomoodally, F., 2018. Antibiotic-potentiating activity, phytochemical profile, and cytotoxicity of *Acalypha integrifolia* Willd. (Euphorbiaceae). Journal of Herbal Medicine 11, 53—59. https://doi.org/10.1016/j.hermed.2017.03.005.

Seebaluck, R., Gurib-Fakim, A., Mahomoodally, F., 2015. Medicinal plants from the genus *Acalypha* (Euphorbiaceae) - a review of their ethnopharmacology and phytochemistry. Journal of Ethnopharmacology 159, 137—157. https://doi.org/10.1016/j.jep.2014.10.040.

Tropicos, 2018. Missouri Botanical Garden. http://www.tropicos.org/Name/12804707?projectid=17.

WCSP, 2018. World Checklist of Selected Plant Species. In: Goaverts, R. (Ed.). https://wscp.science.kew.org/namedetail.do?name_id=734.

Aloe lomatophylloides

Joyce Govinden Soulange[1], Devina Lobine[1],
Mala Ranghoo Sanmukhiya[1], Melanie J.R. Howes[2],
Paul Chazot[3]

[1] Faculty of Agriculture, University of Mauritius, Réduit, Mauritius;
[2] Natural Capital and Plant Health Department, Jodrell Laboratory, Royal
Botanic Gardens, Kew, United Kingdom; [3] Department of Biosciences,
Durham University, Durham, United Kingdom

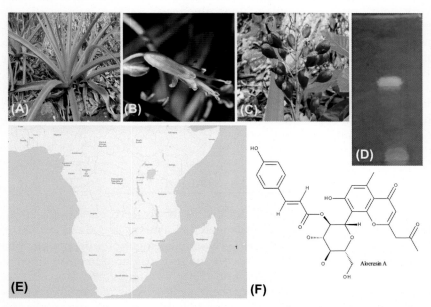

FIGURE 2 *Aloe lomatophylloides* in the wild (A), *A. lomatophylloides* flower (B),
A. lomatophylloides seeds (C), No TLC fingerprint available (D), distribution of
A. lomatophylloides in sub-Saharan Africa (GBIF, 2018) (E), chemical structure of aloeresin A (F)

Underexplored Medicinal Plants from Sub-Saharan Africa
https://doi.org/10.1016/B978-0-12-816814-1.00002-8

1. General description

1.1 Botanical nomenclature

Aloe lomatophylloides Balf. F

1.2 Botanical family

Xanthorrhoeaceae

1.3 Vernacular names

Ananas marron

2. Botanical description

Aloe lomatophylloides has a short stem, often recumbent, and 3—4 cm in diameter. The leaves are very fleshy, little oblique, pale yellowish-green fairly loose rosette of about 50—70 cm long and 8 cm wide at the base, with short prickles running along the margins. The inflorescence is 90—120 cm long with peduncle of 30—45 cm long. The flower is hermaphrodite, pedicellate, and pale-reddish-orange. The bracts are 1—2 mm in length, whereas the pedicles are 1—15 mm long. The perianth is tubular with unequal lobes and ranges from 1.3 to 2 cm in size (Antoine et al., 1978). The fruit is a globose or globose-oblong berry of about 2—2.3 cm long, and translucent green in color (Fig. 9C). The seeds are dark grayish brown and are approximately 3 mm long (Castillon and Castillon, 2010; Gurib-Fakim and Brendler, 2004).

3. Distribution

Aloe lomatophylloides is now limited to the Reserve of "Grande Montagne" of Rodrigues and is endangered (Castillon and Castillon, 2010; Gurib-Fakim and Brendler, 2004). The management of wild populations and natural habitats (in situ conservation) is considered to be an efficient and important way of conservation (Sarasan et al., 2006). However, as natural and man-made disasters are placing species in natural reserves and in unprotected areas under considerable pressure, nowadays the trend has changed to include both ex situ and in situ plant conservation strategies within an integrated conservation program including collaboration among scientific or plant breeding organizations (Khan et al., 2012; Li and Pritchard, 2009).

Given the limited population of *A. lomatophylloides* in Rodrigues, an attempt has been made to conserve this species through in vitro propagation and ex situ conservation. This species has been successfully regenerated in vitro and the true-to-type acclimatized plants have been reintroduced in the endemic garden at the Farm of University of Mauritius, Mauritius Cane Industry Authority Green Space (Réduit), Citadel, Fort Adelaide Green Space (Port Louis), Arboretum of the State House (Réduit), and Park of Mont Choisy (Lobine, 2017).

4. Ethnobotanical usage

The crushed leaves are applied as a poultice to relieve muscle pain, whereas a decoction of the leaves is taken to increase menstrual flow (Gurib-Fakim, 2003; Lobine et al., 2017b).

5. Phytochemical constituents

The first report on the phytochemistry of *A. lomatophylloides* was portrayed by Van Wyk et al. (1995), whereby they reported the presence of eight anthraquinones common to *Aloe vera* in the roots of *A. lomatophylloides*, namely, chrysophanol, asphodelin, aloechrysone, aloesaponarin, laccaic acid D-methyl ester, aloesaponol I, and aloesaponol II. Recently, the aloin and vitexin content of the Mascarene *Aloe*s and *A. vera* were evaluated, and 60.0 nmol/g of aloin and 39.6 nmol/g of vitexin were recorded in the methanolic extract of *A. lomatophylloides* (Lobine et al., 2017a). In another study, the methanolic extract of the *A. lomatophylloides* was analyzed using high-resolution liquid chromatography—ultraviolet tandem mass spectrometry (LC-UV-MS/MS), and compounds belonging to the class of anthraquinones, anthrones, chromones, and flavone C-glycosides were detected.

Furthermore, it was observed that aloesin and 2″-O-*trans*-p-coumaroylaloenin were detected in other Mascarene *Aloe*s (*A. purpurea*, *A. tormentorii*, and *A. macra*) but not in *A. lomatophylloides*, suggesting that the lack of these compounds may be useful to distinguish *A. lomatophylloides* from the other Mascarene *Aloe*s. The gas chromatography—mass spectrometry (GC-MS) analysis of monosaccharides from the Mascarene *Aloe*s revealed the presence of arabinose, fucose, xylose, mannose, and galactose. However, following a general trend, a lower concentration of sugars was observed in *A. lomatophylloides*, and it was hypothesized that the comparatively thinner leaves and firm texture of the inner mesophyll of *A. lomatophylloides* might account for its lower monosaccharide content (Lobine et al., 2017b).

6. TLC fingerprinting of plant extract

Thin layer chromatography fingerprint is not available for this plant.

7. Pharmacological properties

Historically, *Aloe* was used topically to heal wounds and various skin conditions, and orally as a laxative. Today, in addition to these uses, the use of *Aloe* is extended to traditional remedy for a variety of conditions, including diabetes, asthma, epilepsy, and osteoarthritis (Govinden-Soulange, 2014). Recent studies carried out on Mascarene *Aloe*s have revealed new therapeutic properties of *A. lomatophylloides* as described hereunder.

7.1 Antimicrobial properties

Different extracts of *Aloe* leaves were evaluated for antimicrobial activity using broth microdilution techniques, and the extracts were active against *Staphylococcus aureus, Klebsiella pneumoniae,* and *Escherichia coli.* The chloroform:methanol (4:1 v/v) extract was observed to be most effective against the tested bacteria (Ranghoo-Sanmukhiya et al., 2010). In another study, the methanolic extract of *A. tormentorii* was found to be effective against *Bacillus cereus, S. aureus,* and *E. coli,* with minimum inhibitory concentration values ranging between 3.13 and 25 mg/mL (Lobine et al., 2017b).

7.2 Antioxidant properties

Many reports have highlighted the efficacy of antioxidants in preventing or delaying the course of many diseases (Hajhashemi et al., 2010; Zhang et al., 2015). The antioxidant potential of the *A. lomatophylloides* methanolic extract was evaluated by trolox equivalent antioxidant capacity (TEAC) and total antioxidant capacity (copper-reducing equivalent) assay. The scavenging potential of the *A. lomatophylloides* assayed by the TEAC method was 0.440 mm, with this species exhibiting the highest activity compared to the other investigated Mascarene *Aloe*s. However, the extract was also characterized with lower copper-reducing activity with a value of 0.255 mm.

7.3 Neuroprotective properties

Earlier literature has highlighted some of the effects of *A. vera* on neuronal activity (Parihar et al., 2004; Rathor et al., 2014). However, crude methanolic extract of *A. lomatophylloides* displayed differential concentration-dependent neuroprotective characteristics against the toxic effects of hydrogen peroxide (250 µM) in neuronal cells (CAD) cultures with a value of 30% (Lobine et al., 2017a).

8. Additional information

8.1 Therapeutic (proposed) usage

Antimicrobial, antioxidant, and laxative

8.2 Safety data

No toxic effect has been observed on fibroblast cells (MRC 5) and neuronal cells (CAD) at concentrations up to 0.1 mg/mL.

8.3 Trade information

Endangered

8.4 Dosage

Not available

References

Antoine, R., Brenan, J.P.M., Mangenot, G., 1978. Flore Des Mascareignes, La Réunion, Maurice, Rodrigues. Familles 177–188. The Sugar Industry Research Institute, Mauritius.

Castillon, J.B., Castillon, J.P., 2010. In: Castillon, J.P. (Ed.), The Aloes of Madagascar. France and MSM Ltd., Mauritius. Etang Sale; Reunion.

GBIF, 2018. *Aloe lomatophylloides* Balf.f in GBIF Secretariat (2017). GBIF Backbone Taxonomy. Checklist dataset. https://doi.org/10.15468/39omei.

Govinden-Soulange, J., 2014. Healing Aloes from the Mascarenes Islands. In: Gurib-Fakim, A. (Ed.), Novel Plant Bioresources: Applications in Food, Medicine and Cosmetics. John Wiley & Sons, Ltd., Chichester, UK, pp. 205–214.

Gurib-Fakim, A., 2003. An Illustrated Guide to the Flora of Mauritius and the Indian Ocean Islands. Caractère Ltée: Baie du Tombeau, Mauritius.

Gurib-Fakim, A., Brendler, T., 2004. Medicinal and Aromatic Plants of Indian Ocean Islands: Madagascar, Comoros, Seychelles and Mascarenes. Medpharm, Stuttgart, Germany, 567 p.

Hajhashemi, V., Vaseghi, G., Pourfarzam, M., Abodollahi, A., 2010. Are antioxidants helpful for disease prevention? Research in Pharmaceutical Sciences 5 (1), 1–8.

Khan, S., Al-Qurainy, F., Nadeem, M., 2012. Biotechnological approaches for conservation and improvement of rare and endangered plants of Saudi Arabia. Saudi Journal of Biological Sciences 19 (1), 1–11.

Li, D.Z., Pritchard, H.W., 2009. The science and economies of ex-situ plant conservation. Cell Press 14 (11), 614–662.

Lobine, D., 2017. Validation of Biological Properties and Phylogeny of Aloes Endemic to Mascarene Islands. University of Mauritius, Réduit, Mauritius.

Lobine, D., Cummins, I., Govinden-Soulange, J., Ranghoo-Sanmukhiya, M., Lindsey, K., Chazot, P.L., Ambler, C.A., Grellscheid, S., Sharples, G., Lall, N., Lambrechts, I.A., Lavergne, C., Howes, M.J.R., 2017a. Medicinal Mascarene *Aloes*: an audit of their phytotherapeutic potential. Fitoterapia 124, 120–126.

Lobine, D., Howes, M.J.R., Cummins, I., Govinden-Soulange, J., Ranghoo-Sanmukhiya, M., Lindsey, K., Chazot, P.L., 2017b. Bioprospecting endemic Mascarene *Aloes* for potential neuroprotectants. Phytotherapy Research 31 (12), 1926–1934.

Parihar, M.S., Chaudhary, M., Shetty, R., Hemnani, T., 2004. Susceptibility of hippocampus and cerebral cortex to oxidative damage in streptozotocin treated mice: prevention by extracts of *Withania somnifera* and *Aloe vera*. Journal of Clinical Neuroscience 11 (4), 397–402.

Ranghoo-Sanmukhiya, M., Govinden-Soulange, J., Lavergne, C., Khoyratty, S., Da Silva, D., Frederich, M., Kodja, H., 2010. Molecular biology, phytochemistry and bioactivity of three endemic *Aloe* species from Mauritius and Réunion Islands. Phytochemical Analysis 21 (6), 566–574.

Rathor, N., Arora, T., Manocha, S., Patil, A.N., Mediratta, P.K., Sharma, K.K., 2014. Anticonvulsant activity of *Aloe vera* leaf extract in acute and chronic models of epilepsy in mice. Journal of Pharmacy and Pharmacology 66 (3), 477–485.

Sarasan, V., Cripps, R., Ramsay, M.M., Atherton, C., McMichen, M., Prendergast, G., Rowntree, J.K., 2006. Conservation *in vitro* of threatened plants-Progress in the past decade. In vitro Cellular and Developmental Biology-Plant 42 (3), 206–214.

Van Wyk, B.E., Yenesew, A., Dagne, E., 1995. The chemotaxonomic significance of root anthraquinones and pre-anthraquinones in the genus *Lomatophyllum* (asphodelaceae). Biochemical Systematics and Ecology 23 (7), 805–808.

Zhang, Y.J., Gan, R.Y., Li, S., Zhou, Y., Li, A.N., Xu, D.P., Li, H.B., 2015. Antioxidant phytochemicals for the prevention and treatment of chronic diseases. Molecules 20 (12), 21138–21156.

Further reading

Govinden-Soulange, J., Lobine, D., Frederich, M., Kodja, H., Coetzee, M.P.A., Ranghoo-Sanmukhiya, V.M., 2017. Metabolomic and molecular signatures of Mascarene Aloes using a multidisciplinary approach. South African Journal of Botany 108, 137–143.

3

Aloe macra

Joyce Govinden Soulange[1],
Mala Ranghoo Sanmukhiya[1], Devina Lobine[1],
Christophe Lavergne[2], Melanie J.R. Howes[3],
Paul Chazot[4]

[1] Faculty of Agriculture, University of Mauritius, Réduit, Mauritius;
[2] Conservatoire Botanique National de Mascarin, La Reunion, France;
[3] Natural Capital and Plant Health Department, Jodrell Laboratory, Royal Botanic Gardens, Kew, United Kingdom; [4] Department of Biosciences, Durham University, Durham, United Kingdom

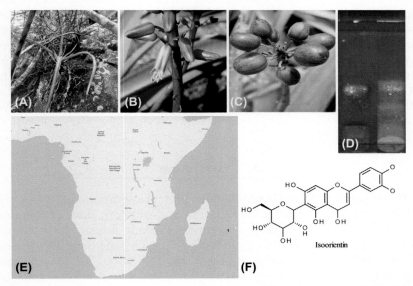

FIGURE 3 *Aloe macra* in the wild (A), *A. macra* flower (B), *A. macra* seeds (C), TLC chromatogram. Lane 1; isoorientin; Lane 2: *A. macra* crude methanolic extracts (D), distribution of *A. macra* in sub-Saharan Africa (GBIF, 2018) (E), chemical structure of isoorientin (F)

13

1. General description

1.1 Botanical nomenclature

Aloe macra Haw (synonyms: *Lomatophyllum macrum* (Haw.) Salm-Dyck, *Phylloma macrum* (Haw.) Sweet, *Lomatophyllum borbonicum* auct. non Willd.)

1.2 Botanical family

Xanthorrhoeaceae

1.3 Vernacular names

Mazambron marron or Mazambron sauvage

2. Botanical description

Aloe macra, traditionally known as Mazambron Marron or Mazambron Sauvage, is endemic to Réunion Island (France) (Govinden-Soulange, 2014) and looks similar to *A. purpurea* but is thinner, acaule, greenish, and lay on a support or down on earth. The leaves are 70 cm long and 2—7 cm wide. Morphologically, *A. macra* can be distinguished from *A. purpurea* by a spindlier character and the absence of red margin on the leaf borders (Govinden-Soulange, 2014). The flowers are brighter than those of *A. purpurea* and are reddish orange at the base and yellow at the top, tips of segments and green outside. The size of the perianth varies from 1.2 to 1.4 cm, and the pedicels are of about 1 cm long. The berry fruit is 1.1—1.5 cm in diameter (Marais and Coode, 1978; Ranghoo-Sanmukhiya et al., 2010).

3. Distribution

The majority of the wild populations of *A. macra* occurs on rocky cliffs and dry forest remnants of the northern and southern sides of Réunion Island, up to 600 m altitude, sometimes 1300 m, commonly in Grand Bassin, Entre-Deux, Mafate, Grande Chaloupe, Morne Saint-Denis, and Rivière des Pluies (Castillon and Castillon, 2010; Riou, 2017). Some rare populations also exist on exposed wet rocky walls from the east (Salazie) and south (Langevin) of the island. *Aloe macra* has been classified on the IUCN Red List of threatened species as "Endangered" (UICN France et al., 2010) because of the drastic decline in the population of *A. macra* as a result of the destruction of its habitat, by alien invasive plants, herbivores, and predators. More than 50% of the populations disappeared in 13 years (Riou, 2017). Lobine et al. (2015) have successfully micropropagated *A. macra* by using in vitro culture methods.

4. Ethnobotanical usage

The leaves of *A. macra* Haw. are used to alleviate minor infections, boils, and constipation and as a general healing substance for external use (Govinden-Soulange, 2014). The term "Mazambron" derived from Malagasy *Mahajamberon*, means who makes a grimace. To wean their children, the mothers used to put the juice of the leaves on their breasts (Lavergne, 1990).

5. Phytochemical constituents

Van Wyk et al. (1995) investigated the presence of nine different anthraquinones and pre-anthraquinones that are all known to be characteristic constituents of the subterranean metabolites of *Aloe*, in the roots of seven species of *Lomatophyllum* (now included in the *Aloe* genus) using thin layer chromatography (TLC) and high-performance liquid chromatography (HPLC) techniques. The results revealed the presence of chrysophanol and asphodelin in addition to the 1-methyl-8-hydroxyanthraquinones aloasaponarin I, aloesaponarin II, and laccaic acid D-methyl ester, together with the corresponding pre-anthraquinones were detected in *A. macra* (formerly known as *L. macrum*). A study conducted by Ranghoo-Sanmukhiya et al. (2010) revealed that in addition to the common compounds reported in Mauritian *Aloes* and *Aloe vera* (namely, anthraquinones, carbohydrates, flavonoids, steroids, sugars, and polysaccharides), other flavonoids, such as apigenin (apigenin-8-C-glucoside) and isoorientin (luteolin-6-C-glucoside) have been identified in *A. macra*. Interestingly, isoorientin was identified only in leaf extracts of *A. macra*. Nonetheless, the study also demonstrated that *A. macra* contained the lowest percentage of anthraquinones as compared with the *Aloe* species from Mauritius (Ranghoo-Sanmukhiya et al., 2010), whereas Lobine et al. (2017b) reported the occurrence of vitexin in the methanolic extract of this species. In another study, several compounds, comprising of mainly anthraquinones, anthrones, chromones, and flavone C-glycosides were detected during the liquid chromatograph—mass spectrometry analysis. The main constituents were caffeoylquinic acid, isoorientin, and isoorientin with a pentose or hexose moiety, aloesin or isomers, aloeresin or isomers, and aloin or nataloin isomer.

6. TLC fingerprinting of plant extract

Leaves of *A. macra* were obtained from Joseph Guého Arboretum, Réduit, inside the Mauritius Sugar Industry Research Institute. The samples were lyophilized and stored in air-tight bottles. The extracts were prepared according to the protocol described by Ranghoo-Sanmukhiya et al. (2010), Govinden-Soulange et al. (2017) and Lobine et al. (2017b) for respective studies. For bioassays: 100 mg of lyophilized samples were extracted in 10 mL of cold 70% methanol, heated under reflux for 1 h, sonicated for 15 min, and centrifuged for 10 min at 5000 rpm. The extract was concentrated to dryness and the residues were resuspended in water and stored in aliquots at −20°C (Lobine et al., 2017b). Two microlitres of filtered crude extract was spotted on the TLC plate and allowed to develop for 1h using ethyl acetate: formic acid: glacial acetic acid: H_2O (100:11:11:26 v/v) as the mobile phase. The developed chromatogram was observed under ultraviolet (UV) light (253 and 366 nm). The developed plate was sprayed with natural products/polyethylene glycol reagent (NP/PEG). Isoorientin and vitexin were used as controls.

7. Pharmacological properties

7.1 Antimicrobial properties

The antibacterial activity of the methanolic leaf extract of *A. macra* was evaluated using the serial dilution method. Ranghoo-Sanmukhiya et al. (2010) reported antibacterial activity of different *A. macra* extracts against *Staphylococcus aureus*, *Klebsiella pneumoniae*, and *Escherichia coli*, with minimum inhibitory concentration values varying between 0.68 and 19.38 mg/mL. Interestingly, *A. macra* was noted to exhibit higher antimicrobial activity against the tested microorganisms than those from other Mascarene *Aloe*s and *A. vera*. The potent antimicrobial activity has been ascribed to the presence of isoorientin, a flavone not detected in other Mascarene aloes or even the *A. vera*. In another study, the methanolic extract has been observed to display antimicrobial activity against five bacterial strains (two Gram-positive, *S. aureus* and *Bacillus cereus*; and three Gram-negative, *E. coli*, *Pseudomonas aeruginosa*, and *K. pneumoniae*) (Lobine et al., 2017b).

7.2 Antiviral properties

Fortin et al. (2002) investigated the effect of methanolic extract of *A. macra* against two viruses: Herpes simplex type 1 virus (HSV-1) and poliovirus type 2 (PV). The results revealed that *A. macra* contained tannins and sterols, and possess antiviral activity against HSV-1.

7.3 Antityrosinase activity

Tyrosinase is a copper-containing monooxygenase enzyme that plays a vital role in the biosynthesis of melanin, a pigment that protects the skin against external stresses such as UV irradiation and oxidative stressors. Overactivity of tyrosinase leads to overproduction of the melanin, which may cause skin disorders such as age spots, ephelides, melasma, and senile lentigines. Inhibition of the tyrosinase enzyme activity has been proved to be an effective approach of managing overproduction of melanin (Mapunya et al., 2011; Zaidi et al., 2014). In this study, the tyrosinase inhibitory activity of the Mascarene *Aloes* was evaluated according to the protocol described by Momtaz et al. (2008). Among all the tested *Aloe* extracts, only *A. macra* showed inhibitory activity against the enzyme, exhibiting 50% tyrosinase inhibition at 0.95 mg/mL, as compared to the positive control kojic acid, 0.003 mg/mL (Lobine et al., 2017b). The result suggested that *A. macra* need to be further investigated for their ability to inhibit melanin production, for exploring its potential use in cosmetics.

7.4 Antioxidant properties

The antioxidant properties of *A. macra* have been recently portrayed (Lobine et al., 2017a,b). The methanolic extract has been observed to display moderate free radical scavenging potential diphenylpicrylhydrazyl (DPPH) assay: 50% inhibitory concentration (IC_{50}) value of 0.389 mg/mL, when compared to the activity of 0.110 mg/mL for the reference antioxidant standard and Trolox equivalent antioxidant capacity assay: 0.360 mM compared to Trolox equivalents. The result for the total antioxidant capacity (copper-reducing equivalent) assay indicated that this species possess notable reducing potency (Govinden-Soulange et al., 2017; Lobine et al., 2017b).

8. Additional information

8.1 Therapeutic (proposed) usage

Antibacterial, antioxidant, and skin protection

8.2 Safety data

Survival of Cath.-a-differentiated (CAD) cells was assessed after 24 h pretreatment with *Aloe* extracts (0.01 and 0.1 mg/mL [w/v]) followed by 24 h posttreatment with 250 μM H_2O_2 (i.e., *Aloe* extracts—containing media was removed before addition of H_2O_2—preconditioning protocol). All the treatments were performed in triplicates *A. macra* extract elicited a significant delayed cytotoxicity against CAD cells.

8.3 Trade information

Endangered

8.4 Dosage

Not available

References

Castillon, J.B., Castillon, J.P., 2010. In: Castillon, J.P. (Ed.), The Aloes of Madagascar. France and MSM Ltd., Mauritius. Etang Salé; Réunion.

Fortin, H., Vigor, C., Lohézic-Le Dévéhat, F., Robin, V., Le Bossé, B., Boustie, J., Amoros, M., 2002. *In vitro* antiviral activity of thirty-six plants from La Réunion Island. Fitoterapia 73 (4), 46−350.

GBIF, 2018. *Aloe macra* Haw. In GBIF Secretariat (2017). GBIF Backbone Taxonomy. Checklist dataset. https://doi.org/10.15468/39omei.

Govinden-Soulange, J., 2014. Healing aloes from the Mascarenes Islands. In: Gurib-Fakim, A. (Ed.), Novel Plant Bioresources: Applications in Food, Medicine and Cosmetics. John Wiley & Sons, Ltd., Chichester, UK, pp. 205−214.

Govinden-Soulange, J., Lobine, D., Ranghoo-Sanmukhiya, M., Coetzee, M., Frederich, M., Kodja, H., 2017. Metabolomic and molecular profiles of Mascarene *Aloes* using a multidisciplinary approach. South African Journal of Botany 108, 137−143.

Lavergne, R., 1990. Fleurs de Bourbon, tome 9. Imprimerie Cazal, Sainte-Clotilde, 262 p.

Lobine, D., Govinden-Soulange, J., Ranghoo-Sanmukhiya, V.M., Lavergne, C., 2015. A tissue culture strategy towards the rescue of endangered Mascarene Aloes. ARPN Journal of Agricultural and Biological Science 10 (1), 28−38.

Lobine, D., Cummins, I., Govinden-Soulange, J., Ranghoo-Sanmukhiya, M., Lindsey, K., Chazot, P.L., Ambler, C.A., Grellscheid, S., Sharples, G., Lall, N., Lambrechts, I.A., Lavergne, C., Howes, M.J.R., 2017a. Medicinal Mascarene Aloes: an audit of their phytotherapeutic potential. Fitoterapia 124, 120−126.

Lobine, D., Howes, M.J.R., Cummins, I., Govinden-Soulange, J., Ranghoo-Sanmukhiya, M., Lindsey, K., Chazot, P.L., 2017b. Bioprospecting endemic Mascarene Aloes for potential neuroprotectants. Phytotherapy Research 31 (12), 1926−1934.

Mapunya, M.B., Hussein, A.A., Rodriguez, B., Lall, N., 2011. Tyrosinase activity of *Greyia flanaganii* (Bolus) constituents. Phytomedicine 18, 1006−1012.

Marais, W., Coode, M.J.E., 1978. 183. Liliacées. In: Bosser, J., Cadet, T., Guého, J., Marais, W. (Eds.), Flore des Mascareignes, La Réunion, Maurice, Rodrigues. Sugar Industry Research Institute, Mauritius, Institut de Recherche pour le Développement (IRD), Paris. Royal Botanic Gardens, Kew.

Momtaz, S., Lall, N., Basson, A., 2008. Inhibitory activities of mushroom tyrosine and DOPA oxidation by plant extracts. South African Journal of Botany 74, 577−582.

Ranghoo-Sanmukhiya, M., Govinden-Soulange, J., Lavergne, C., Khoyratty, S., Da Silva, D., Frederich, M., Kodja, H., 2010. Molecular biology, phytochemistry and bioactivity of three endemic *Aloe* species from Mauritius and Réunion islands. Phytochemical Analysis 21 (6), 566−574.

Riou, A., 2017. Le Plan Directeur de Conservation d'*Aloe macra* (Haw.): un outil Réunionnais pour conserver une espèce endémique et menacée. Mémoire de stage d'ingénieur en horticulture. AgroParisTech, Montpellier, 43 p. + annexes.

UICN France, MNHN, FCBN, CBNM, 2010. La Liste rouge des espèces menacées en France - Chapitre Flore vasculaire de La Reunion. UICN France, Paris, 23 p.

Van Wyk, B.E., Yenesew, A., Dagne, E., 1995. The chemotaxonomic significance of root anthraquinones and pre-anthraquinones in the genus *Lomatophyllum* (Asphodelaceae). Biochemical Systematics and Ecology 23 (7), 805—808.

Zaidi, K.U., Ali, A.S., Ali, S.A., Naaz, I., 2014. Microbial tyrosinases: promising enzymes for pharmaceutical, food bioprocessing, and environmental Industry. Biochemistry Research International 1—16.

Aloe purpurea

Mala Ranghoo Sanmukhiya[1],
Joyce Govinden Soulange[1], Devina Lobine[1],
Melanie J.R. Howes[2], Paul Chazot[3]

[1] Faculty of Agriculture, University of Mauritius, Réduit, Mauritius;
[2] Natural Capital and Plant Health Department, Jodrell Laboratory, Royal
Botanic Gardens, Kew, United Kingdom; [3] Department of Biosciences,
Durham University, Durham, United Kingdom

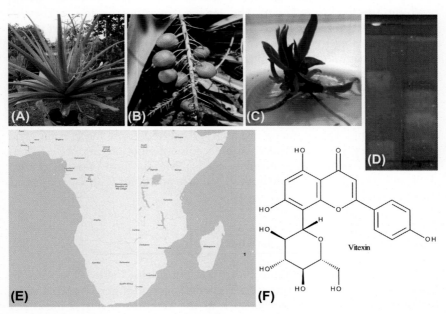

FIGURE 4 Acclimatized *Aloe purpurea* plant (A), *A. purpurea* seeds (B), In vitro regenerated *A. purpurea* plantlet (C), TLC chromatogram, Lane 1; vitexin, Lane 2; *A. purpurea* extract (D), distribution of *A. purpurea* in sub-Saharan Africa (GBIF, 2018) (E), chemical structure of vitexin (F).

Underexplored Medicinal Plants from Sub-Saharan Africa
https://doi.org/10.1016/B978-0-12-816814-1.00004-1

21

1. General description

1.1 Botanical nomenclature

Aloe purpurea Lam

1.2 Botanical family

Xanthorrhoeaceae

1.3 Vernacular names

Mazambron marron, Mazambron sauvage, and Socotrine du pays.

2. Botanical description

Aloe purpurea is the only Mascarene Aloe that forms a shrub (Govinden-Soulange, 2014), with a solitary trunk reaching 3 m in height and 7—10 cm diameter at the base. It has fleshy leaves, borne in a terminal rosette reaching up to 1 m × 12 cm. The leaves are more or less recurved, concave, dark green, or tinted with brown margins bearing short spiny, narrowly bordered with pink or red. The short spines are close to each other at the base and spaced at the tip. The panicle of the inflorescence is 20—30 cm long with a branched and flattened peduncle. The branches arise from about the same point. The flowers occur in bunches, with more or less tubular perianth (1.7—1.8 cm long), of reddish orange color. The tube is 7—9 mm long, and the lobes are little spread, unequal and of 8—10 mm long. The stamens are slightly exerted from the corolla. The fruit is a berry, which is fleshy, indehiscent, subglobular, and 1.7—1.2 cm in diameter, containing angular seeds (Marais and Coode, 1978). *A. purpurea* is highly variable both in leaf size and color (Gurib-Fakim and Brendler, 2004).

3. Distribution

Aloe purpurea is endemic to Mauritius but is also believed to exist in Réunion Island. *Aloe purpurea* is regarded as endangered and can be found growing in nature parks such as the Yemen forest and the Black River Gorges and a few private gardens around the island (Govinden-Soulange, 2014).

Aloes present a typical conservation challenge, requiring protection of taxa that are rare, endemic, and/or exploited (Grace, 2011). In view of the various "bottlenecks" associated with the propagation of *Aloe* species, plant tissue culture has been proposed as an alternative for the mass propagation of endemic Mascarene *Aloes* toward sustainable use including future research toward commercial development. A system for the in vitro regeneration of Mascarene *Aloes* was successfully developed using immature seedling explants, cultured in Murashige and Skoog (MS) medium supplemented with different plant growth regulators. The in vitro regenerated *A. purpurea* plants were acclimatized and are now cultivated in different regions of Mauritius. The genetic integrity of the regenerated and acclimatized plantlets was also confirmed by employing random amplification of polymorphic DNA, inter-simple sequence repeat, and inter-retrotransposon amplified polymorphism marker assays, and results indicated that all the tissue culture—derived plants are true-to-type (Lobine et al., 2015; Lobine, 2017).

4. Ethnobotanical usage

In the Mascarenes, the leaf sap of *A. purpurea* is applied to the breast to encourage weaning, and the leaves are also used internally as antispas-modic (Gurib-Fakim, 2003).

5. Phytochemical constituents

The chemical profile of the *A. purpurea* has been described. Preliminary phytochemical screening of *A. purpurea* leaves has revealed the presence of anthraquinones, phenols, and flavonoids and possibly alkaloids, coumarins, tannins, saponins, and terpenes in the species (Ranghoo-Sanmukhiya et al., 2010). The anthraquinone and pre-anthraquinone content of the roots of *A. purpurea* (formerly known as *Lomatophyllum purpurea*) have been investigated by Van Wyk et al. (1995) using thin layer chromatography (TLC) and high-performance liquid chromatography (HPLC) techniques. Results have confirmed the presence of six anthra-quinones namely, chrysophanol, asphodelin, aloechrysone, laccaic acid D-methyl ester, aloesaponol I, and aloesaponol II. In the study, it was also observed that *A. purpurea* leaf extracts contained the highest anthraqui-none (1.13% barbaloin) levels as compared with the other investigated Mascarene *Aloes*, *A. macra*, and *A. tormentorii*. HPLC analyses performed using the methanolic extract of *A. purpurea* has revealed the presence of aloin and vitexin at a concentration of 182.2 nmol/g and 27.6 nmol/g, respectively (Lobine et al., 2017b). Liquid chromatography—mass spec-trometry (LC-MS) and gas chromatography—mass spectrometry (GC-MS) analysis identified aloesin, aloeresin A, 2″-O-*trans*-p-coumaroyl aloenin, vitexin, isovitexin, isoorientin, and 6′-O-malonylnataloin or isomer. The GC-MS analysis also revealed the presence of arabinose, fucose, xylose, mannose, and galactose in the whole leaf methanolic extract of *A. purpurea* (Lobine et al., 2017b).

6. TLC fingerprinting of plant extract

Leaves of *A. purpurea* were collected from Joseph Guého Arboretum, Réduit, inside the Mauritius Sugar Industry Research Institute. The samples were lyophilized and stored in air-tight bottles. The extracts were prepared according to the protocol described by Ranghoo-Sanmukhiya et al. (2010), Govinden-Soulange et al. (2017), and Lobine et al. (2017a,b) for the respective study. For bioassays: 100 mg of lyophilized samples were extracted in 10 mL of cold 70% methanol, heated under reflux for 1 h, sonicated for 15 min, and centrifuged for 10 min at 5000 rpm. The extract was concentrated to dryness and the residues were resuspended in water and stored in aliquots at −20°C.

Two microlitres of the filtered crude extract was spotted on the TLC plate and allowed to develop for 1 h using ethyl acetate: formic acid: glacial acetic acid: H_2O (100: 11:11:26 v/v) as the mobile phase. The developed chromatogram was observed under ultraviolet (UV) light (253 and 366 nm). The developed plate was sprayed with natural products/polyethylene glycol reagent (NP/PEG). Isoorientin and vitexin were used as the reference compounds. Fluorescent spots showed the presence of flavonoids. NP/PEG: (1:1) aminoethanol diphenyl borate (10 g/L) in methanol + macrogol (PEG) solution 400R at 50 g/L in methanol.

7. Pharmacological properties

Recent in vitro studies have demonstrated a wide range of useful pharmacological properties of *A. purpurea*, which highlight the necessity to carry out further investigation for considering its potential to be used as phytomedicines.

7.1 Antibacterial properties

The use of *Aloe* leaves to treat microbial infections is perhaps the most popular application in this genus (Lobine et al., 2017b). The antibacterial property of *A. purpurea* was first reported by Ranghoo-Sanmukhiya et al. (2010). The different tested extracts (dichloromethane:methanol (1:1), chloroform, chloroform:methanol (4:1) and (1:1), and methanol) have shown notable activity against *Staphylococcus aureus*, *Klebsiella pneumoniae*, and *Escherichia coli*. In another activity guided study, the methanolic extract of *A. purpurea* was used to exhibit activity against *Bacillus cereus*, *S. aureus*, and *E. coli* (Lobine et al., 2017b).

7.2 Antioxidant properties

Aloe purpurea extract from Mauritius possesses potent antioxidant activity. Methanolic extract of *A. purpurea* showed remarkable scavenging potency when diphenylpicrylhydrazyl and Trolox equivalent antioxidant capacity methods were used to analyze its antioxidant potential (Govinden-Soulange et al., 2017; Lobine et al., 2017a). The methanolic extract of *A. purpurea* has also exhibited notable reducing power for copper equivalent assay. Furthermore, the methanolic extract was observed to increase the superoxide dismutase activity in differentiated Cath.-a-differentiated (CAD) cells (Lobine et al., 2017b).

7.3 Wound healing properties

In this study, the wound healing activity of *A. purpurea* was investigated by employing scratch assay on human keratinocyte (HaCaT) cells to monitor the effect of *A. purpurea* extract on fibroblast migration and proliferation into the wounded monolayer. The extract was tested at a concentration of 0.1 mg/mL, and the stimulation rate was expressed as a percentage of the closed area. The closed area with extract of *A. purpurea* was 74.1% as compared to the control (modified Eagle's medium), with 64.9% closed area, which indicated the ability of *A. purpurea* extract to reduce the damaged area after physical injury (Lobine et al., 2017b).

7.4 Neuroprotective properties

The neuroprotective property was investigated by treating CAD neuronal cells exposed to hydrogen peroxide (250 µM), with crude extracts of *A. purpurea* (0.01 and 0.1 mg/mL) for 24 h. The results demonstrated that the *A. purpurea* elicited differential significant levels of neuroprotection ranging from approximately 53% to 58% (Lobine et al., 2017a,b).

8. Additional information

8.1 Therapeutic (proposed) usage

Antibacterial, antioxidant, and wound healing

8.2 Safety data

In this study, cytotoxicity and neuroprotective characteristics of *A. purpurea* methanolic extract were measured by applying different concentrations of the extract (0.0001, 0.001, 0.01, and 0.1 mg/mL) for 24 h to CAD cell cultures. Cell viability was assessed using a standard MTT assay. *A. purpurea* extract showed no toxic effect on CAD cells.

8.3 Trade information

Endangered

8.4 Dosage

Not available

References

GBIF, 2018. *Aloe purpurea* Lam. In GBIF Secretariat (2017). GBIF Backbone Taxonomy. https://doi.org/10.15468/39omei. Checklist dataset. GBIF.org.

Govinden-Soulange, J., Lobine, D., Ranghoo-Sanmukhiya, M., Coetzee, M., Frederich, M., Kodja, H., 2017. Metabolomic and molecular profiles of Mascarene *Aloes* using a multidisciplinary approach. South African Journal of Botany 108, 137—143.

Govinden-Soulange, J., 2014. Healing Aloes from the Mascarenes islands. In: Gurib-Fakim, A. (Ed.), Novel Plant Bioresources: Applications in Food, Medicine and Cosmetics. John Wiley & Sons, Ltd., Chichester, UK, pp. 205—214.

Grace, O.M., 2011. Current perspectives on the economic botany of the genus *Aloe* L. (Xanthorrhoeaceae). South African Journal of Botany 77 (4), 980—987.

Gurib-Fakim, A., Brendler, T., 2004. Medicinal and Aromatic Plants of Indian Ocean Islands: Madagascar, Comoros, Seychelles and Mascarenes. Medpharm, Stuttgart, Germany, 567 p.

Gurib-Fakim, A., 2003. An Illustrated Guide to the Flora of Mauritius and the Indian Ocean Islands. Caractère Ltée, Baie du Tombeau, Mauritius.

Lobine, D., Govinden-Soulange, J., Ranghoo Sanmukhiya, M., Lavergne, C., 2015. A tissue culture strategy towards the rescue of endangered Mascarene Aloes. ARPN Journal of Agricultural and Biological Science 10 (1), 28—38.

Lobine, D., Cummins, I., Govinden-Soulange, J., Ranghoo-Sanmukhiya, M., Lindsey, K., Chazot, P.L., Ambler, C.A., Grellscheid, S., Sharples, G., Lall, N., Lambrechts, I.A., Lavergne, C., Howes, M.J.R., 2017a. Medicinal Mascarene *Aloes*: an audit of their phytotherapeutic potential. Fitoterapia 124, 120—126.

Lobine, D., Howes, M.J.R., Cummins, I., Govinden-Soulange, J., Ranghoo-Sanmukhiya, M., Lindsey, K., Chazot, P.L., 2017b. Bioprospecting endemic Mascarene *Aloes* for potential neuroprotectants. Phytotherapy Research 31 (12), 1926—1934.

Lobine, D., 2017. Validation of Biological Properties and Phylogeny of Aloes Endemic to Mascarene Islands. University of Mauritius, Réduit, Mauritius.

Marais, W., Coode, M.J.E., 1978. 183. Liliacées. In: Bosser, J., Cadet, T., Guého, J., Marais, W. (Eds.), Flore des Mascareignes, La Réunion, Maurice, Rodrigues. Sugar Industry Research Institute, Mauritus, Institut de Recherche pour le Développement (IRD), Paris. Royal Botanic Gardens, Kew.

Ranghoo-Sanmukhiya, M., Govinden-Soulange, J., Lavergne, C., Khoyratty, S., Da Silva, D., Frederich, M., Kodja, H., 2010. Molecular biology, phytochemistry and bioactivity of three endemic *Aloe* species from Mauritius and Réunion Islands. Phytochemical Analysis 21 (6), 566—574. https://doi.org/10.1002/pca.1234.

Van Wyk, B.E., Yenesew, A., Dagne, E., 1995. The chemotaxonomic significance of root anthraquinones and pre-anthraquinones in the genus *Lomatophyllum* (Asphodelaceae). Biochemical Systematics and Ecology 23 (7), 805—808.

Further reading

Castillon, J.B., Castillon, J.P., 2010. In: Castillon, J.P. (Ed.), The *Aloes* of Madagascar. France and MSM Ltd., Mauritius. Etang Salé; Reunion.

Aloe spicata

Bianca Fibrich, Namrita Lall

Department of Plant and Soil Sciences, University of Pretoria, Pretoria, Gauteng, South Africa

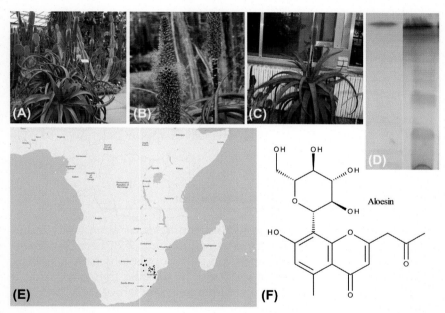

FIGURE 5 *Aloe spicata* in Botanischer Garten Dresden (BotBln, 2007) (A), *A. spicata* flower (Wolf, 2008) (B), *A. spicata* with a single flower spike (Karelj, 2008) (C), TLC chromatogram, Lane 1; *A. spicata* prevanalin spray, Lane 2; *A. spicata* postvanalin spray (D), distribution of *A. spicata* in sub-Saharan Africa (GBIF, 2018) (E), chemical structure of aloesin (F).

29

1. General description

1.1 Botanical nomenclature

Aloe spicata L.f
Synonyms: *Aloe sessiliflora* Pole-Evans, *Aloe tauri* L.C. Leach

1.2 Botanical family

Xanthorrhoeaceae

1.3 Vernacular names

Gazaland aloe, bottle brush aloe, lebombo aloe (English)
Lebombo-aalwyn (Afrikaans)
Inhlaba (isiZulu)
Tshikhopha (Tshivenda)

2. Botanical description

Aloe spicata is a multistemmed aloe, reaching heights of up to 2 m. The yellow flowers are visually similar to bottle brushes; however, they lack a stalk (Van Wyk and Smith, 1996). The leaves appear pale green to gray and are arranged as a rosette.

3. Distribution

Aloe spicata is distributed throughout South Africa, abundantly found in the Lowveld to the southern part of Limpopo, Northern KwaZulu-Natal, and southern Mpumalanga. Disjunct populations have also been identified in Northern parts of Limpopo. In addition to South Africa, it has also been identified in Mozambique and Zimbabwe (Van Wyk and Smith, 1996).

4. Ethnobotanical usage

Aloe spicata has been reported to be of ethnoveterinary use for the treatment of coccidiosis, fowl typhoid, and Newcastle disease (Mwale et al., 2005). The fruit and stem have been reportedly used for applications in skin care. Traditional claims have also been made pertaining to the skin lightning effects of *A. spicata*, however, scientific exploration by Mapunya et al. (2012) could not confirm this. *A. spicata* has been reportedly used as a laxative (Watt and Breyer-Brandwijk, 1962).

5. Phytochemical constituents

Several compounds have been isolated and identified including acetylated mannans, polymannans, anthraquinones, and anthraquinone glycosides, anthrones, and lectins. The presence of aloesin, aloin A and B, and 6-O-coumaroylaloesin have been confirmed by high-performance liquid chromatography (Cock, 2015; Van Zyl et al., 2002).

6. TLC fingerprinting of plant extract

To observe the separation of compounds present within *A. spicata*, 2 mg of the ethanolic leaf extract was weighed out and dissolved in 200 μL of ethanol. The separation of compounds present within the crude extract of *A. spicata* was observed using silica gel 60 F254 thin layer chromatography (TLC) plates. The plates were cut to size and, using a soft pencil, a line was drawn 1 cm from both the bottom and top of the plate. On the bottom line, samples were spotted approximately 1 cm apart using a capillary. The spots were allowed to dry completely and the TLC plate placed in a TLC chamber containing the eluent. Before the addition of the TLC plate, the chamber was left briefly to allow the mobile phase to totally saturate the chamber. For this experiment, 10 mL of eluent (7:3 dichloromethane: methanol [v/v]) was used. The samples were then allowed to separate until the solvent front reached the line drawn at the top of the TLC plate. After this, the TLC plate was observed under short and long wavelengths of ultraviolet light, as well as after spraying with freshly prepared vanillin.

7. Pharmacological properties

A. spicata has been reported for its antityrosinase activity, antimalarial, and antiinflammatory activity.

7.1 Antiplasmodial activity

In a study by Viljoen (1999) the plant material was dried at 28°C and powdered and extracted with methanol for 24 h. Filtered extract was dried, and their efficacy was investigated using *Plasmodium falciparum* chloroquine-resistant Gambian FCR-3 strain. Parasitized erythrocytes were cultured in vitro and the antimalarial activity determined through the titrated hypoxanthine incorporation assay for a single (48 h) and double (78 h) cycle of parasite growth. The results were compared to untreated parasites and uninfected red blood cells. Following 24 h of incubation, labeled 3H-hypoxanthine was added and the inhibition of 50% of the parasite growth was determined using a sigmoidal dose—response curve that was generated. The results revealed *A. spicata* to have antiplasmodial activity as it exhibited 92.18% inhibition at a concentration of 50 μg/mL after 24 h (single growth phase) and 63.95% after 48 h (Van Zyl et al., 2002).

7.2 Antiinflammatory

Leaf material was collected from the National Botanical Institute in Pretoria and extracted with methanol. The cyclooxygenase-I inhibitory activity was investigated by preparing cycloxygenase-I from seminal seep vesicle microsome fractions. The percentage inhibition was determined by measuring the formation of prostaglandins as compared to a solvent blank. The methanolic extract showed 92% inhibition of cyclooxygenase-I, at a concentration of 100 μg/mL (Lindsey et al., 2002).

7.3 Antityrosinase

Leaf material was collected from the Manie van der Schijff Botanical Garden of the University of Pretoria in July 2006 and ethanolic extracts were prepared. The tyrosinase inhibitory potential was determined by measuring the conversion of L-tyrosine or L-3,4-dihydroxyphenylalanine (L-DOPA), and the results were compared to that of the positive control, kojic acid. At a concentration of 500 μg/mL *A. spicata* showed poor activity as it inhibited only 13% of tyrosinase activity when L-tyrosine was used as a substrate and showed no inhibition at all when L-DOPA was used as the substrate, suggesting that it may act on the monophenolase activity of tyrosinase as a mechanism of action (Mapunya et al., 2012).

8. Additional information

8.1 Therapeutic (proposed) usage

Antimalarial, antiinflammatory, wound healing, and as a laxative

8.2 Safety data

No official safety data are available; however, Magee (2005) reported that side effects or adverse reactions may be observed when taken orally; it may damage intestinal mucosa, may induce nephrotoxicity and cardiovascular hyperactivity, and may reduce the efficacy of drugs when used in combination.

8.3 Trade information

Not threatened, not endangered, and abundant

8.4 Dosage

Not available

References

BotBln, 2007. Species: *Aloe sessilifora*; Genus: Category: Aloe; Familia: Category: Xanthorrhoeaceae Habitus and Inflorescence. Botanischer Garten Dresden. Available online: https://commons.wikimedia.org/wiki/File:Aloe_sessilifora_BotGardDresden070219_ HabitusInflorescenceB.jpg (CC BY-SA 3.0).

Cock, I.E., 2015. The genus Aloe; phytochemistry and therapeutic uses including treatments for gastrointestinal conditions and chronic inflammation. In: Rainsford, K.D. (Ed.), Novel Natural Products: Therapeutic Effects in Pain, Arthritis, and Gastro-Intestinal Diseases, twentieth ed. Springer, pp. 179–235. ISSN 0071-786x.

GBIF, 2018. *Aloe spicata* L.f. in GBIF Secretariat (2017). GBIF Backbone Taxonomy. Checklist dataset. https://doi.org/10.15468/39omei.

Karelj, 2008. *Aloe spicata*. The Botanical Gardens of Charles University, Prague, Czech Republic. Available online: https://commons.wikimedia.org/wiki/File:Aloe_spicata_Pr.jpg. The copyright holder of this work, release this work into the public domain. This applies worldwide.

Lindsey, K.K., Jager, A.K., Viljoen, A.M., 2002. Cyclooxygenase inhibitory activity of *Aloe* species. South African Journal of Botany 68, 47–50.

Magee, K.A., 2005. Herbal therapy: a review of potential health risks and medical interactions. Orthodontic and Craniofacial Research 8, 60–74.

Mapunya, M.B., Nikolova, R.V., Lall, N., 2012. Melanogenesis and antityrosinase activity of selected South African plants. Evidence-Based Complementary and Alternative Medicine 2012, 1-1-6. https://doi.org/10.1155/2012/374017.

Mwale, M., Bhebhe, E., Chimonyo, M., Halimani, T.E., 2005. Use of herbal plants in poultry health management in the Mushagashe small-scale commercial farming area in Zimbabwe. International Journal of Applied Research in Veterinary Medicine 3 (2), 163–170.

Van Wyk, B.-E., Smith, G., 1996. Guide to the Aloes of South Africa. Briza Publications, Pretoria.

Van Zyl, R.L., Viljoen, A.M., Jager, A.K., 2002. *In vitro* activity of *Aloe* extracts against *Plasmodium falciparum*. South African Journal of Botany 68, 101–110.

Viljoen, A.M., 1999. A chemotaxonomic study of phenolic leaf compounds in the genus Aloe. PhD thesis. Rand Afrikaans University, Johannesburg, South Africa.

Watt, J.M., Breyer-Brandwijk, M.G., 1962. The Medicinal and Poisonous Plants of Southern Africa and Eastern Africa: Being an Account of Their Medicinal and Other Uses, Chemical Composition, Pharmacological Effects and Toxicology in Man and Animal. Livingston.

Wolf, M., 2008. *Aloe sessilifora* im Botanischen Garten Dresden. Available online: https://commons.wikimedia.org/wiki/File:Aloe_sessilifora_Detail_01.jpg. (CC BY-SA 3.0).

CHAPTER

6

Aloe tormentorii

Devina Lobine[1], Mala Ranghoo Sanmukhiya[1],
Joyce Govinden Soulange[1], Kersley Pynee[2],
Melanie J.R. Howes[3], Paul Chazot[4]

[1] Faculty of Agriculture, University of Mauritius, Réduit, Mauritius; [2] The
Mauritius Herbarium, Ministry of Agro Industry and Food Security,
Mauritius; [3] Natural Capital and Plant Health Department, Jodrell
Laboratory, Royal Botanic Gardens, Kew, United Kingdom; [4] Department of
Biosciences, Durham University, Durham, United Kingdom

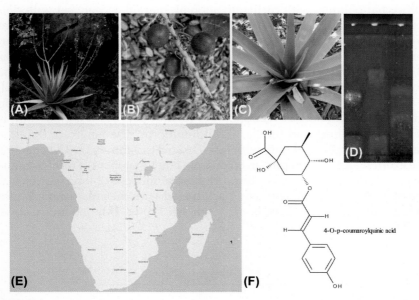

FIGURE 6 *Aloe tormentorii* in the wild (A), *A. tormentorii* berries (B), close-up of *A. tormentorii* leaves (Molteno, 2014) (C), TLC chromatogram, Lane 1; isoorientin, Lane 2; vitexin' Lane 3; *A. tormentorii* extract (D), distribution of *A. tormentorii* in sub-Saharan Africa (GBIF, 2018) (E), chemical structure of 4-O-p-coumaroylquinic acid (F).

1. General description

1.1 Botanical nomenclature

Aloe tormentorii (Marais) L.E. Newton and G.D. Rowley

1.2 Botanical family

Xanthorrhoeaceae

1.3 Vernacular names

Mazambron vert

2. Botanical description

Commonly known as "Mazambron vert" (Govinden-Soulange, 2014), *A. tormentorii* is a stemless or short-stemmed plant, of dense rosette type and not erect, but lying with few suckers. The leaves are 60 cm long and 15 cm wide, mainly at the base, channelled, rigid, ovate-acuminate, and somewhat oblique, with cartilaginous pink margin, closely set with deltoid spines. The leaves are pale green or greenish blue and can turn bronze in color when exposed to the sun. The inflorescence is 90−120 cm long, with the main peduncle of 30−35 cm long. The primary branches (3−7) are 30−60 cm long. The main raceme is up to 30 cm long, and the flowers are orange-red, green tipped. The bracts are minute, deltoid, 1−2 mm long, and the pedicels are of 1.3−2 mm long and salmon pink in color. The anthophore is very short (1−1.5 mm long), and the perianth is of 1.4−1.7 cm long and tubular-infundibuliform. The length of the tube varies between 7 and 9 mm, with lobes from 5 to 9 mm long. The stamens are exerted and salmon pink in color. Like other members of former genus *Lomatophyllum*, *A. tormentorii* bears globose or globose-oblong berries that are of 2−2.3 cm in diameter and dark-tinged with purple, turning bright orange after shedding, seeds dark grayish brown (Marais and Coode, 1978).

3. Distribution

Aloe tormentorii grows only on two small rocky islands (Round Island and Gunner's coin) in the north of Mauritius, in a much drier and sunnier area than usually assigned to species of the former genus *Lomatophyllum* (Castillon and Castillon, 2010; Marais and Coode, 1978).

Most *Aloe* species, except *A. vera*, are protected by the Convention on International Trade in Endangered Species (CITES, 2015) and are described as Endangered Species of Wild Fauna and Flora (CITES, 2015) and the International Union for Conservation of Nature (IUCN, 2015) Red List of Threatened Species. Because the natural coastal habitats of islands have been severely degraded and invaded by invasive alien exotic species, *A. tormentorii* was edging on the brink of extinction and henceforth an efficient strategy for the conservation of this endemic species has been developed. *A. tormentorii* was successfully regenerated using tissue culture techniques, and the acclimatized plantlets were cultivated into different regions. The true-to-type nature of the in vitro regenerated endemic *A. tomentorii* plants was unveiled using random amplification of polymorphic DNA, inter-simple sequence repeat, and inter-retrotransposon amplified polymorphism analysis, which is vital for any plant conservation and/or reintroduction program (Lobine et al., 2015; Lobine, 2017).

4. Ethnobotanical usage

The leaves of *A. tormentorii* are used to treat cutaneous bacterial infections and boils (Gurib-Fakim, 2003) and also used internally as antispasmodics and to relieve discomfort associated with menstruation.

5. Phytochemical constituents

Ranghoo-Sanmukhiya et al. (2010) reported the occurrence of alkaloids, anthraquinones, terpenes, phenols, flavonoids, coumarins, saponins, and tannins in leaf extracts of *A. tormentorii*, and the flavonoids detected in this species is thought to be of apigenin type. It was observed that Mauritian Aloes are richer in anthraquinone (0.95% expressed as barbaloin for *A. tormentorii* leaf extracts) than the Réunion *Aloe* sp *A. macra*. During high-performance liquid chromatography analysis of Mascarene Aloes and *A. vera*, aloin and vitexin were detected in significant amounts, with a superior concentration of vitexin in *A. tormentorii* (67.3 nmol/g) (Lobine et al., 2017b). Furthermore, spectral data obtained from liquid chromatography—mass spectrometry analysis indicated the presence of caffeoyl- and coumaroyl-quinic acid derivatives, flavonoids, chromones, anthrones, and anthraquinones in the *A. tormentorii*. Nonetheless, 4-O-p-coumaroylquinic acid and microdontin A or B were detected in *A. tormentorii* when compared to the other investigated *Aloe* species, and this compound may be considered as a biochemical marker to differentiate *A. tormentorii* from other Mascarene Aloes (Lobine et al., 2017a).

The sugar content of *A. tormentorii* has also been evaluated using gas chromatography—mass spectrometry technique, and the results revealed the presence of arabinose, fucose, xylose, mannose, and galactose, with arabinose as the predominant monosaccharide present in this species.

6. TLC fingerprinting of plant extract

Leaves of *A. tormentorii* were obtained from Joseph Guého Arboretum, Réduit, inside the Mauritius Sugar Industry Research Institute. The samples were lyophilized and stored in air-tight bottles. The extracts were prepared according to the protocol described by Ranghoo-Sanmukhiya et al. (2010), Govinden-Soulange et al. (2017), and Lobine et al. (2017a,b) for respective studies. For bioassays 100 mg of lyophilized samples were extracted in 10 mL of cold 70% methanol, heated under reflux for 1 h, sonicated for 15 min, and centrifuged for 10 min at 5000 rpm. The extract was concentrated to dryness and the residues were resuspended in water and stored in aliquots at $-20°C$ (Lobine et al., 2017a,b). Two microlitres of the filtered crude extract were loaded on the thin layer chromatography (TLC) plate and allowed to develop for 1 h using ethyl acetate:formic acid: glacial acetic acid: H_2O (100:11:11:26 v/v) as the mobile phase. The developed chromatogram was observed under ultraviolet (UV) (253 and 366 nm) light. The plate was sprayed with natural products/polyethylene glycol reagent. Isoorientin and vitexin were used as controls.

7. Pharmacological properties

Aloe tormentorii is often mistaken for *A. vera* and is hence used in the folk medicine of the Mascarene Islands to treat several ailments known to be relieved by *A. vera*. However, a few medicinal properties of *A. tormentorii* have recently been validated.

7.1 Antimicrobial properties

Serial dilution technique was used to determine the minimum inhibitory concentration (MIC) for antibacterial activity of the *A. tormentorii* extracts. In the study by Ranghoo-Sanmukhiya et al. (2010), it was found that the different tested extracts displayed noteworthy antibacterial potential against *Staphylococcus aureus*, *Klebsiella pneumoniae*, and *Escherichia coli*, with MIC values varying between 4.1 mg/mL and 21.6 mg/mL, with the chloroform:methanol (4:1) extract showing the lowest MIC values (Ranghoo-Sanmukhiya et al., 2010). *A. tormentorii* methanolic extract has also been reported to exhibit antimicrobial potential against *Bacillus cereus, S. aureus,* and *E. coli,* with MIC values varying between 3.13 and 25 mg/mL (Lobine et al., 2017a).

7.2 Antioxidant properties

A multiple assay system was employed to provide a comprehensive prediction of the antioxidant efficacy of the *A. tomentorii* extracts. The antioxidant activities of the methanolic *A. tormentorii* extract based on diphenylpicrylhydrazyl (DPPH), Trolox equivalent antioxidant capacity (TEAC), and total antioxidant capacity (TAC) (copper-reducing equivalent) revealed that this *Aloe* species possesses significant radical scavenging and reducing potential. For the DPPH assay, the 50% inhibitory concentration (IC_{50}) values (0.413 mg/L) of the crude extracts was comparable to the activity of 0.110 mg/mL for the reference antioxidant standard (quercetin), and for the TEAC method, the scavenging potential was 0.38 mM, as compared to Trolox equivalents (Govinden-Soulange et al., 2017; Lobine et al., 2017b). *A. tormentorii* was characterized by moderate copper-reducing activity with a value of 0.311 mM (Lobine et al., 2017b).

7.3 Neuroprotective properties

In this study, the healing Mascarene Aloes were evaluated for their neuroprotective properties of relevant neurodegenerative diseases. The results also revealed that 0.01 mg/mL of the *A. tormentorii* extract demonstrated differential concentration-dependent neuroprotective characteristics (74% neuroprotection) against the toxic effects of hydrogen peroxide (250 µM) in Cath.-a-differentiated (CAD) cell cultures (Lobine et al., 2017b).

8. Additional information

8.1 Therapeutic (proposed) usage

Antibacterial and wound healing

8.2 Safety data

In vitro cytotoxicity screening using the MTT assay indicated that the crude methanolic extract of *A. tormentorii* elicited no toxic effect on CAD neuronal cells at concentrations up to 0.1 mg/mL.

8.3 Trade information

Endangered

8.4 Dosage

Not available

References

Castillon, J.B., Castillon, J.P., 2010. In: Castillon, J.P., Sale, E. (Eds.), The Aloes of Madagascar. France and MSM Ltd., Mauritius. Réunion.

CITES, 2015 (Online). https://cites.org/sites/default/files/eng/app/2015/E-Appendices-2015-02-05.pdf.

GBIF, 2018. Aloe tormentorii (Marais) L.E.Newton & G.D.Rowley in GBIF Secretariat (2018). GBIF Backbone Taxonomy. Checklist dataset. https://doi.org/10.15468/39omei, accessed via GBIF.org.

Govinden-Soulange, J., 2014. Healing Aloes from the Mascarenes islands. In: Gurib-Fakim, A. (Ed.), Novel Plant Bioresources: Applications in Food, Medicine and Cosmetics. John Wiley & Sons, Ltd., Chichester, UK, pp. 205–214.

Govinden-Soulange, J., Lobine, D., Ranghoo-Sanmukhiya, M., Coetzee, M., Frederich, M., Kodja, H., 2017. Metabolomic and Molecular profiles of Mascarene Aloes using a multidisciplinary approach. South African Journal of Botany 108, 137–143.

Gurib-Fakim, A., 2003. An Illustrated Guide to the Flora of Mauritius and the Indian Ocean Islands. Caractère Ltée, Baie du Tombeau, Mauritius.

IUCN, 2015. Red List of Threatened Species (Online). http://www.iucnredlist.org.

Lobine, D., 2017. Validation of Biological Properties and Phylogeny of *Aloes* Endemic to Mascarene Islands. University of Mauritius, Réduit, Mauritius.

Lobine, D., Govinden-Soulange, J., Ranghoo Sanmukhiya, M., Lavergne, C., 2015. A tissue culture strategy towards the rescue of endangered Mascarene Aloes. ARPN Journal of Agricultural and Biological Science 10 (1), 28–38.

Lobine, D., Cummins, I., Govinden-Soulange, J., Ranghoo-Sanmukhiya, M., Lindsey, K., Chazot, P.L., Ambler, C.A., Grellscheid, S., Sharples, G., Lall, N., Lambrechts, I.A., Lavergne, C., Howes, M.J.R., 2017a. Medicinal Mascarene Aloes: an audit of their phytotherapeutic potential. Fitoterapia 124, 120–126.

Lobine, D., Howes, M.J.R., Cummins, I., Govinden-Soulange, J., Ranghoo-Sanmukhiya, M., Lindsey, K., Chazot, P.L., 2017b. Bioprospecting endemic Mascarene Aloes for potential neuroprotectants. Phytotherapy Research 31 (12), 1926–1934.

Marais, W., Coode, M.J.E., 1978. 183. *Liliacées*. In: Bosser, J., Cadet, T., Julien, H.R., Marais, W. (Eds.), *Flore des Mascareignes - La Réunion, Maurice, Rodrigues. 177. Iridacées* à 188. *Joncacées*, pp. 1–41. Institut de Recherche pour le Développement, Paris; Mauritius Sugar Industry Research Institute, Ile Maurice; The Royal Botanic Gardens, Kew.

Molteno, S., 2014. Aloe Tormentorii - Ile Aux Aigrettes - Mauritius. Species Previously Classed as Lomatophyllum Tormentorii. Available online: https://commons. wikimedia.org/wiki/File:Aloe_tormentorii_-_Ile_aux_aigrettes_-_3.jpg. The copyright holder of this work, release this work into the public domain. This applies worldwide.

Ranghoo-Sanmukhiya, M., Govinden-Soulange, J., Lavergne, C., Khoyratty, S., Da Silva, D., Frederich, M., Kodja, H., 2010. Molecular biology, phytochemistry and bioactivity of three endemic *Aloe* species from Mauritius and Réunion Islands. Phytochemical Analysis 21 (6), 566–574.

Bauhinia galpinii

Joseph O. Erhabor[1,2], Lyndy Joy McGaw[1]

[1] Phytomedicine Programme, Department of Paraclinical Sciences, Faculty of Veterinary Sciences, University of Pretoria, Pretoria, Gauteng, South Africa; [2] Phytomedicine Unit, Department of Plant Biology and Biotechnology, University of Benin, Benin City, Nigeria

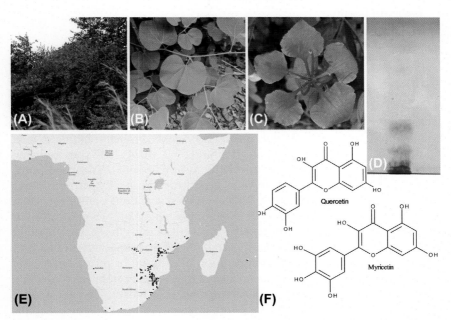

FIGURE 7   Aerial plant parts of *Bauhinia galpinii* (Bernard, 2015) (**A**), leaves of *B. galpinii* (Vengolis, 2017) (**B**), flowers of *B. galpinii* (Rulkens, 2010) (**C**), TLC chromatogram, fingerprint of *B. galpinii* (**D**), distribution of *B. galpinii* in sub-Saharan Africa (GBIF, 2018) (**E**), chemical structures of quercetin and myricetin (**F**).

1. General description

1.1 Botanical nomenclature

Bauhinia galpinii N.E.Br

1.2 Botanical family

Fabaceae

1.3 Vernacular names

Pride of De Kaap; Pride of the Cape; Lowveld Bauhinia, red bauhinia (English).
Vlam-van-die-Vlakte; Beesklou-klimop (Afrikaans).
Kisololo (Siswati).
Motshiwiriri (Sesotho sa Leboa).
Tswiriri (Tswana).
Mutswiriri (Tshivenda).
Umvangatane, Umvangatane Usololo, Umhuwa (Zulu).

2. Botanical description

B. galpinii is a leguminous plant from the Fabaceae family. The genus was named after the Bauhin brothers, Swiss—French botanists Jean Bauhin (1541—1612) and Gaspard Bauhin (1560—1624). The species name *'galpinii'* was in commemoration of the famous South African botanist, Ernest Edward Galpin. *B. galpinii* is a pantropical, hardy, drought, and frost-resistant shrub or climber. This evergreen scandent plant grows fast and climbs into surrounding trees reaching a height of 3—5 m or more. It has broad leaves borne on short stalks with entire margins that are bilobed at the tip. The leaves are alternately arranged, often folded lengthwise and appear like the double-leaf configuration of a heart, or more commonly like a butterfly wing. The upper surface of the leaves is glabrous (hairless), whereas the underside is puberulent (sparsely hairy). The terracotta-coloured flowers (orange to dark red flowers) have five brown sepals, five to eight large spade-shaped petals, and three stamens. Flowering occurs throughout the year, but mostly during late spring and summer (i.e., from November to March). The elongated fruit pod has large seeds that are dark reddish-brown in color (Akhter et al., 2012; Anonymous, 2018; Lorraine, 2011; Shakya et al., 2016).

3. Distribution

B. galpinii is an evergreen rambling shrub endemic to eastern and southern Africa, where it is popularly called the Pride of De Kaap (Shakya et al., 2016). This common popular name, Pride of De Kaap, was derived from the De Kaap valley in the south of Nelspruit in Mpumalanga, northeastern region of South Africa, where it is extensively widespread (Hankey, 2001). This indigenous South African plant common in the bushveld areas of the country can also be found in Swaziland, Zimbabwe, Mozambique, Egypt, and India (Lorraine, 2011). It is commonly cultivated in the warm areas of the United States and Mexico where it has naturalized without any significant threat of invasiveness.

4. Ethnobotanical usage

Generally, *Bauhinia* species including those native to South Africa are used in folk medicine across the world to treat an array of diseases such as diabetes, inflammation, pain, gastrointestinal tract disorders, and infectious diseases (Ahmed et al., 2012; Filho, 2009). Traditionally, *B. galpinii* leaves are used for the treatment of epilepsy and convulsions (Risa et al., 2004) while the bark and leaves are utilized to treat diarrhea and infertility (Mabogo, 1990; Samie et al., 2010). The seeds of this ornamental plant can also be used to treat amenorrhea (Van Wyk and Gericke, 2000), the bark and root are used against stomach spasms, and the root is used to manage infertility (Arnold and Gulumian, 1984). The tuber of red bauhinia is also reported for treating pneumonia, venereal diseases, and diarrhea (Van Wyk and Gericke, 2000). A decoction of the root is used for improving sexual performance and for treating stomach worms while a soft porridge of the root mixture/concoction can be utilized to alleviate stomach pains (Mahwasane et al., 2013). The indigenous people of South Africa use the long flexible branches for weaving baskets and for constructing roof trusses for their huts (Hankey, 2001). The flowers are very attractive to bees, butterflies, birds, and other insects, providing pollen that is of great value to pollinators. The shrubby and sheltering habit of this plant make it a common nesting site for small birds. The leaves and twigs are very good forage for sheep and goats (Lorraine, 2011; Watt and Breyer Brandwijk, 1962).

5. Phytochemical constituents

Three major compounds, the flavonoid glycosides quercetin-3-O-galactopyranoside, myricetin-3-O-galactopyranoside, and 2″-O-rhamnosylvitexin, were previously isolated and identified from the leaves of *B. galpinii* (Aderogba et al., 2007). In a PhD study, four bioactive compounds (β-3 ethoxy sitosterol, isoetin 2′-methyl ether or isoetin 4′-methyl ether, 3, 5, 7, 3′, 4′-pentahydroxyflavone (quercetin), and 3, 5, 7, 3′, 4′, 5′hexahydroxyflavone (myricetin)) and two previously isolated compounds (quercetin-3-O-β-galactopyranoside and myricetin-3-O-β-galactopyranoside) were identified and characterized from the leaves (Ahmed, 2013). Farag et al. (2015) also identified nine compounds from the leaves and shoots of *B. galpinii*, whereas three other compounds and one unidentified compound were found only in the leaf. The identified compounds include (epi)catechin dimer, (epi)catechin, (epi)catechin trimer, (epi)afzelechin—(epi)catechin dimer, luteolin-C-hexoside, rutin, apigenin-C-hexoside, quercetin-3-O-hexoside (isoquercetin), kaempferol-3-O-rutinoside, isorhamnetin-3-O-rutinoside, quercetin-3-O-rhamnoside, and isorhamnetin-3-O-hexoside. No compound thus far has been isolated from the seed, tuber, flower, stem bark, or root.

6. TLC fingerprinting of plant extract

For the separation of *B. galpinii*, 100 mg of the 70% ethanolic extract was weighed and dissolved in 10 mL of either acetone or methanol. For the thin layer chromatography (TLC) analysis of *B. galpinii* crude extract, TLC silica gel 60 F_{254} plates were used to observe the separation of the compounds present within the extract. Ten microliters of the sample was spotted onto the TLC plate. The spots were allowed to dry completely and placed in a TLC tank, which contained a 10 mL eluent 8:2:1 ethyl acetate:methanol:formic acid solvent system. The sample was allowed to separate until the solvent system reached 1 cm from the top of the TLC plate. A freshly prepared vanillin (0.1 g) dissolved in methanol (28 mL) and 1 mL sulfuric acid was used to detect the bands on the TLC plate, and the plate was observed under ultraviolet (UV) light (254 nm).

7. Pharmacological properties

Pharmacological activity studies on *B. galpinii* have been predominantly conducted on the leaves with very few reports on the root bark and apical bud. Biological activity studies on the shoot, flower, stem, and tuber are also yet to be reported. Following the ethnomedical reports, extensive usage and wide distribution in South Africa and in the tropics of *B. galpinii*, there is still much opportunity for it to be explored in future research and development.

7.1 Antimicrobial activity

A previous study revealed that the acidified 70% acetone leaf extract, fractions, and isolated compounds were active against a range of common bacterial and fungal strains. In the study, enhanced polyphenolic-rich acetone crude extract showed moderate activity against the Gram-positive bacteria (*Staphylococcus aureus* American Type Culture Collection [ATCC] 29213, *Enterococcus faecalis* ATCC 29212) and Gram-negative bacteria (*Pseudomonas aeruginosa* ATCC 27853, *Escherichia coli* ATCC 25922) with minimum inhibitory concentrations (MIC) values ranging from 156 to 625 µg/mL. Of the five fractions (butanol, hexane, ethyl acetate, dichloromethane, and water), the hexane fraction showed excellent antibacterial activity with MIC value of 39 µg/mL against *E. coli* and *S. aureus*. Similarly, noteworthy activity was also observed with the dichloromethane and ethyl acetate fractions against *E. faecalis* and *S. aureus* with MIC of 39 µg/mL against both organisms. The isolated compounds (3β-ethoxyl sitosterol, quercetin-3-O-β-galactopyranose, myricetin-3-O-β-galactopyranose, quercetin, and myricetin) tested against the four microorganisms were found to be active with MIC values ranging from 7.8 to 125 µg/mL. The compound 3,5,7,3′,4′,5′-hexahydroxyflavone (myricetin) showed the best antibacterial activity against *E. faecalis* with an MIC of 7.8 µg/mL. On the other hand, the crude extract, fractions, and isolated compounds were also found to be active against the fungal organisms. The acidified phenolic-rich crude extract of *B. galpinii* leaf had excellent antifungal activity against *Cryptococcus neoformans* (MIC of 7.8 µg/mL), whereas *Aspergillus fumigatus* (MIC of 625 µg/mL) was most resistant against it. The butanol fraction with an MIC of 39 µg/mL had the best antifungal activity against *C. neoformans* while the isolated compounds quercetin and myricetin had excellent antifungal activity against both clinical isolates (M0825, 1051604, 1051608) and ATCC (10231) strains of *Candida albicans* (Ahmed et al., 2012; Ahmed, 2013).

In another study, the acetone root bark extract was tested against 110 clinical strains of *Campylobacter*. It was found that the acetone extract of *B. galpinii* root bark had good anticampylobacter activity (MIC of 0.75 mg/mL) against three of the isolates representing 2.7% of the 110 *Campylobacter* strains. The extract was also active against 78 isolates of the 110 clinical strains of *Campylobacter* (71% of the strains) with an MIC of 1.5 mg/mL, whereas at MICs of 3 mg/mL and 6 mg/mL, it was active against 23 isolates (21% of the strains) and 6 isolates (5.4% of the strains) respectively (Samie et al., 2009).

7.2 Antidiabetic and antiinflammatory activities

In 2015, Farag and colleagues evaluated the antidiabetic activity of lyophilized 70% methanolic extract of *B. galpinii* leaves using the alpha-glucosidase enzyme inhibition assay. The leaves were sourced from Orman Botanical garden, Giza, Egypt, and a lyophilized 70% methanolic extract was prepared. The lyophilized extract had outstanding inhibitory activity against the alpha-glucosidase enzyme (50% inhibitory concentration (IC_{50}) of 20 µg/mL). In another study conducted by Shakya and coworkers, the antidiabetic activity of the ethanolic extract of *B. galpinii* leaves was determined using alloxan-induced diabetic rats. The ethanolic extract at 250 and 500 mg/kg displayed a significant dose-dependent antihyperglycemic activity with fasting blood glucose levels of 252.06 and 189.83 mg/dL against base values of 284.48 and 287.48 mg/dL, respectively (Shakya et al., 2016).

The antiinflammatory activity of *B. galpinii* leaves was assessed against cyclooxygenase-1 (COX-1), cyclooxygenase-2 (COX-2), and 15-lipoxygenase enzymes by Ahmed et al. (2012). It was found that the phenolic-rich acetone leaf extract had inhibitory activity against the COX-1 and 15-lipoxygenase (15-LOX) enzymes but showed no inhibition against the COX-2 enzyme. The extract at a concentration of 377.66 µg/mL inhibited 50% of the COX-1 enzyme, whereas at 25 µg/mL it had moderate percentage inhibitory activity against the 15-LOX enzyme with 56.31% inhibition and an IC_{50} value of 4.10 µg/mL (Ahmed et al., 2012; Ahmed, 2013).

7.3 Antioxidant activity

In a previous study, Aderogba et al. (2007) quantitatively determined the radical scavenging potential of the crude extracts, solvent fractions, and isolated compounds from *B. galpinii* leaf. The leaves were collected from the MEDUNSA campus of the University of Limpopo, South Africa. The air-dried powdered leaves were initially extracted with methanol and the marc re-extracted with 10% aqueous methanol. The fractions were obtained by sequential extraction of the combined extracts suspended in distilled water with the various extracting solvents (hexane, dichloromethane, ethyl acetate, and butanol) to get the corresponding fractions. Furthermore, the antioxidant capacity of the extract, fractions, and isolated compounds (obtained via column chromatography on silica gel and Sephadex LH-20) were tested using the diphenylpicrylhydrazyl (DPPH) radical scavenging assay. Myricetin-3-O-galactopyranoside had the best inhibitory activity (IC_{50} of 11.33 µM) in the DPPH free radical scavenging assay as compared to quercetin-3-O-galactopyranoside (IC_{50} of 20.52 µM) and 2″-O-rhamnosylvitexin (IC_{50} not determined, as it failed to scavenge

50% of the DPPH radical at the tested concentrations). Although the crude extract showed considerable DPPH radical scavenging capacity with an IC_{50} value of 31.73 µg/mL, the butanol fractions among the tested fractions gave the best antioxidant activity with an IC_{50} value of 28.85 µg/mL.

In another study, Kaur and Arora (2010) revealed that the methanol extract of *B. galpinii* bark and leaf had moderate inhibitory activity (45.45% and 50.60%) against the superoxide anion radical at 700 and 800 µg/mL, respectively. In a separate investigation conducted by Ahmed (2013) it was found that the phenolic-enriched crude extract and fractions of *B. galpinii* leaves had strong antioxidant activity in a concentration-dependent manner against DPPH and 2,2′-azinobis-3-ethylbenzothiazoline-6-sulfonic acid (ABTS) radical as well as a strong ferric ion reducing capacity. Of the extract and fractions, the butanol fraction showed the best antiradical activity against the DPPH (IC_{50} of 1.02 µg/mL) and ABTS (IC_{50} of 0.89 µg/mL) radicals. It also exhibited the strongest ferric ion reducing capacity (32.70). Farag et al. (2015) in their investigation of the lyophilized 70% methanolic extract of *B. galpinii* leaves, revealed that the extract had moderate inhibitory activity (49.6 µg/mL) against the DPPH radical.

8. Additional information

8.1 Therapeutic (proposed) usage

Antibacterial, antifungal, antidiabetic, and antiinflammatory

8.2 Safety data

The dichloromethane and 90% methanolic extract of *B. galpinii* leaves had strong antigenotoxic properties in the Ames and Vitotox tests or assays (Verschaeve and Van Staden, 2008). In a cytotoxicity test (1-(4,5-dimethylthiazol-2-yl)-3,5-diphenylformazan [MTT] viability assay) conducted on three isolated compounds from the leaves of *B. galpinii* by Aderogba et al. (2007), it was found that myricetin-3-O-galactopyranoside was cytotoxic to Vero cells (IC_{50} of 74.68 µg/mL) and bovine dermis cells (IC_{50} of 30.69 µg/mL), whereas quercetin-3-O-galactopyranoside and 2-O-rhamnosylvitexin were noncytotoxic to both cells. The acetone bark extract in another cytotoxicity study was found to be very toxic to Vero cells (IC_{50} of 2.71 µg/mL) in the MTT-formazan viability assay (Samie et al., 2009). Ahmed et al. (2012) using the MTT assay showed that the phenolic-enriched acidified 70% acetone leaf extract had a concentration-dependent low cytotoxic effect on Vero African monkey kidney cells with an IC_{50} value of 35.68 µg/mL. Lastly, the apical bud of the plant was found not to possess any hydroxynitrile lyase activity and was noncyanogenic (Kassim et al., 2014).

8.3 Trade information

Not threatened, not endangered, and abundant.

8.4 Dosage

Not available

References

Aderogba, M., McGaw, L.J., Ogundaini, A., Eloff, J., 2007. Antioxidant activity and cytotoxicity study of the flavonol glycosides from *Bauhinia galpinii*. Natural Product Research 21, 591–599.

Ahmed, A.S., 2013. Biological Activities of Extracts and Isolated Compounds from *Bauhinia Galpinii* (Fabaceae) and *Combretum Vendae* (Combretaceae) as Potential Antidiarrhoeal Agents. University of Pretoria (Doctoral dissertation.

Ahmed, A.S., Elgorashi, E.E., Moodley, N., McGaw, L.J., Naidoo, V., Eloff, J.N., 2012. The antimicrobial, antioxidative, anti-inflammatory activity and cytotoxicity of different fractions of four South African *Bauhinia* species used traditionally to treat diarrhoea. Journal of Ethnopharmacology 143, 826–839.

Akhter, M.S., Rahman, S.M.M., Rahman, M.H., 2012. Micropropagation of *Bauhinia acuminata* L. International Research Journal of Applied Life Sciences 1 (3), 35–43.

Anonymous, 2018. Red bauhinia, Bauhinia galpinii. Brisbane City Council. Available at: https://weeds.brisbane.qld.gov.au/weeds/red-bauhinia.

Arnold, H.-J., Gulumian, M., 1984. Pharmacopoeia of traditional medicine in Venda. Journal of Ethnopharmacology 12, 35–74.

Bernard, D., 2015. S110 Road East of Berg-en-Dal. Kruger NP, South Africa. Available online: https://commons.wikimedia.org/wiki/File:Red_Bauhinia_(Bauhinia_galpinii)_(16510446185).jpg.(CCBY-SA2.0).

Farag, M.A., Sakna, S.T., El-fiky, N.M., Shabana, M.M., Wessjohann, L.A., 2015. Phytochemical, antioxidant and antidiabetic evaluation of eight *Bauhinia* L. species from Egypt using UHPLC–PDA–qTOF-MS and chemometrics. Phytochemistry 119, 41–50.

Filho, V.C., 2009. Chemical composition and biological potential of plants from the genus *Bauhinia*. Phytotherapy Research 23, 1347–1354.

GBIF, 2018. *Bauhinia galpinii* N.E.Br. In GBIF Secretariat (2017). GBIF Backbone Taxonomy. Checklist dataset. https://doi.org/10.15468/39omei.

Hankey, A., 2001. Bauhinia galginii. Plantza Africa. Available online. http://pza.sanbi.org/bauhinia-galpinii.

Kassim, M.A., Sooklal, S.A., Archer, R., Rumbold, K., 2014. Screening for hydroxynitrile lyase activity in non-commercialised plants. South African Journal of Botany 93, 9–13.

Kaur, P., Arora, S., 2010. Comparison of antioxidant activity of different methanol extract of Cassia and *Bauhinia* sp. Journal of Chinese Clinical Medicine 5, 457–462.

Lorraine, S., 2011. Bauhinia galpinii. A database of Indigenous South African Flora. Available at: https://kumbulanursery.co.za/plants/bauhinia-galpinii.

Mabogo, D.E.N., 1990. The Ethnobotany of the Vhavenda. University of Pretoria. PhD thesis.

Mahwasane, S.T., Middleton, L., Boaduo, N., 2013. An ethnobotanical survey of indigenous knowledge on medicinal plants used by the traditional healers of the Lwamondo area, Limpopo province, South Africa. South African Journal of Botany 88, 69–75.

Risa, J., Risa, A., Adsersen, A., Gauguin, B., Stafford, G.I., Van Staden, J., Jäger, A.K., 2004. Screening of plants used in southern Africa for epilepsy and convulsions in the GABAA-benzodiazepine receptor assay. Journal of Ethnopharmacology 93, 177–182.

Rulkens, T., 2010. Flower of *Bauhinia galpinii*, Growing in the Wild Close to Chimoio. Mozambique. Available online. https://commons.wikimedia.org/wiki/File:Bauhinia_galpinii_2.jpg. (CC BY-SA 2.0.

Shakya, P.C., Irchhaiya, R., Alok, S., 2016. Antidiabetic activity ethanolic leaves extract of *Bauhinia galpinii* linn. alloxan induced diabetic in rats. International Journal of Pharmacognosy 3, 281–287.

Samie, A., Obi, C.L., Lall, N., Meyer, J.J.M., 2009. *In vitro* cytotoxicity and antimicrobial activities, against clinical isolates of Campylobacter species and *Entamoeba histolytica*, of local medicinal plants from the Venda region, in South Africa. Annals of Tropical Medicine and Parasitology 103, 159–170.

Samie, A., Tambani, T., Harshfield, E., Green, E., Ramalivhana, J., Bessong, P., 2010. Antifungal activities of selected Venda medicinal plants against *Candida albicans*, *Candida krusei* and *Cryptococcus neoformans* isolated from South African AIDS patients. African Journal of Biotechnology 9 (20), 2965–2976.

Van Wyk, B.-E., Gericke, N., 2000. People's Plants: A Guide to Useful Plants of Southern Africa. Briza Publications.

Vengolis, 2017. Lalbag. Available online. https://commons.wikimedia.org/wiki/File:Bauhinia_galpinii_11.jpg. (CC BY-SA 3.0).

Verschaeve, L., Van Staden, J., 2008. Mutagenic and antimutagenic properties of extracts from South African traditional medicinal plants. Journal of Ethnopharmacology 119, 575–587.

Watt, J., Breyer Brandwijk, M., 1962. Medicinal and Poisonous Plants of Southern and Eastern Africa, second ed. E. & S. Livingstone Ltd., Edinburgh & London. 1457 pp.

Bruguiera gymnorhiza

Nabeelah Sadeer[1], Nadeem Nazurally[2],
Rajesh Jeewon[1], Mohamad Fawzi Mahomoodally[1]

[1] Department of Health Sciences, Faculty of Science, University of Mauritius,
Réduit, Mauritius; [2] Department of Agricultural and Food Science, Faculty of
Agriculture, University of Mauritius, Réduit, Mauritius

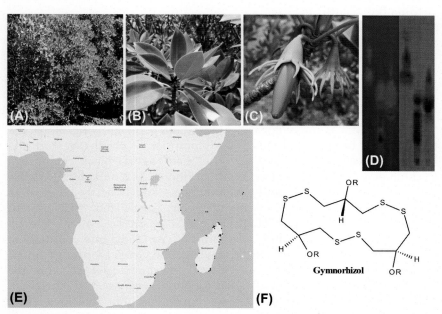

FIGURE 8 *Bruguiera gymnorhiza* growing along the coast (A), flower of *B. gymnorhiza* (B), fruit of *B. gymnorhiza* (C), TLC chromatogram, Lane 1; extract under ultraviolet light (365 nm), Lane 2; extract sprayed with 10% H_2SO_4 (D), distribution of *B. gymnorhiza* in sub-Saharan Africa (GBIF, 2018) (E), chemical structure of gymnorhizol (F).

Underexplored Medicinal Plants from Sub-Saharan Africa
https://doi.org/10.1016/B978-0-12-816814-1.00008-9

51

1. General description

1.1 Botanical nomenclature

Bruguiera gymnorhiza (L.) Lam

1.2 Botanical family

Rhizophoraceae

1.3 Vernacular names

Black mangrove, Burma mangrove (English)
Manglier, Paletuvier, Mangrove (Mauritius)
Honkalahy, Voandrano (Madagascar)
Swartwortelboom (Afrikaans)
Isi Hlobane (Zulu)
Isi Khangathi (Xhosa)
Muia (kiSwahili)
M'tumansi, Setaca (Mozambique)
Mhonko (Comoros)
Grand manglier, Mangrove latte, Mangrove (Seychelles)

2. Botanical description

B. gymnorhiza is an ecologically important plant growing along the coastlines of tropical and subtropical countries. It originates from the Rhizophoraceae family and is classified as a black mangrove (Nebula et al., 2013). *B. gymnorhiza* is considered as a halophyte because the plant lives in high-salinity environments and is easily adapted to harsh coastal conditions owing to their specialized root system (Kathiresan and Bingham, 2001). The genus was named after a French physician, zoologist, and explorer, Jean-Guillaume Bruguière (1750–1799). "Gymnorhiza" originates from the Greek words "gymnos" meaning naked or bare and "rhiza" meaning root or rhizome (Gurib-Fakim and Brendler, 2004). It is a glabrous tree reaching a height of 5–8 m covered with reddish-brown bark. The tree develops short prop-roots also called pneumatophores as compared to *Rhizophora mucronata* Lam., which develops rhizophores (buttress, stilt roots) as root systems. Leaves are opposite, apple green when young, glossy, elliptic to oblong with reddish petioles of 30–45 mm long, dotted with minute black spots on the inferior surface, pointed without spins. Flowers solitary, reddish in color about 10–25 mm long, 8–18 sepals, and petals are creamy white about 10–12 mm long. The tree germinates fruits of 20 mm long, 15—20 mm thick, cylindrical in shape, obtuse at the extremity. The plant is protected in South Africa (Gurib-Fakim and Brendler, 2004, PlantZafrica, 2005).

3. Distribution

B. gymnorhiza has a unique feature in terms of its propagules, which float in water and is the main reason behind the widely extended distribution of the plant to Central and South America from India through East Africa (Yong, 2018). The plant is native to many countries namely Southern and East Africa, Australia, and Asia (Yi et al., 2015; Barik et al., 2016). This mangrove species can also be found along the muddy and rocky shores of Comoros, Seychelles, and Mauritius in protected zones (Gurib-Fakim and Brendler, 2004). The approximate coverage of *B. gymnorhiza* in KwaZulu-Natal and Eastern Cape are estimated to be 16.79 and 2.23 km^2, respectively (Naidoo, 2016).

4. Ethnobotanical usage

B. gymnorhiza has many potential and promising therapeutic values as reported by many ethnomedicinal studies. Generally, *B. gymnorhiza* is the most common mangrove species used in folklore medicine followed by other species namely *Rhizophora mucronata* and *Acanthus ilicifolius* L (Sadeer et al., 2019). In Comoros and Mauritius, a decoction made from 15 cm of the root of *B. gymnorhiza* and 5—7 leaves of *Piper borbonense* (Miq.) C. DC. can be drunk twice a day to manage diabetes, hypertension, and haemorrhage (Gurib-Fakim and Brendler, 2004). Additionally, in India, the bark and leaves are used against diarrhea and fever (Ahmed et al., 2007; Karimulla and Kumar, 2011), whereas in China, the fruit instead is used against the same ailments (Bamroongrugsa, 1999). According to known literature, India is recognized as the prime country using *B. gymnorhiza* as a traditional remedy; however, no report has mentioned the traditional usage of this plant in Africa (Sadeer et al., 2019).

5. Phytochemical constituents

Phytochemical profiling of *B. gymnorhiza* has not been done extensively, thus only a few studies are available. Nonetheless, the few screenings performed revealed the presence of many biologically active metabolites. For instance, Rahman et al. (2011) detected the presence of flavonoids, reducing sugars, gums, saponins and tannins from the methanolic root extract. Sun and Guo (2004) reported the isolation of one compound, gymnorrhizol from the methanolic shoot extract. Barik et al. (2016) isolated a flavone, 5, 7-dihydroxy-2- [3-hydroxy-4, 5-dimethoxy-phenyl]-chromen-4-one, from the methanolic leaf extract using spectroscopic techniques. Han et al. (2005) isolated three novel pimaren diterpenoids, ent-8(14)-pimarene-15R, 16-diol, ent-8(14)-pimarene-1a, 15R, 16-triol, and (5R, 9S, 10R, 13S, 15S)-ent-8(14)-pimarene-1-oxo-15R, 16-diol from the methanolic stem extract using ^1H and ^{13}C nuclear magnetic resonance. Sur et al. (2016) reported the isolation of polyphenols namely gallic acid, quercetin, and coumarin isolated from the methanolic leaf extract.

6. TLC fingerprinting of plant extract

Fruits were selected as the testing materials for thin layer chromatography (TLC). They were allowed to dry at room temperature before the extraction procedure. The dried plant material was ground and extracted with methanol in a sample to solvent ratio of 1:4 (w/v) by maceration. After 2 weeks of maceration, the sample was filtered and the latter was evaporated in vacuo in a rotary evaporator at 40°C. The concentrated sample was freeze-dried to obtain a powdered methanolic extract (Sudirman et al., 2014). The bioactive compounds of the methanolic fruit freeze-dried extract were separated by TLC. Markings on the TLC plate were made with a pencil, and glass capillaries were used for spotting of extract. The plate was then placed in a TLC tank filled with 10 mL of n-hexane and ethyl acetate (4:1) as a solvent system. The samples were allowed to separate until the solvent system reached 1 cm from the top of the plate. The spots were viewed under ultraviolet (UV) light irradiation at wavelengths 254 and 365 nm, and the plate was sprayed with 10% H_2SO_4 (Handayani et al., 2015; Sudirman et al., 2014)

7. Pharmacological properties

There is a significant shortage of knowledge regarding the pharmacological values of the plant. For instance, it is considered as a rather important plant in the medical lore to cure diabetes, fever, and diarrhea but has not been properly pharmacologically validated yet. Till date, very few studies such as antioxidant, antinociceptive, antiinflammatory, antimicrobial, toxicity, and hepatoprotective have been conducted, and there has been only one report on the in vivo antidiabetic inhibitory activity of this plant.

7.1 Antioxidant activity

Barik et al. (2016) conducted diphenylpicrylhydrazyl (DPPH) antioxidant test on the methanolic leaf extract, which reported a percentage inhibition of 68% and 59% at 2 and 1 mg/mL respectively. The leaf samples were collected in West Bengal, India, and subjected to maceration for extraction before the antioxidant inhibition activity. Another study conducted by Haq et al. (2011) on the methanolic leaf and bark extracts 50% inhibitory concentration (IC_{50}) values of 0.038 ± 0.003 and 0.025 ± 0.003 µg/mL respectively. Sur et al. (2016) conducted a series of antioxidant assays on the methanolic leaf extracts collected in the mangrove forest in West Bengal, India. The IC_{50} values of the reducing capacities of DPPH, nitric oxide, hydroxyl, superoxide, and ABTS radical scavenging assays were reported to be 0.355 ± 0.005, 0.305 ± 0.004, 0.311 ± 0.004, 0.356 ± 0.007, and 0.056 ± 0.0003 µg/mL, respectively. The authors concluded in the chapter that the leaves rich in polyphenols contribute to healing injuries of hepatic tissue because of its good antioxidant effects.

Furthermore, Banerjee et al. (2008) screened the methanolic leaf, stem bark, and root extracts, resulting in IC_{50} values of 2052.20 ± 172.01, 254.69 ± 21.26, and 1532.71 ± 46.32 µg/mL of dry material, respectively. When comparing this to the positive control (ascorbic acid) with IC_{50} values of 12.5 ± 0.03, 2.85 ± 0.09, and 1.55 ± 0.16 mg/g of dry material, it was concluded that the extracts were not significantly potent, and the authors related the low reducing capacity with the extraction solvent used in the experiment. Importantly, in contrast to the studies done by Haq et al. (2011) and Sur et al. (2016), lower IC_{50} values were recorded showing extracts were more active although the same extraction solvent was used (methanol) as Banerjee et al. (2008). *B. gymnorhiza* naturally consists of a large pool of antioxidants, which makes it a good candidate for future drug development (Lee et al., 2003), thus further antioxidant tests should be conducted for a conclusive validation of the plant.

7.2 Antimicrobial activity

Antimicrobial activity test was conducted by Haq et al. (2011) on the methanolic, ethanolic, and chloroform leaf extracts. Results showed that ethanolic leaf extracts showed more significant inhibition against *Escherichia coli* (9.91 mm), *Staphylococcus aureus* (15.85 mm), *Pseudomonas aeruginosa* (8.90 mm), and *Bacillus cereus* (14.56 mm) as compared to the methanolic leaf extracts. Additionally, Seepana et al. (2016) tested the ethanol and aqueous leaf extracts against *Salmonella typhi* using agar well diffusion, which showed inhibition zones of 18 and 11 mm, respectively. No activity was recorded against *E. coli*, *Shigella flexneri*, and *Klebsiella pneumonia*. The authors concluded that *B. gymnorhiza* can be a potential candidate for developing antimicrobial drugs against clinical pathogens.

8. Additional information

8.1 Therapeutic (proposed) usage

Antioxidant, antimicrobial, and anticancer

8.2 Safety data

The water leaf extract showed moderate activity against breast ductal carcinoma cells namely MDA-MB-435S and AGS with IC_{50} values of 1.38 and > 2.50 mg/mL. However, no activity was reported for methanolic leaf extracts (Uddin et al., 2011).

8.3 Trade information

Not threatened

8.4 Dosage

Not available

References

Ahmed, F., Shahid, I., Gain, N., Reza, M., Sadhu, S., 2007. Antinociceptive and antidiarrhoeal activities of *Bruguiera gymnorrhiza*. Oriental Pharmacy and Experimental Medicine 7 (3), 280–285.

Bamroongrugsa, N., 1999. Bioactive substances from the mangrove resource. Songklanakarin Journal of Science and Technology 21.

Banerjee, D., Chakrabarti, S., Hazra, A.K., Banerjee, S., Ray, J., Mukherjee, B., 2008. Antioxidant activity and total phenolics of some mangroves in Sundarbans. African Journal of Biotechnology 7 (6), 805–810.

Barik, R., Sarkar, R., Biswas, P., Bera, R., Sharma, S., Nath, S., Karmakar, S., Sen, T., 2016. 5, 7-dihydroxy-2-(3-hydroxy-4, 5-dimethoxy-phenyl)-chromen-4-one-a flavone from *Bruguiera gymnorrhiza* displaying anti-inflammatory properties. Indian Journal of Pharmacology 48 (3), 304.

GBIF, 2018. *Bruguiera gymnorhiza* (L.) Lam. In: GBIF Secretariat (2017). GBIF Backbone Taxonomy. Checklist dataset. https://doi.org/10.15468/39omei.

Gurib-Fakim, A., Brendler, T., 2004. Medicinal and Aromatic Plants of Indian Ocean Islands: Madagascar, Comoros, Seychelles and Mascarenes. Medpharm GmbH Scientific Publishers.

Han, L., Huang, X., Sattler, I., Dahse, H.M., Fu, h., Grabley, S., Lin, W., 2005. Three pimaren diterpenoids from marine mangrove plant, *Bruguiera gymmorhiza*. Die Pharmazie 60, 705–707.

Handayani, S., Yuwono, S.S., Suprayitno, A.E., 2015. Isolation and identification structure antioxidant active compounds of ethyl acetate fraction hypokotil *Bruguiera gymnorhiza* (L) Lamk. International Journal of ChemTech Research 8 (4), 1858-187.

Haq, M., Sani, W., Hossain, A.B.M.S., Taha, R.M., Monneruzzaman, K.M., 2011. Total phenolic content, antioxidant and antimicrobial activities of *Bruguiera gymnorhiza*. Journal of Medicinal Plants Research 5 (17), 4112–4118.

Karimulla, S., Kumar, B., 2011. Antidiabetic and antihyperlipidemic activity of bark of *Bruguiera gymnorrhiza* on streptozotocin induced diabetic rats. Asian Journal of Pharmaceutical Sciences 1, 4–7.

Kathiresan, K., Bingham, B.L., 2001. Biology of mangroves and mangrove ecosystems. Advances in Marine Biology 40, 81–251.

Lee, S.E., Hyun, J.H., Ha, J.S., Jeong, H.S., Kim, J.H., 2003. Screening of medicinal plant extracts for antioxidant activity. Life Sciences 73, 167–179.

Naidoo, G., 2016. The mangroves of South Africa: an ecophysiological review. South African Journal of Botany 107, 101–113.

Nebula, M., Harisankar, H., Chandramohanakumar, N., 2013. Metabolites and bioactivities of Rhizophoraceae mangroves. Natural Products and Bioprospecting 3 (5), 207–232.

PlantZafrica, 2005. *Bruguiera gymnorhiza* [Online] Available on: http://pza.sanbi.org/bruguiera-gymnorhiza.

Rahman, M., Ahmed, A., Shahid, I., 2011. Phytochemical and pharmacological properties of *Bruguiera gymnorrhiza* roots extract. International Journal of Pharmaceutical Research 3, 63–67.

Sadeer, N.B., Jeewon, R., Nazurally, N., Rengasamy, K.R.R., Mahomoodally, F., 2019. Ethnopharmacology, phytochemistry, and global distribution of mangroves-a comprehensive review. Marine Drugs Journal 17 (4), 231.

Seepana, R., Perumal, K., Kada, N.M., Chatragadda, R., Raju, M., Annamalai, V., 2016. Evaluation of antimicrobial properties from the mangrove *Rhizophora apiculata* and *Bruguiera gymnorrhiza* of Burmanallah coast, South Andaman, India. Journal of Coastal Life Medicine 4 (6), 475–478.

Sudirman, S., Nurjanah, Jacoeb, A.M., 2014. Proximate compositions, bioactive compunds and antioxidant activity from large-leafed mangrove (*Brugueira gymnorhiza*) fruit. International Food Research Journal 21 (6), 2387–2391.

Sun, Y.Q., Guo, Y.W., 2004. Gymnorrhizol, an unusual macrocyclic polydisulfide from the Chinese mangrove *Bruguiera gymnorhiza*. Tetrahedron Letters 45 (28), 5533–5535.

Sur, T.K., Hazra, A., Hazra, A.K., Bhattacharyya, D., 2016. Antioxidant and hepatoprotective properties of Indian Sunderban mangrove *Bruguiera gymnorrhiza* L. leave. Journal of Basic and Clinical Pharmacy 7 (3), 75.

Uddin, S.J., Grice, I.D., Tiralongo, E., 2011. Cytotoxic effects of Bangladeshi medicinal plant extract. Evidence-Based Complementery and Alernative Medicine 578092, 1–7.

Yi, X.X., Deng, J.G., Gao, C.H., Hou, X.T., Li, F., Wang, Z.P., Hao, E.W., Xie, Y., Du, Z.C., Huang, H.X., 2015. Four new cyclohexylideneacetonitrile derivatives from the hypocotyl of mangrove (*Bruguiera gymnorrhiza*). Molecules 20 (8), 14565–14575.

Yong, J., 2018. Origin of Mangroves & Mangrove Diversity.

Further reading

Hamilton, S.E., Casey, D., 2016. Creation of a high spatio-temporal resolution global database of continuous mangrove forest cover for the 21st century (CGMFC-21). Global Ecology and Biogeography 25 (6), 729–738.

Mainga, V.N., 2005. *Bruguiera gymnorhiza* (L.) Savigny [Online] Available from: https://www.prota4u.org/database/protav8.asp?g=pe&p=Bruguiera+gymnorhiza+(L.)+Savigny.

Buddleja saligna

Danielle Twilley, Namrita Lall

Department of Plant and Soil Sciences, University of Pretoria, Pretoria, Gauteng, South Africa

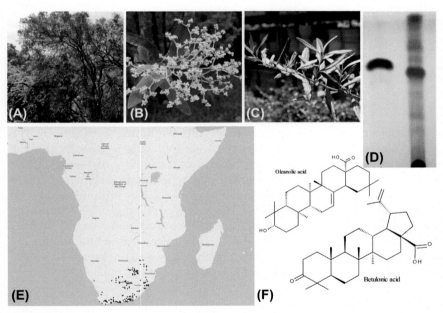

FIGURE 9 Aerial plant parts of *Buddleja saligna* (JMK, 2014) (A), flower buds of *B. saligna* (JMK, 2013) (B), leaves of *B. saligna* (Shawka, 2010) (C), TLC chromatogram, Lane 1; oleanolic acid, Lane 2: *B. saligna* extract (D), distribution of *B. saligna* in sub-Saharan Africa (GBIF, 2018) (E), chemical structures of oleanolic acid and betulonic acid (F).

Underexplored Medicinal Plants from Sub-Saharan Africa
https://doi.org/10.1016/B978-0-12-816814-1.00009-0

1. General description

1.1 Botanical nomenclature

Buddleja saligna Willd

1.2 Botanical family

Buddlejaceae

1.3 Vernacular names

False olive (English)
Witolien (Afrikaans)
umBatacwepe (Siswati)
Lelothwane (South Sotho)
Mothlware (Tswana)
unGqeba (Xhosa)
iGqebaelimhlope (Zulu)

2. Botanical description

Buddleja saligna is an evergreen plant from the Buddlejaceae family. The genus was named after amateur botanist, Rev. Adam Buddle, and the species name *"saligna"* was given because of the willow-like leaves. It can be classified as a large shrub or small tree, which can reach heights up to 10m. The leaves are petiolate, narrow, and hairless with a dark green surface and a whitish underside. The leaves of *B. saligna* look similar to those of an olive tree, and therefore, the common name of the plant is "false olive." From August to January, small creamy to white flowers are borne on the ends of the branches, which possess a faint honey-like scent (Aubrey, 2002; PlantZAfrica, 2015).

3. Distribution

Buddleja saligna is a common evergreen shrub, which is distributed throughout Southern Africa from coastal to inland regions as well as parts of the Kalahari, and it is also found in Zimbabwe (Aubrey, 2002). It naturally occurs in the bushvelds, grassland, forests, and woody and rocky areas.

4. Ethnobotanical usage

Buddleja saligna is traditionally widely used in southern Africa for its medicinal properties. It is used for the treatment of colic, colds, and urinary problems and to relieve coughs and sore eyes. For these symptoms, a bark or leaf decoction is generally prepared. It is used as purgatives and, therefore, also known as a laxative. It is used for diabetes, tuberculosis, thrush and sores, anasarca (widespread swelling of the skin), and chest pains, and the leaves are used as soap (Adedapo et al., 2009; Chukwujekwu et al., 2014; Hutchings et al., 1996; Scott et al., 2004; Van Wyk et al., 1997).

5. Phytochemical constituents

There have only been five compounds previously isolated from the leaves and stems of *B. saligna*: oleanolic acid, betulonic acid, betulone, ursolic acid and α-spinasterol. The flowers have not yet been studied for any biological activity, and there has been no report of compounds isolated from the flowers (Bamuamba et al., 2008; Chukwujekwu et al., 2015; Singh et al., 2017).

From the collected leaves and stems, 100% methanol extracts were prepared to obtain a methanolic leaf and a methanolic stem extract. For the phytochemical analysis, the extracts were tested for total phenolic, total flavonoids, total flavonols, and total proanthocyanidins. Both extracts showed the presence of all the tested phytochemicals; however, the leaf extract had a higher content of flavonoids and flavonols, whereas the stem extract had a higher content of phenolics and proanthocyanidins (Adedapo et al., 2009).

6. TLC fingerprinting of plant extract

For the separation of *B. saligna*, 2 mg of the ethanolic extract was weighed out and dissolved in 200 μL of ethanol. For the standard, oleanolic acid (Sigma—Aldrich Co. St Louis, MO, USA) was weighed out in the same manner as the extract and dissolved in 600 μL of ethanol. For the thin layer chromatography (TLC) analysis of *B. saligna* crude extract, silica gel 60 F254 TLC plates were used to observe the separation of the compounds present in the extract. Plate markings were made with a soft pencil, and glass capillaries were used to spot the samples onto the TLC plate. Reference standard oleanolic acid was spotted to determine whether it is present in the extract. The spots were left to dry completely and placed in a TLC tank, which contained a 10 mL eluent 9:1 chloroform: methanol solvent system. The samples were allowed to separate until the solvent system reached 1 cm from the top of the TLC plate. The plate was observed under ultraviolet (UV light) (long and short wavelength) and sprayed with freshly prepared vanillin to detect the bands on the TLC plate.

7. Pharmacological properties

Buddleja saligna has not been extensively researched for its in vitro and in vivo medicinal properties. Although it is a widely distributed and well-known plant in South Africa, there is still an opportunity for research and development on this plant.

7.1 Antibacterial activity

In a previous study, the leaves and stems of *B. saligna* were collected in autumn from Cape Town, South Africa. Two separate extracts were prepared, an aqueous infusion and a 4:1 acetone:water extract. The 4:1 acetone:water extract was partitioned into hexane, chloroform, and ethyl acetate fractions. The aqueous crude extract showed no activity against *Escherichia coli* American type culture collection (ATCC) 25922, *Staphylococcus aureus* ATCC 25923, or *Mycobacterium aurum* A+, whereas the 4:1 acetone/water extract and its subsequent hexane partition showed significant activity. The hexane partition then underwent chromatographic separation using silica to yield oleanolic acid, which furthermore showed significant activity against *Mycobacterium tuberculosis* H37Rv, *M. avium* ATCC 25291, *M. scrofulaceum* ATCC 19981, and *M. microti* ATCC 19422 (Bamuamba et al., 2008).

In another study, the methanolic shoot and leave extracts were tested for their antibacterial activity against 5 g-positive bacteria (*Bacillus cereus, Staphylococcus epidermidis, S. aureus, Micrococcus kristinae, Streptococcus pyogenes*) and 5 g-negative bacteria (*E. coli, Salmonella poona, Serratia marcescens, Pseudomonas aeruginosa, Klebsiella pneumoniae*). It was found that the antibacterial activity of the leaf extract was generally higher than that of the stem extract. Further, the leaf extract was active against all the bacteria except for *Serratia marcescens* at 2.5 and 5 mg/mL. The opposite was found for the stem extract where antibacterial activity was only seen on *B. cereus, S. pyogenes*, and *P. aeruginosa* at the same concentrations (Adedapo et al., 2009).

7.2 Antidiabetic and antiplasmodial activity

In a study conducted by Chukwujekwu et al. (2015), the antidiabetic and antiplasmodial activity of *B. saligna* was evaluated. The leaves were collected from Kwa-Zulu Natal, South Africa. An 80% methanol extract was prepared and liquid—liquid partitioning was performed to obtain a hexane, dichloromethane, and water partition respectively. The hexane partition was tested for alpha-glucosidase inhibitory activity (50% inhibitory concentration [IC_{50}] of 260 µg/mL), in vitro antiplasmodial activity (IC_{50} of 8.5 µg/mL), and cytotoxicity against Chinese hamster ovarian (CHO) cells (IC_{50} of 1.7 µg/mL). The hexane partition then underwent chromatographic separation to obtain three pure compounds: betulonic acid, betulone, and α-spinasterol. All three compounds showed IC_{50} values smaller than 27 µg/mL for alpha-glucosidase inhibitory activity and IC_{50} values lower than 14 µg/mL for antiplasmodial activity (Chukwujekwu et al., 2015).

7.3 Antioxidant activity

In another study, the leaves and stems of *B. saligna* were collected in the Eastern Cape, South Africa. From the collected leaves and stems, 100% methanol extracts were prepared to obtain a methanolic leaf and a methanolic stem extract. The extracts were tested for their antioxidant activity using the 2,2′-azinobis-3-ethylbenzothiazoline-6-sulfonic acid (ABTS) and diphenylpicrylhydrazyl (DPPH) radical scavenging assays as well as their total antioxidant activity using the ferric reducing ability of plasma (FRAP) assay. The stem extract showed a high inhibition of the DPPH free radical than that of the leaf extract with 94.9% and 93.8% inhibition respectively at 0.1 mg/mL. The opposite was observed in the ABTS assay when 100% and 98.8% inhibition were observed for the leaf and stem extract, respectively. However, when considering the total antioxidant activity, the leaf extract showed higher activity in the FRAP assay than the stem extract with 490.98 ± 38.89 µmol Fe (II)/g and 1546.98 ± 63.67 µmol Fe (II)/g respectively (Adedapo et al., 2009).

8. Additional information

8.1 Therapeutic (proposed) usage

Antibacterial, antiplasmodial, antidiabetic, and anticancer

8.2 Safety data

Oleanolic acid showed low cytotoxicity against CHO cells with a IC_{50} greater than 100 µg/mL (Bamuamba et al., 2008). Betulonic acid and betulone showed IC_{50} values smaller than 51 µg/mL on CHO cells, whereas α-spinasterol showed an IC_{50} value greater than 100 µg/mL (Chukwujekwu et al., 2015).

8.3 Trade information

Not threatened, not endangered, and abundant

8.4 Dosage

Not available

References

Adedapo, A.A., Jimoh, F.O., Koduru, S., Masika, P.J., Afolayan, A.J., 2009. Assessment of the medicinal potentials of the methanol extracts of the leaves and stems of *Buddleja saligna*. BMC Complementary and Alternative Medicine 91, 21. https://doi.org/10.1186/1472-6882-9-21.

Aubrey, A., 2002. Buddleja Saligna Willd. Online. Available at: http://www.plantzafrica.com/plantab/buddlesalig.htm.

Bamuamba, K., Gammon, D.W., Meyers, P., DijouxFranca, M.G., Scott, G., 2008. Antimycobacterial activity of five plant species used as traditional medicines in the Western Cape Province (South Africa). Journal of Ethnopharmacology 117, 385–390.

Chukwujekwu, J.C., Amoo, S.O., de Kock, C.A., Smith, P.J., Van Staden, J., 2014. Antiplasmodial, acetylcholinesterase and alpha-glucosidase inhibitory and cytotoxicity properties of Buddleja saligna. South African Journal of Botany 94, 6–8.

Chukwujekwu, J.C., Rengasamy, K.R.R., de Kock, C.A., Smith, P.J., Poštová Slavětíbská, L., Van Staden, J., 2015. Alpha-glucosidase inhibitory and antiplasmodial properties of terpenoids from the leaves of *Buddleja saligna* Willd. Journal of Enzyme Inhibition and Medicinal Chemistry. https://doi.org/10.3109/14756366.2014.1003927.

GBIF, 2018. *Buddleja saligna* Willd. stdterms.in GBIF Secretariat (2017). GBIF Backbone Taxonomy. Checklist dataset. https://doi.org/10.15468/39omei.

Hutchings, A., Scott, A.H., Lewis, G., Cunningham, A.B., 1996. Zulu Medicinal Plants: An Inventory. University of Natal Press, Scottsville, p. 240.

JMK, 2013. Flower Buds of a False Olive at Skeerpoort, on the Southern Slope of the Magaliesberg. South Africa. Available online: https://commons.wikimedia.org/wiki/File:Buddleja_saligna,_blomknoppe,_Skeerpoort,_a.jpg. (CC BY-SA 3.0).

JMK, 2014. Habit of a false olive in a valley of the Magaliesberg, near Skeerpoort. South Africa. Available online: https://commons.wikimedia.org/wiki/File:Buddleja_saligna,_habitus,_Skeerpoort.jpg. (CC BY-SA 3.0).

PlantZAfrica, 2015. *Buddleja saligna* Herba. Online. Available at: http://www.plantzafrica.com/medmonographs/buddlejasaligna.pdf.

Scott, G., Springfield, E.P., Coldrey, N.A., 2004. Pharmacognostic study of 26 South African plant species used as traditional medicines. Pharmaceutical Biology 42, 186–213.

Shawka, A., 2010. Leaves of Buddleja Saligna — the Sand Olive. Photo Taken in Cape Town. Available online:. The copyright holder of this work, release this work into the public domain. This applies worldwide. https://commons.wikimedia.org/wiki/File: Buddleja_saligna_-_Cape_Town_6.jpg.

Singh, A., Venugopala, K.N., Khedr, M.A., Pillay, M., Nwaeze, K.U., Coovadia, Y., Shode, F., Odhav, B., 2017. Antimycobacterial, docking and molecular dynamic studies of pentacyclic triterpenes from Buddleja saligna leaves. Journal of Biomolecular Structure and Dynamics 35 (12), 2654–2664.

Van Wyk, B., Palgrave, K.C., Van Wyk, P., 1997. Field Guide to Trees of Southern Africa. Struik Publishers, Cape Town, pp. 223–237.

Combretum molle

Sunelle Rademan, Namrita Lall

Department of Plant and Soil Sciences, University of Pretoria, Pretoria, Gauteng, South Africa

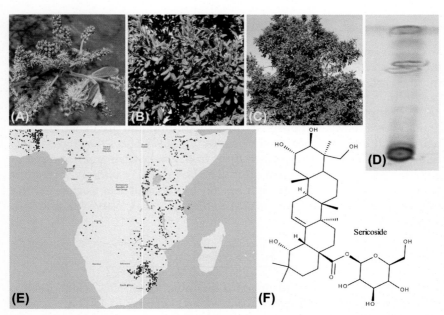

FIGURE 10 Flowers of *Combretum molle* (Coetzee, 2015) (A), aerial parts of *C. molle* (JMK,2016a; JMK, 2016b) (B, C), TLC chromatogram, fingerprint of *C. molle* (D), distribution of *C. molle* in sub-Saharan Africa (GBIF, 2018) (E), chemical structure of sericoside (F).

1. General description

1.1 Botanical nomenclature

Combretum molle R.Br. ex G.Don.

Underexplored Medicinal Plants from Sub-Saharan Africa
https://doi.org/10.1016/B978-0-12-816814-1.00010-7

1.2 Botanical family

Combretaceae

1.3 Vernacular names

Velvet Bush willow; Velvet Leaf willow (English)
Basterrooibos; Fluweelboswilg (Afrikaans)
Mokgwethe (North Sotho)
iNkukutwane (Siswati)
Xikhukhutsane (Tsonga)
Modubatshipi; Moduba (Tswana)
Mugwiti (Venda)
umBondwe (Zulu)

2. Botanical description

C. molle, more commonly known as the velvet bush willow, is a small to medium-sized tree from the Combretaceae family that can grow up to 13 m. The bark of *C. molle* is gray when the tree is still young and becomes gray-brown to black for mature trees. The leaves of *C. molle* varies from narrow elliptic to circular in form, usually a dark green in summer and green with a reddish to purplish tinge in autumn and are generally very hairy on the lower side of the leaves. *C. molle* bears 4-winged fruit, referred to as samara fruit, which turns from a yellowish green and red to a golden reddish brown when dried. The leaves of *C. molle* have secretory scales of which the density is high on the abaxial leaf surface in the intervein regions (Naidoo et al., 2012; Masupa, 2011; Van Wyk and Van Wyk, 2013).

3. Distribution

C. molle is widespread in Mozambique; Namibia; South Africa; Zimbabwe; and tropical Africa from sea level to around 1500 m. *C. molle* occurs naturally in open woodlands, rocky areas, and bushveld commonly associated with quartzite formations (Masupa, 2011; Van Wyk and Van Wyk, 2013).

4. Ethnobotanical usage

C. molle is known to be used in traditional medicine for various ailments including fever, pain, wounds, cough, and colds and a range of infections including HIV/AIDS. The roots of *C. molle* are mostly used as a wound dressing and as a decoction for the treatment of hookworm, snake bites, leprosy, general body swellings, fever, stomach pains, constipation, sterility, and abortion (Drummond and Coates-Palgrave, 1973; Watt and Breyer-Brandwijk, 1962; Kokwaro, 1976; Chhabra et al., 1989). The stem bark part of *C. molle* has been reported to be used for the treatment of angina and stomach problems (Kerharo, 1974; Watt and Breyer-Brandwijk, 1962). The leaves of *C. molle* are commonly used in traditional medicine as wound dressing, antidiarrheal, anthelmintic, and for the treatment of dropsy and chest complaints, whereas it is also used as an aid in childbirth (Drummond and Coates-Palgrave, 1973; Haerdi, 1964; Kokwaro, 1976; Kerharo, 1974). Although the fruits of *C. molle* are thought to be toxic, it is also traditionally used as an aid in childbirth (Watt and Breyer-Brandwijk, 1962). Only one African species of the *Combretum* genus is traditionally used as an anticancer agent, namely, *Combretum zeyheri* (Fyhrquist et al., 2002). Although most of the species in the Combretaceae family are traditionally used for infections and pain-related ailments, the discovery of combretastatin compounds, in particular, Combretastatin A4, has implicated the potential of Combretaceae species as possible anticancer agents. Combretastatin compounds are thought to occur throughout the Combretaceae family and Combretastatin A4 is known to be active against colon, leukemia, and lung cancers. Combretastatin A1 and A4 have been isolated from the bark of *Combretum caffrum* (Cragg and Newman, 2005; Mohammad, 2006).

5. Phytochemical constituents

A study by Naidoo et al. (2012) reported that the secretory scales of *C. molle* contain a variety of secondary metabolites including lipids, terpenoids, phenolics, flavonoids, and alkaloids, which most likely offer protection against microbial and herbivore attacks. There have been a few compounds isolated from different plant parts of *C. molle*. Most of the isolated compounds from *C. molle* have been isolated from the stem bark including: β-D-glucopyranosyl 2α,3β,6β-trihydroxy-23-galloylolean-12-en-28-oate, arjugenin, arjunglucoside I and II, combregenin, combreglucoside (Ponou et al. 2008), punicalagin, and sericoside (Asres et al. 2001). The compounds: mollic acid, mollic acid 3ß-O-arabinoside, mollic acid 3ß-O-glucoside, and mollic acid 3ß-O-xyloside have all been isolated from the leaves of *C. molle* (Pegel and Rogers, 1985), whereas the combretene compounds (combretene A and B) have been isolated from the aerial plant parts of *C. molle* (Bahar et al. 2004). Other compounds isolated from *C. molle* include the phenanthrene compounds: 2,6-dihydroxy-2,3,6-trimethoxyphenanthrene, 2,6-dihydroxy-4,7-trimethoxy-9,10-dihydrophenanthrene, 3,4-dihydroxy-4,5-dimethoxybibenzyl

(Letcher et al. 1972), 3,6-dihydroxy-2,4,7-trimethoxyphenanthrene, and 6,7-dihydroxy-2,3,4-trimethoxy-9,10-dihydrophenanthrene (Kovács et al. 2008).

6. TLC fingerprinting of plant extract

For the separation of *C. molle*, 2 mg of an ethanolic extract was weighed out and dissolved in 200 µL ethanol. For the thin layer chromatography (TLC) analysis of *C. molle* crude extract, silica gel 60 F254 TLC plates were used to observe the separation of the compounds present in the extract. Plate markings were made with a soft pencil, and glass capillaries were used to spot the samples onto the TLC plate. The spots were left to dry completely before placing in a TLC tank, which contained 10 mL of the eluent (Polar: 8 mL Ethyl acetate/1.8 mL Methanol/0.8 mL Water; Intermediate: 5 mL Chloroform/4 mL Ethyl acetate/1 mL Formic acid; Nonpolar: 9 mL Benzene/1 mL Ethanol/0.1 mL Hexane) (Masoko and Eloff, 2006). The samples were allowed to separate until the solvent system reached 1 cm from the top of the TLC plate. The plate was observed under ultraviolet (UV light) (long and short wavelength), followed by spraying with freshly prepared vanillin to detect the bands on the TLC plate.

7. Pharmacological properties

The biological activity of *C. molle* has been researched for a wide range of ailments. These include activity against pathogenic microorganisms, parasitic worms, protozoa, viruses and activity against inflammation, cancerous cell growth, reactive oxygen species, and snake venom. The following sections elaborate on the in vitro biological activity found for the different plant parts of *C. molle*.

7.1 Anthelmintic activity

Leaf extracts of *C. molle* have been reported to have activity against roundworms *Caenorhabditis elegans* var. *bristol* (McGaw et al. 2001) and *Haemonchus contortus* (Ademola and Eloff, 2010; Simon et al. 2012; Suleiman et al. 2013) and the flatworm *Schistosoma haematobium* (Asres et al. 2001) species.

7.2 Antimicrobial activity

Different plant parts of *C. molle* have been investigated for their antibacterial and antifungal activities. The majority of the antimicrobial research was found on the bark, leaf, and stem bark *C. molle* extracts. Bark extracts have been found to exhibit antibacterial activity against *Actinomyces viscosus* (Khan et al. 2000), *Mycobacterium tuberculosis* (Lall and Meyer, 1999), *Staphylococcus aureus* (Regassa and Araya, 2012), *Streptococcus mutans* (Khan et al. 2000), and antifungal activity against *Candida albicans* (Khan et al. 2000). Leaf extracts from *C. molle* have shown to be active against a variety of fungi including: *Aspergillus fumigatus* (Masoko et al. 2007), *C. albicans* (Baba-Moussa et al. 1999; Khan et al. 2000; Masoko et al. 2007), *Candida krusei* (Mangoyi et al. 2014), *Candida neoformans* (Masoko et al. 2007), *Epidermophyton floccosum* (Baba-Moussa et al. 1999), *Microsporum canis* (Masoko et al. 2007), *Microsporum gypseum* (Baba-Moussa et al. 1999), *Sporothrix schenckii* (Masoko et al. 2007), *Trichophyton mentagrophytes* (Baba-Moussa et al. 1999), and *Trichophyton rubrum* (Baba-Moussa et al. 1999), whereas it has been found to be active against three bacterial species namely, *S. aureus* (Eloff, 1998; Regassa and Araya, 2012), *Streptococcus agalactiae* (Regassa and Araya, 2012), and *Streptococcus pyogens*.

Stem bark extracts have been reported to have activity against a wide range of bacteria including, *Bacillus cereus* (Geyid et al. 2005), *Helicobacter pylori* (Njume et al. 2011; Nyenje and Ndip, 2012), *Pleisomonas shigelloides* (Nyenje and Ndip, 2012), *Pseudomonas aeruginosa* (Nyenje and Ndip, 2012), *S. aureus* (Asres et al., 2001; Geyid et al., 2005), and *S. pyogens* (Nyenje and Ndip, 2012). Other plant parts, including root (*S. aureus* and *C. albicans* (Steenkamp et al. 2007)), seed (*S. aureus* (Regassa and Araya, 2012), and *Histoplasma capsulatum* var. *farciminosum* (Wondmnew and Teshome, 2016)), stem (*S. aureus* (Regassa and Araya, 2012)), and wood (*A. viscosus* (Khan et al. 2000)) extracts, have also been reported to have antimicrobial activity.

7.3 Antiprotozoal activity

C. molle extracts have shown to possess antileishmanial, antimalarial, and antitrypanosomal activity. Stem bark extracts have been reported to be active against *Leishmania donovani* (Asres et al. 2001) and *Trypanosoma brucei rhodesiense* (Asres et al. 2001). Antimalarial activity against the causal agent, *Plasmodium falciparum*, has been reported for stem bark (Asres et al. 2001), stem (Ares and Balcha, 1998), and leaf (Gansané et al. 2010; Traoré-Coulibaly et al., 2013) extracts.

7.4 Antiviral activity

Methanolic and aqueous root extracts of *C. molle* have been shown to possess activity against HIV/AIDS (Human Immunodeficiency Virus/ Acquired Immune Deficiency Syndrome) by targeting HIV-1 reverse transcriptase through their effects on RNA (ribonucleic acid)-dependent-DNA (deoxyribonucleic acid)-polymerase (RDDP) and ribonuclease H (RNase H) (Bessong et al. 2005).

7.5 Anti-inflammatory activity

Various leaf extracts from *C. molle* have been reported to possess anti-inflammatory activity. Water, acetone, and ethyl acetate extracts have been shown to act against inflammation through the inhibition of the cyclooxygenase-1 (COX-1) enzyme (McGaw et al. 2001). Additionally, another study reported that the acetone and ethanolic leaf extracts have anti-inflammatory activity via targeting hematopoietic prostaglandin D2 synthase in *Escherichia coli* (Moyo et al. 2014).

7.6 Antioxidant activity

An ethanolic leaf extract of *C. molle* has been reported to possess free radical scavenging activity against the diphenylpicrylhydrazyl (DPPH) free radical and reactive nitric species scavenging through scavenging nitric oxide (NO) (Koevi et al. 2015). Furthermore, a study by McGaw et al. (2001) reported that the acetone, ethyl acetate, and methanolic leaf extracts of *C. molle* do not have any DNA-damaging activity in *E. coli*.

7.7 Anti—snake venom activity

Ethanolic ethanolic and aqueous leaf extracts of *C. molle* have been reported to have in vitro activity that can support its usage in the treatment of snake bites, moreover snake venom. These extracts have been shown to inhibit hyaluronidase, phospholipase A2, and proteolytic activity against the venom of *Bitis arietans*, whereas inhibition of hyaluronidase was reported against the venom of *Naja nigricollis* (Molander et al. 2014, 2015).

Although it is a well-known plant in Southern Africa, which has been scientifically validated for many of its medicinal uses in traditional medicine, there is still an opportunity for research regarding its mechanism of action for its pharmacological activities.

8. Additional information

8.1 Therapeutic (proposed) usage

Anthelmintic, antibacterial, antifungal, anti-inflammatory, anti-leishmaniasis, antimalarial, antischistosomal, anti—snake venom, anti-trypanosomal, antiviral, and anticancer.

8.2 Safety data

C. molle extracts have been reported to possess antiproliferative activity on a variety of cancerous cell lines. Leaf extracts have been found to be moderately active against the HeLa (cervical carcinoma), K5625 (chronic myeloid leukemia), and MCF-7 (hormone-dependent breast adenocarcinoma), while being highly active against the T24 (urinary bladder transitional cell carcinoma) cell line (Fyhrquist et al. 2006; Gansané et al. 2010). Similar observations have been made for the root extract of *C. molle*; with moderate activity against the HeLa and MCF-7 cell lines and potent activity against the T24 cell line (Fyhrquist et al. 2006). A stem bark extract has also been shown to possess moderate activity against the KB-HeLa (cervical carcinoma cell line infected with the Human Papillomavirus) subline (Asres et al. 2001).

A water extract prepared from the leaves of *C. molle* was found to be toxic to the neuromuscular system in rats when administered intraperitoneally (50% lethal dose of 700 mg/kg), though oral administration of the same preparation was found to be nontoxic with no signs of poisoning or mortality up to a concentration of 8000 mg/kg (Yeo et al., 2012).

8.3 Trade information

Least concern (SANBI, 2010—2012), not endangered, and abundant

8.4 Dosage

Not available

References

Ademola, I.O., Eloff, J.N., 2010. *In vitro* anthelmintic activity of *Combretum molle* (R. Br. ex G. Don) (Combretaceae) against *Haemonchus contortus* ova and larvae. Veterinary Parasitology 169, 198—203.

Asres, K., Balcha, F., 1998. Phytochemical screening and *in vitro* antimalarial activity of the stem bark of *Combretum molle*. R. Br. ex G. Don Ethiopian Pharmaceutical Journal 16, 25—33.

Asres, K., Bucar, F., Knauder, E., Yardley, V., Kendrick, H., Croft, S.L., 2001. *In vitro* antiprotozoal activity of extract and compounds from the stem bark of *Combretum molle*. Phytotherapy Research 15, 613—617.

Baba-Moussa, F., Akpagana, K., Bouchet, P., 1999. Antifungal activities of seven West African Combretaceae used in traditional medicine. Journal of Ethnopharmacology 66, 335—338.

Bahar, A., Tawfeq, A.A.H., Passreiter, C.M., Jaber, S.M., 2004. Combretene A and B, Two new triterpenes from *Combretum molle*. Pharmacien Biologiste 42, 109—113.

Bessong, P.O., Obi, C.L., Andréola, M.L., Rojas, L.B., Pouységu, L., Igumbor, E., Meyer, J.J.M., Quideau, S., Litvak, S., 2005. Evaluation of selected South African medicinal plants for inhibitory properties against human immunodeficiency virus type 1 reverse transcriptase and integrase. Journal of Ethnopharmacology 99, 83—91.

Chhabra, S.C., Mahunnah, R.L.A., Mshiu, E.N., 1989. Plants used in traditional medicine in Eastern Tanzania. II. Angiosperms (Capparidaceae — Ebenaceae). Journal of Ethnopharmacology 25, 339—359.

Coetzee, B., 2015. *Combretum Molle* R.Br. Ex G.Don - Flowers and Flower Buds - White River. South Africa. Available online: https://commons.wikimedia.org/w/index.php?curid=43115208. (CC BY-SA 3.0).

Cragg, G.M., Newman, D.J., 2005. Plants as a source of anticancer agents. Journal of Ethnopharmacology 100, 72—79.

Drummond, R.B., Coates-Palgrave, K., 1973. Common Trees of the Highweld (ISBN, Rhodesia).

Eloff, J.N., 1998. A sensitive and quick microplate method to determine the minimal inhibitory concentration of plant extracts for bacteria. Planta Medica 64, 711—713.

Fyhrquist, P., Mwasumbi, L., Hæggström, C.-A., Vuorela, H., Hiltunen, R., Vuorela, P., 2002. Ethnobotanical and antimicrobial investigation on some species of *Terminalia* and *Combretum* (Combretaceae) growing in Tanzania. Journal of Ethnopharmacology 79, 169—177.

Fyhrquist, P., Mwasumbi, L., Vuorela, P., Vuorela, H., Hiltunen, R., Murphy, C., Adlercreutz, H., 2006. Preliminary antiproliferative effects of some species of *Terminalia, Combretum* and *Pteleopsis* collected in Tanzania on some human cancer cell lines. Fitoterapia 77, 358—366.

Gansané, A., Sanon, S., Ouattara, L.P., Traoré, A., Hutter, S., Ollivier, E., Azas, N., Traore, A.S., Guissou, I.P., Sirima, S.B., 2010. Antiplasmodial activity and toxicity of crude extracts from alternatives parts of plants widely used for the treatment of malaria in Burkina Faso: Contribution for their preservation. Parasitology Research 106, 335—340.

GBIF, 2018. *Combretum Molle* R.Br. Ex G.Don. Checklist Dataset. https://www.gbif.org/occurrence/map?taxon_key=7961582 on 2018-08-16.

Geyid, A., Abebe, D., Debella, A., Makonnen, Z., Aberra, F., Teka, F., Kebede, T., Urga, K., Yersaw, K., Biza, T., 2005. Screening of some medicinal plants of Ethiopia for their antimicrobial properties and chemical profiles. Journal of Ethnopharmacology 97, 421—427.

Haerdi, F., 1964. Die Eingeborenen-Heilpflanzen des Ulanga-Distriktes Tanganjikas (Ostafrika). Acta Tropica Supplement 8, 1—278.

JMK, 2016a. Combretum Molle R.Br. Ex G.Don. Foliage and Fruit of Velvet Bushwillow on the Bronberg Near Pretoria. Available online: https://commons.wikimedia.org/w/index.php?curid=49435727 (CC BY-SA 4.0).

JMK, 2016b. Combretum molle R.Br. ex G.Don. Foliage and fruit tree of Velvet bushwillow on the Bronberg near Pretoria. https://commons.wikimedia.org/w/index.php?curid=49435772. (CC BY-SA 4.0).

Kerharo, J., 1974. La Pharmacopée Sénégalaise traditionelle- Plantes médicinales et toxiques. Vigot Freres Edn., Paris.

Khan, M.N., Ngassapa, O., Matee, M.I.N., 2000. Antimicrobial activity of Tanzanian chewing sticks against oral pathogenic microbes. Pharmacien Biologiste 38, 235—230.

Koevi, K.A., Millogo, V., Hzounda Fokou, J.B., Sarr, A., Ouedraogo, G.A., Bassene, E., 2015. Phytochemical analysis and antioxidant activities of *Combretum molle* and *Pericopsis laxiflora*. International Journal of Biological and Chemical Sciences 9, 2423—2431.

Kokwaro, O., 1976. Medicinal Plants of East Africa. East African Literature, Nairobi.

Kovács, A., Vasas, A., Hohmann, J., 2008. Natural phenanthrenes and their biological activity. Phytochemistry 69, 1084—1110.

Lall, N., Meyer, J.J.M., 1999. *In vitro* inhibition of drug-resistant and drug-sensitive strains of *Mycobacterium tuberculosis* by ethnobotanically selected South African plants. Journal of Ethnopharmacology 66, 347—354.

Letcher, R.M., Nhamo, L.R.M., Gumiro, I.T., 1972. Chemical constituents of the Combretaceae. Part II. Substituted phenanthrenes and 9,10-dihydrophenanthrenes and a substituted bibenzyl from the heartwood of *Combretum molle*. Journal of the Chemical Society, Perkin Transactions 1, 206—210.

Mangoyi, R., Chitemerere, T., Chimponda, T., Chirisa, E., Mukanganyama, S., 2014. In: Gurib-Fakim, A. (Ed.), Novel Plant Bioresources: Applications in Food, Medicine and Cosmetics, first ed. JohnWiley & Sons, Ltd., pp. 179–191 (Chapter 14).

Masoko, P., Eloff, J.N., 2006. Bioautography indicates the multiplicity of antifungal compounds from twenty-four southern African *Combretum* species (Combretaceae). African Journal of Biotechnology 5, 1625–1647.

Masoko, P., Picard, J., Eloff, J.N., 2007. The antifungal activity of twenty-four Southern African *Combretum* species (Combretaceae). South African Journal of Botany 73, 173–183.

Masupa, T., 2011. Combretum Molle R.Br. Ex G.Don. Available at: http://www.plantzafrica.com/plantcd/combretummolle.htm.

McGaw, L.J., Rabe, T., Sparg, S.G., Jager, A.K., Eloff, J.N., Van Staden, J., 2001. An investigation on the biological activity of *Combretum* species. Journal of Ethnopharmacology 75, 45–50.

Mohammad, S., 2006. Anticancer agents from medicinal plants. Bangladesh Journal of Pharmacology 1, 35–41.

Molander, M., Nielsen, L., Søgaard, S., Staerk, D., Rønsted, N., Diallo, D., Chifundera, K.Z., van Staden, J., Jäger, A.K., 2014. Hyaluronidase, phospholipase A2 and protease inhibitory activity of plants used in traditional treatment of snakebite-induced tissue necrosis in Mali, DR Congo and South Africa. Journal of Ethnopharmacology 157, 171–180.

Molander, M., Staerk, D., Mørck Nielsen, H., Brandner, J.M., Diallo, D., Chifundera, K.Z., van Staden, J., Jäger, A.K., 2015. Investigation of skin permeation, *ex vivo* inhibition of venom-induced tissue destruction, and wound healing of African plants used against snakebites. Journal of Ethnopharmacology 165, 1–8.

Moyo, R., Chimponda, T., Mukanganyama, S., 2014. Inhibition of hematopoietic prostaglandin D2 Synthase (H-PGDS) by an alkaloid extract from *Combretum molle*. BMC Complementary and Alternative Medicine 14, 221.

Naidoo, Y., Heneidak, S., Gairola, S., Nicholas, A., Naidoo, G., 2012. The leaf secretory scales of *Combretum molle* (Combretaceae): morphology, ultrastructure and histochemistry. Plant Systematics and Evolution 298, 25–32.

Njume, C., Jide, A.A., Ndip, R.N., 2011. Aqueous and organic solvent-extracts of selected South African medicinal plants possess antimicrobial activity against drug-resistant strains of *Helicobacter pylori*: inhibitory and bactericidal potential. International Journal of Molecular Sciences 12, 5652–5665.

Nyenje, M.E., Ndip, R.N., 2012. Bioactivity of the acetone extract of the stem bark of *Combretum molle* on selected bacterial pathogens: preliminary phytochemical screening. Journal of Medicinal Plants Research 6, 1476–1481.

Pegel, K.H., Rogers, C.B., 1985. The characterisation of mollic acid 3β-D-xyloside and its genuine aglycone mollic acid, two novel 1α-hydroxycycloartenoids from *Combretum molle*. Journal of the Chemical Society, Perkin Transactions 1, 1711–1715.

Ponou, B.K., Barboni, L., Teponno, R.B., Mbiantcha, M., Nguelefack, T., Park, H.J., Lee, K.T., Tapondjou, L.A., 2008. Polyhydroxyoleanane-type triterpenoids from *Combretum molle* and their anti-inflammatory activity. Phytochemistry Letters 1, 183–187.

Regassa, F., Araya, M., 2012. *In vitro* antimicrobial activity of *Combretum molle* (Combretaceae) against *Staphylococcus aureus* and *Streptococcus agalactiae* isolated from crossbred dairy cows with clinical mastitis. Tropical Animal Health and Production 44, 1169–1173.

SANBI, 2010–2012. Combretum Molle R.Br. Ex G.Don. Available at: http://redlist.sanbi.org/species.php?species=2039-32.

Simon, M.K., Ajanusi, O.J., Abubakar, M.S., Idris, A.L., Suleiman, M.M., 2012. The anthelmintic effect of aqueous methanol extract of *Combretum molle* (R. Br. x. G. Don) (Combretaceae) in lambs experimentally infected with *Haemonchus contortus*. Veterinary Parasitology. https://doi.org/10.1016/j.vetpar.2011.12.022.

Steenkamp, V., Fernandes, A.C., Van Rensburg, C.E.J., 2007. Antibacterial activity of Venda medicinal plants. Fitoterapia 78, 561–564.

Suleiman, M.M., Simon, M.K., Ajanusi, O.J., Idris, A.L., Abubakar, M.S., 2013. In vitro anthelmintic activity of the stem-bark of Combretum molle R. Br. x. G. Don (Combretaceae) against *Haemonchus contortus*. Journal of Medicinal Plants Research 7, 952–956.

Traoré-Coulibaly, M., Paré-Toé1, L., Sorgho, H., Koog, C., Kazienga, A., Dabiré, K.R., Gouagna, L.C., Dakuyo, P.Z., Ouédraogo, J.B., Guissou, I.P., Guiguemdé, T.R., 2013. Antiplasmodial and repellent activity of indigenous plants used against malaria. Journal of Medicinal Plants Research 7, 3105–3111.

Van Wyk, B., Van Wyk, P., 2013. Field Guide to Trees of Southern Africa, second ed. Random House Struik (Pty) Ltd.

Watt, J.M., Breyer-Brandwijk, M.G., 1962. The Medicinal and Poisonous Plants of Southern and Eastern Africa. E. and S. Livingstone Ltd, London, p. 194.

Wondmnew, K., Teshome, D., 2016. The effect of *Combretum molle* seed extracts on the growth of the mycelial form of *Histoplasma capsulatum var farciminosum*-an *in vitro* trial. Virology & Mycology 5, 1.

Yeo, D., Bouagnon, R., Djyh, B.N., Tuo, C., N'guessan, J.D., 2012. Acute and subacute toxic study of aqueous leaf extract of *Combretum molle*. Tropical Journal of Pharmaceutical Research 11, 217–223.

CHAPTER

11

Commelina benghalensis

Bianca Fibrich, Namrita Lall

Department of Plant and Soil Sciences, University of Pretoria, Pretoria, Gauteng, South Africa

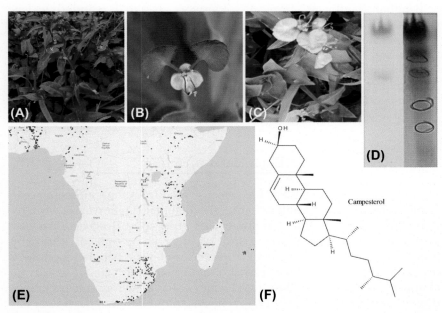

FIGURE 11 Aerial plant parts of *Commelina benghalensis* (A), flower of *C. benghalensis* (ARS, 2006) (B), flower and leaves of *C. benghalensis* (C), TLC chromatogram, Lane 1; *C. benghalensis* prevanillin spray, Lane 2; *C. benghalensis* postvanillin spray (D), distribution of *C. benghalensis* in sub-Saharan Africa (GBIF, 2018) (E), chemical structure of campesterol (F).

Underexplored Medicinal Plants from Sub-Saharan Africa
https://doi.org/10.1016/B978-0-12-816814-1.00011-9

1. General description

1.1 Botanical nomenclature

Commelina benghalensis L.
Synonyms: *C. canescens* Vahl (from Yemen); *C. cucullata* L. (from India); *C. nervosa* Burm.f., *C. mollis* Jacq., *C. turbinate* Vahl., *C. procurrens* Schlechtend, *C. prostrata* Regel, and *C. delicatula* Schlectend

1.2 Botanical family

Commelinaceae

1.3 Vernacular names

Benghal dayflower, tropical spiderwort, Benghal wandering Jew (English)
Blouselblommetjie (Afrikaans)
Lala-tau, Khopo-e-nyenyane (Sesotho)
Uhlotshane (isiXhosa)
Idambiso, idemadema, idlebendlele, idangbane (isiZulu)
Ndamba (Tshivenda)
Indabane (Ndebele)

2. Botanical description

Commelina benghalensis is a herbaceous weed from the Commelinaceae family. The common English name, the Benghal dayflower, is fittingly derived from the fact that the flowers are quite short-lived because they open quite early in the morning and, however, show signs of wilting by midday (Webster et al., 2005). In tropical climates the Benghal dayflower occurs as a perineal; however, with a hexaploid life cycle, in temperate climates associated with the United States, it has been found to occur as a diploid annual (Holm et al., 1977). The hexaploid Benghal dayflower has rarely been noted to produce subterranean flowers, whereas the diploid Benghal dayflower has been noted to produce subterranean flowers, an almost unique feature belonging to *C. benghalensis* (Faden and Hafliger, 1982; Holm et al., 1977; Maheshwari and Maheshwari, 1955; Maheshwari and Singh, 1934). These flowers are born on leafy bracts in both aerial and subterranean cases. However, the aerial flowers are typically chasmogamous, consisting of three petals, two of which are pale blue to lilac and placed above the third, which may be more pale or white, while the subterranean flowers are cleistogamous. The dichotomously branched succulent stems allow the Benghal dayflower to creep distances of 20—90 cm in length, forming roots at the nodes, and ascend to heights of 30 cm when supported. Like the stems, the leaves too are pubescent and can be identified through parallel venation as well as entire leaf margins (Faden and Hafliger, 1982). A distinguishing characteristic of *C. benghalensis* when compared to approximately 170 species of the same genus is that it is vegetatively distinct (Faden, 1992). For *C. benghalensis* found in the United States, these characteristics include the presence of long hairs at the summit of the leaf sheath, proportionally long and short leaf blade, rhizomes, and an annual growth habit (Webster et al., 2005). Pollination may occur through self-pollination or insects; although the flowers lack nectar, they are quite showy (Faden, 1992). The fruit is a pyriform two-valved capsule comprised of five dimorphic seeds, one large and four small seeds per aerial fruit, or one large and two small per subterranean fruit. The blackish brown seeds produced by *C. benghalensis* are rectangular and have a nettled appearance (Faden and Hafliger, 1982; Reed, 1977). A cap present over the embryo is dislodged during germination (Webster et al., 2005).

3. Distribution

Commelina benghalensis is considered a weed as it affects at least 25 crops in 29 different countries including bananas, corn, soybean, wheat, pastures, and cotton (Holm et al., 1977; Wilson, 1981). It is natively present throughout many tropical regions including Asia and Africa and the current distribution includes Australia, South America, the West Indies and North America (including Mexico), and the Pacific islands (Faden, 1992; Faden and Hafliger, 1982; Webster et al., 2005). Approximately 16 species are found in Southern Africa.

4. Ethnobotanical usage

Commelina benghalensis has been reported for medicinal uses within the Zulu culture, specifically as a poultice and remedy for hypertension. Sotho people have also reported it for the treatment of infertility in women, sore throats and eyes, burns, rashes, leprosy, and dysentery. The mucilage obtained from flowering plants has been reported to treat infant's thrush. In Eastern Africa, the juice is used for ophthalmia, burns, and sore throats (Ibrahim et al., 2010). In Southern Nigeria, a poultice is prepared for the treatment of sore feet (Ibrahim et al., 2010). In Cameroon, it has been reported for wound healing (Burkill, 2000). In the Philippines, it is also used for sore eyes as in African practices as well as for the treatment of urethral pain. In India, it is used as a demulcent, emollient, depressant, bitter, refrigerant, and laxative (Hassan et al., 2009). In Madagascar, leaf decoctions have been reported to be effective for Malaria. It also offers feeding value and is used for animal fodder or is eaten as a vegetable, such as spinach (Webster et al., 2005).

Although some compounds such as n-octacosanol, n-triocotanol, stigmasterol, campesterol, and hydrocyanic acid have been reported to have been isolated from both the vegetative and flowering parts of the whole plant, there is no report in literature on the type of useful secondary metabolites contained in the plant as it is considered a weed (Burkill, 2000; Jayvir et al., 2002)

5. Phytochemical constituents

Compounds reported to have been isolated from *C. benghalensis* include n-triocotanol, stigmasterol, n-octacosanol, campesterol, and hydrocyanic acid. Phytochemical investigations have revealed the presence of anthocyanins, steroids, iridoids, terpenoids, lignans, dammarane, sterols, hydrocyanic acid and campesterol, flavonoids, aliphatic alcohols, polyols, phenolic acids, volatile waxes, n-octacosanol, n-trioctanol with lutein, and β-carotene found to be present in high quantity (Hassan et al., 2009; Khan et al., 2011; Raju et al., 2007; Tiwari et al., 2013).

6. TLC fingerprinting of plant extract

For the separation of compounds present within *C. benghalensis*, 2 mg of the ethanolic extract was weighed out and dissolved in 200 μL ethanol and observed using silica gel 60 F254 thin layer chromatography (TLC) plates. The plates were cut to size and, using a soft pencil, a line was drawn 1 cm from both the bottom and top of the plate. On the bottom line, samples were spotted approximately 1 cm apart using a capillary. The spots were allowed to dry completely and the TLC plate placed in a TLC chamber containing the eluent. Before the addition of the TLC plate, the chamber was left briefly to allow the mobile phase to totally saturate the chamber. For this experiment, 10 mL of eluent (9:5 dichloromethane: methanol) was used. The samples were allowed to separate until the solvent front reached the line drawn at the top of the TLC plate. After this, the TLC plates were observed under short and long wavelengths of ultraviolet light, followed by spraying with freshly prepared vanillin/sulfuric acid (1%).

7. Pharmacological properties

Commelina benghalensis has been researched for its in vitro propensity as an antidiarrheal, anthelmintic, antimicrobial, anxiolytic, antioxidant, antitumor, anticancer, and thrombolytic agent (Ahmad et al., 1998; Hassan et al., 2009; Kabir et al., 2016; Mbazima et al., 2008). Its prominence in all nine South African provinces identifies it as a promising medicinal plant holding many opportunities for more extensive research and development endeavors.

7.1 Antidiarrheal activity

Leaves of *C. benghalensis* were taxonomically identified and collected from Chittagong, Bangladesh, in October 2014. The material was dried and a methanolic extract prepared. Using a Swiss albino mouse model, the therapeutic efficacy of the extract as an antidiarrheal was evaluated. Castor oil was administered at concentrations of 200 mg/kg and 400 mg/kg to induce diarrhea, at which the methanolic leaf extract was found to produce notable antidiarrheal effects. This was concluded by measuring the total number of wet feces, which decreased on administration of the extract. Other parameters that were assessed include enteropooling and gastrointestinal motility. The effect of the extract on enteropooling was assessed, as the administration of castor oil resulted in the accumulation of water and electrolytes in the fecal matter of the test subjects, which was found to be significantly reduced at the test concentrations when *C. benghalensis* was administered. Intestinal transit was evaluated using the gastrointestinal motility test, which found that intestinal motility was drastically reduced in the test group treated with *C. benghalensis* (Kabir et al., 2016).

7.2 Anthelmintic activity

Leaf material was collected from Chittagong, Bangladesh, in October 2014 and methanolic and water extracts (using double distilled water) were prepared. An aquarium worm, *Tubifex tubifex* was collected from a local aquarium shop in Chittagong, Bangladesh, and authenticated. The anthelmintic activity was evaluated by considering the time of paralysis and time of death of the worms postadministration. Dose-dependant anthelmintic activity was observed for the methanolic extract with the time taken for paralysis at 10 mg/mL being 12.38 min, 16.25 min at 5 mg/mL, and 22.17 min at 2.5 mg/mL. The time taken for death at each of the concentrations mentioned above was 21.39, 45.64, and 57.25 min, respectively (Kabir et al., 2016).

7.3 Anticarcinogenic activity

Methanolic extracts of *C. benghalensis* were prepared, and their anticarcinogenic activity was evaluated using Jurkat T cells. The parameters considered were growth inhibition and the ability of the extract to induce apoptosis. The cells were treated with the extract at a range of concentrations ($0-600$ µg/mL), the results showed a dose-dependent reduction in cellular proliferation and a decrease in cell viability. By considering morphological and biochemical features, the study concluded that the cytotoxic effects were the result of apoptosis. The conclusions indicated that the crude methanolic extract of *C. benghalensis* contains bioactive compounds useful for the treatment of malignant growths (Mbazima et al., 2008).

7.4 Antioxidant activity

The propensity of *C. benghalensis* extract to scavenge diphenylpicrylhydrazyl (DPPH) free radicals was evaluated by Hassan et al. (2009). The aerial parts were collected from different regions of Bangladesh and authenticated, and hydromethanolic extracts prepared. The results indicated *C. benghalensis* to be a good antioxidant agent where the 50% inhibitory concentration (IC_{50}) value was found to be 21.53 µg/mL (Hassan et al., 2009).

7.5 Antibacterial activity

Authenticated aerial parts of *C. benghalensis* were supplied by the Himalaya Drug Company, New Delhi, from which ethanolic, hexane, and aqueous extracts were prepared. The antibacterial activity of *C. benghalensis* against *Bacillus subtilis*, *Escherichia coli*, *Proteus vulgaris*, *Salmonella typhimurium*, *Pseudomonas aeruginosa*, and *Staphylococcus aureus* was evaluated, and no antibacterial action was observed for any of the extracts (Ahmad et al., 1998). In another study, Gothandam et al. (2010) collected fresh leaves of *C. benghalensis* from Vellore, Tamil Nadu, India, for antimicrobial investigation. Crude methanolic extracts were prepared and the antibacterial activity was evaluated using the disc diffusion method. Of the pathogens tested, *Bacillus cereus*, *Bacillus megaterium*, *Micrococcus leuteus*, *S. aureus*, *Streptococcus lactis*, *Enterobacter aerogenes*, *E. coli*, *Klebsiella pneumoniae*, *P. aeruginosa*, *S. lactis*, *E. aerogenes*, and *S. typhimurium*, only slight zones of inhibition were observed (Gothandam et al., 2010).

7.6 Analgesic activity

The aerial parts of *C. benghalensis* were collected from Old Elephant Road, Eskaton Garden, Dhaka, authenticated, and an extract was prepared using a mixture of methanol and water (7:3 v/v). From the extract, petroleum ether, chloroform, hydromethanolic, and n-butanol fractions were collected, and their analgesic property was evaluated using the hotplate and tail immersion method. Peripheral pharmacological actions utilizing acetic acid–induced writhing test were also performed. All fractions were tested at concentrations of 200 and 400 mg/kg body weight and showed significant analgesic effects for the two models tested. All fractions caused a significant increase in the latency time in the hotplate and tail immersion method, whereas the acetic acid–induced writhing test showed a significant reduction in the writhing response, with the responses decreasing by 48% for the petroleum ether fraction, 68.8% for the chloroform fraction, 61.9% for the n-butanol fraction, and 52.8% for the hydromethanol fraction (Hassan et al., 2010).

8. Additional information

8.1 Therapeutic (proposed) usage

Anticancer, antidiarrheal, and anthelmintic.

8.2 Safety data

Leaves of *C. benghalensis* were taxonomically identified and collected from Chittagong, Bangladesh, in October 2014. The material was dried and a methanolic extract prepared. To evaluate the acute toxicity of *C. benghalensis*, 40 Albino Swiss mice were used. In this study, various doses of the crude methanol extract were administered by stomach tube and the mice observed for general toxicity symptoms. No behavioral, physical, or neurological changes were noted for the duration of the observation period when considering motor activity convulsions, restlessness, coma, lacrimation, and diarrhea as parameters. The median lethal dose (LD_{50}) was thus concluded to be greater than the highest concentration tested (4000 mg/kg) (Kabir et al., 2016).

8.3 Trade information

Not threatened, not endangered, and abundant

8.4 Dosage

Not available

References

Ahmad, I., Mehmood, Z., Mohammad, F., 1998. Screening of some indian medicinal plants for their antimicrobial properties. Journal of Ethnopharmacology 62, 183–193.

ARS, 2006. Agricultural Research Service, United States Department of Agriculture. 2006. Tropical spiderwort (*Commelina benghalensis*)- ID D577-1. Available online: https://commons.wikimedia.org/wiki/Commelina_benghalensis#/media/File:ARS_-_Commelina_benghalensis.jpg. Public domain.

Burkill, H.M., 2000. The Useful Plants of West Tropical Africa, vol. 1. Royal Botanic Gardens, Kew, pp. 429–430.

Faden, R.B., 1992. Proposal to conserve *Commelina benghalensis* (Commelinaceae) with a conserved type under Art. 69.3. Taxon 41, 341–342.

Faden, R.B., Hafliger, E., 1982. Commelinaceae. In: Hafliger, E. (Ed.), Monocot Weeds. Ciba-Geigy, Basel, Switzerland, pp. 100–111.

GBIF, 2018. *Commelina benghalensis* L. In GBIF secretariat (2017). GBIF Backbone Taxonomy. Checklist dataset. https://doi.org/10.15468/39omei. accessed via GBIF.org on 2018-08-20.

Gothandam, K.M., Aishwarya, R., Karthikeyan, S., 2010. Preliminary screening of antimicrobial properties of few medicinal plants. Journal of Phytology 2, 1–6.

Hassan, S., Hossain, M.M., Akter, R., Jamila, M., Mazumder, M.E.H., Rahman, S., 2009. DPPH Free radical scavenging activity of some Bangladeshi medicinal plants. Journal of Medicinal Plants Research 3, 875–879.

Hassan, S., Hossain, M.M., Akter, R., Jamila, M., Mazumder, M.E.H., Alam, M.A., Faraque, A., Rana, S., Rahman, S., 2010. Analgesic activity of different fractions of the aerial parts of *Commelina benghalensis* Linn. International Journal of Pharmacology 6, 63–67.

Holm, L.G., Plucknett, D.L., Pancho, J.V., Herberger, J.P., 1977. The World's Worst Weeds: Distribution and Biology. University of Hawaii, Honolulu, p. 609.

Ibrahim, J., Ajaegbu, V.C., Egharevba, H.O., 2010. Pharmacognostic and phytochemical analysis of *Commelina benghalensis* L. Ethnobotanical Leaflets 14, 610–615.

Jayvir, A., Minoo, P., Gauri, B., Ripal, K., 2002. Nature Heals: A Glossary of Selected Indigenous Medicinal Plant of India, second ed. SRIST Innovations, Ahmedabad, India, p. 22.

Kabir, M.S.H., Hasanat, A., Chowdhury, T.A., Rashid, M.M.U., Hossain, M.M., Ahmed, S., 2016. Study of antidiarrheal and anthelmintic activity of methanol extract of *Commelina benghalensis* leaves. African Journal of Pharmacy and Pharmacology 10, 657–664.

Khan, M.A.A., Islam, M.T., Rahman, M.A., Ahsan, Q., 2011. Antibacterial activity of different fractions of *Commelina benghalensis* L. Der Pharmacia Sinica 2, 320–326.

Maheshwari, P., Maheshwari, J.K., 1955. Floral dimorphism in *Commelina forskalaei* Vahl. And *C. benghalensis* L. Phytomorphology 5, 413–422.

Maheshwari, P., Singh, B., 1934. A preliminary note on the morphology of the aerial and underground flowers of *Commelina benghalensis*, Linn. Current Science 3, 158–160.

Mbazima, V.G., Mokgotho, M.P., February, F., Rees, D.J.G., Mampuru, L.J.M., 2008. Alteration of Bax-to-Bcl-2 ratio modulates the anticancer activity of methanolic extract of *Commelina benghalensis* (Commelinaceae) in Jurkat T cells. African Journal of Biotechnology 7, 3569—3576.

Raju, M., Varakumar, S., Lakshminarayana, R., Krishnakantha, T.P., Baskaran, V., 2007. Carotenoid composition and vitamin A activity of medicinally important green leafy vegetables. Food Chemistry 101, 1598—1605. https://doi.org/10.1016/j.foodchem.2006.04.015.

Reed, C.F., 1977. Economically important foreign weeds: potential problems in the United States. In: Agriculture Handbook 498. Washington D.C.: U.S. Government Printing Office, USDA—Agricultural Research Service/APHIS, 746 pp.

Tiwari, S.K., Lahkar, M., Dash, S., Samudrala, P.K., Thomas, J.M., Augistine, B.B., 2013. Preliminary phytochemical, toxicity and anti-inflammatory evaluation of *Commelina benghalensis*. International Journal of Green Pharmacy 201—205.

Webster, T.M., Burton, M.G., Culpeper, A.S., York, A.C., Prostko, E.P., 2005. Tropical spiderwort (*Commelina benghalensis*): a tropical invader threatens agroecosystems of the southern United States. Weed Technology 19, 501—508.

Wilson, A.K., 1981. Commelinaceae—a review of the distribution, biology, and control of the important weeds belonging to this family. Tropical Pest Management 27, 405—418.

Further reading

PlantZAfrica, 2015. *Commelina benghalensis* L. Online Available at: http://pza.sanbi.org/commelina-benghalensis.

Elaeodendron transvaalense

Thilivhali E. Tshikalange, Fatimah Lawal

Department of Plant and Soil Sciences, University of Pretoria, Pretoria, Gauteng, South Africa

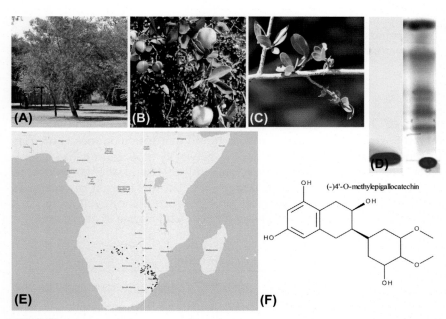

FIGURE 12 A tree of *Elaeodendron transvaalense* (Becking, 2018a) (A), fruit of *E. transvaalense* (Hyde, 2005) (B), leaves of *E. transvaalense* (Becking, 2018b) (C), TLC chromatogram, Lane 1; epigallocatechin, Lane 2; *E. transvaalense* extract (D), distribution map of *E. transvaalense* in sub-Saharan Africa (GBIF, 2017) (E), chemical structure of methyl-epigallocatechin (F).

Underexplored Medicinal Plants from Sub-Saharan Africa
https://doi.org/10.1016/B978-0-12-816814-1.00012-0

1. General description

1.1 Botanical nomenclature

Elaeodendron transvaalense (*Burtt Davy*) R.H. Archer

1.2 Botanical family

Celastraceae

1.3 Vernacular names

Bushveld saffron (English)
Bosveldsaffraan, Lepelhout (Afrikaans)
Monamane (Sotho)
nGcotfo (Swati)
Ximapana (Tsonga)
Mulumanama, Mukuvhazwivhi, Mukundadivhu (Venda)
Ingwavuma, uMgugudo (Zulu)

2. Botanical description

Elaeodendron transvaalense is a small- to medium-sized, bushy tree (about 6—8 m high) occurring in forests and quite often on rocky outcrops in mountainous regions. The bark is generally smooth and has a gray color. Leaves are often clustered on reduced lateral shoots, oblong in shape, about 50 mm long and 20 mm wide. The leaf margin is sometimes toothed. The flowers are greenish and produce oblong, yellow to dark orange, berry-like fruits, which are edible (Tshikalange et al., 2008a).

3. Distribution

The species is widely distributed in the north-eastern parts of South Africa. It grows in KwaZulu-Natal, Swaziland, Mpumalanga, Gauteng through Limpopo province into Mozambique, Zimbabwe, and Zambia extending to Botswana, Angola and Namibia (Van Wyk and Gericke, 2000; PlantZAfrica, 2007).

4. Ethnobotanical usage

Elaeodendron transvaalense is widely used in traditional medicine to treat various ailments including cough, diarrhea, stomach ailments, rash, gout, and sexually associated diseases. Infusions or decoctions are prepared from the stem bark, which is either administered orally or used as an enema. Other traditional uses include the treatment of hemorrhoids, menorrhagia, swellings, and skin diseases (Bessong et al., 2005; Mabogo, 1990; Van Wyk and Gericke, 2000).

5. Phytochemical constituents

Elaeodendron species are rich in terpenoids, gallotannins and proanthocyanidin and a few other phenolic compounds. Triterpenoids and epigallocatechin have been isolated from *E. transvaalense* (Tshikalange and Hussein, 2010). Other compounds isolated from this plant include elaeocyanidin, β-sitosterol, ψ-taraxastanonol, lup-20(30)-ene-3,29-diol, (3α)-(9Cl), and lup-20(29)-ene-30-hydroxy-(9Cl) (Tshikalange, 2007).

6. TLC fingerprinting of plant extract

Stem bark of *E. transvaalense* was collected and left to dry at room temperature for 2 weeks. The dried powder stem bark was placed in a container and soaked in ethanol. The container was closed and left in the dark for 3 days at room temperature before the extract was filtered and concentrated to dryness under reduced pressure. *Elaeodendron transvaalense* ethanolic extract and one pure compound, (−)4′-O-methylepigallocetechin as a reference compound, were spotted on a thin layer chromatography (TLC) plate (silica gel 60 F254), which was developed in a tank containing hexane and ethyl acetate (3:7). The bands on the TLC plate were observed under ultraviolet (UV) light (long and short wavelength) and also sprayed with freshly prepared vanillin/sulfuric acid (2%).

7. Pharmacological properties

Although *E. transvaalense* is a widely used and well-known plant in South Africa, it has not been extensively researched for its biological properties.

7.1 Antimicrobial activity

Ethanol and Chloroform extracts of *E. transvaalense* powdered root were tested for their inhibitory activity against 4 g-positive and

6 g-negative bacteria using the agar dilution method. The results showed that the ethanol extract had some degree of antibacterial activity against *Bacillus cereus*, *Bacillus pumilis*, *Bacillus subtilis*, and *Staphylococcus aureus*, and chloroform extract had no activity against all the tested microorganisms (Tshikalange et al., 2005).

7.2 Hypoglycaemic activity

Stem bark of *E. transvaalense* was collected in Venda (Limpopo Province), and an acetone extract was prepared from the ground plant material. The results revealed the hypoglycemic activity of the *E. transvaalense* extract, but it was toxic to Chang liver cells. The extract also displayed α-glucosidase and α-amylase inhibition activity with 50 % inhibitory concentration (IC_{50}) values of 50.62 and 1.12 µg/mL, respectively (Deutschländer et al., 2009).

7.3 Anti-HIV-1 activity

Dried powdered stem bark of *E. transvaalense* was extracted with several solvents (chloroform, ethyl acetate, and 70% acetone). The extracts were evaluated for their inhibition against α-glycohydrolase, reverse transcriptase, and viral proteins (NF-kB and Tat), which play a significant role in the human immunodeficiency virus (HIV) life cycle. All the extracts of *E. transvaalense* showed little or no significant inhibition against the tested enzymes. The ethyl acetate extracts exhibited the most potent inhibitory activity in both the NF-kB and Tat assays with inhibitory activity of 76% and 75%, respectively, at a concentration of 15 mg/mL. The acetone and chloroform extracts showed moderate activity (Tshikalange et al., 2008a). In another study by Tshikalange et al. (2008b), the ethanol root extract (IC_{50} of 0.01 ng/mL) showed significant anti-HIV activity with little or no toxicity on the CCK5 cell line at the lowest concentration tested (0.1 ng/mL).

8. Additional information

8.1 Therapeutic (proposed) usage

Antimicrobial, anti-HIV, and antidiabetic

8.2 Safety data

Not available

8.3 Trade information

According to Red data list of South African plants, *E. transvaalense* is on a Near Threatened (NT A4ad) status due to over-harvesting of its bark (Williams et al., 2013).

8.4 Dosage

Not available

References

Becking, D., 2018a. *Elaeodendron Transvaalense* 472 2018.04.25 Nylsvley NR. Available online: https://treesa.org/elaeodendron-transvaalense/.

Becking, D., 2018b. 457 2018.04.25 Nylsvley NR. Available online: https://treesa.org/elaeodendron-transvaalense/.

Bessong, P.O., Obi, C.L., Andréola, M., Rojas, L.B., Pouységu, L., Igumbor, E., Meyer, J.J.M., Quideau, S., Litvak, S., 2005. Evaluation of selected South African medicinal plants for inhibitory properties against human immunodeficiency virus type 1 reverse transcriptase and integrase. Journal of Ethnopharmacology 99, 83—91.

Deutschländer, M.S., van de Venter, M., Roux, S., Louw, J., Lall, N., 2009. Hypoglycaemic activity of four plant extracts traditionally used in South Africa for diabetes. Journal of Ethnopharmacology 124, 619—624.

GBIF, 2017. Elaeodendron Transvaalense (Burtt Davy) R.H.Archer in GBIF Secretariat (2017). GBIF Backbone Taxonomy. Checklist dataset. https://doi.org/10.15468/39omei.

Hyde, M.A., 2005. Tree, with Pendulous Branches, Covered in Fruit. Fruit Whitish-Yellow. Although This Was in a Garden, as Far as Is Known the Tree Was Not Planted. Available online: https://www.mozambiqueflora.com/speciesdata/image-display.php?species_id=137070&image_id=1.

Mabogo, D.E.N., 1990. The Ethnobotany of the Vhavenda. M.Sc. thesis. University of Pretoria.

PlantZAfrica, 2007. Elaeodendron Transvaalense (Burtt Davy) R.H.Archer. Online. Available at: http://www.pza.sanbi.org/elaeodendron-transvaalense.

Tshikalange, T.E., Meyer, J.J.M., Hussein, A.A., 2005. Antimicrobial activity, toxicity and the isolation of a bioactive compound from plants used to treat sexually transmitted diseases. Journal of Ethnopharmacology 96, 515—519.

Tshikalange, T.E., Hussein, A., 2010. Cytotoxicity activity of isolated compounds from *Elaeodendron transvaalense* ethanol extract. Journal of Medicinal Plants Research 4 (16), 1695—1697.

Tshikalange, T.E., 2007. In Vitro Anti-HIV-1 Properties of Ethnobotanically Selected South African Plants Used in the Treatment of Sexually Transmitted Diseases. PhD. Dissertation. University of Pretoria, South Africa, 57 pp.

Tshikalange, T.E., Meyer, J.J.M., Lall, N., Muñoz, E., Sancho, R., Van de Venterc, M., Oosthuizen, V., 2008a. *In vitro* anti-HIV-1 properties of ethnobotanically selected South African plants used in the treatment of sexually transmitted diseases. Journal of Ethnopharmacology 119 (3), 478—481.

Tshikalange, T.E., Meyer, J.J.M., Hattori, T., Suzuki, Y., 2008b. Anti-HIV screening of ethnobotanical selected South African plants. South African Journal of Botany 74 (2), 391.

Van Wyk, B.E., Gericke, N., 2000. People's Plants: A Guide to Useful Plants of Southern Africa. Briza Publications, Pretoria, South Africa, 351 pp.

Williams, V.L., Victor, J.E., Crouch, N.R., 2013. Red Listed medicinal plants of South Africa: status, trends, and assessment challenges. South African Journal of Botany 86 (23), 23—35.

Equisetum ramosissimum

Karina Szuman, Namrita Lall

Department of Plant and Soil Sciences, University of Pretoria, Pretoria, Gauteng, South Africa

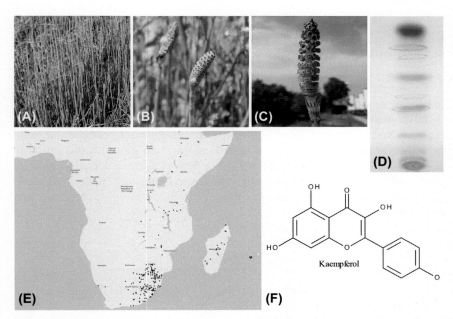

FIGURE 13   Aerial plant parts of *Equisetum ramosissimum* (Filippov, 2005) (A), branch with whorl at node (Martin, 2010) (B), flower spike of *E. ramosissimum* (Adrian, 2012) (C), TLC chromatogram, fingerprint of *E ramosissimum* (D), distribution of *E. ramosissimum* in sub-Saharan Africa (GBIF, 2018) (E), chemical structure of kaempferol (F).

Underexplored Medicinal Plants from Sub-Saharan Africa
https://doi.org/10.1016/B978-0-12-816814-1.00013-2

1. General description

1.1 Botanical nomenclature

Equisetum ramosissimum Desf

1.2 Botanical family

Equisetaceae

1.3 Vernacular names

African horsetail (English)
Bewerasiegras (Afrikaans)
Ishobalehashi (Zulu)
Mohlakaphotwane (South Sotho)

2. Botanical description

Equisetum ramosissimum is a perennial fern from the Equisetaceae family. The plant grows best in moist soils. A black subterranean stem is usually vertical, branching horizontally. Aerial stems are hollow and lie erect above the ground, growing up to 1 meter. Thinner branches emerge in whorls at each node along the length of the stem giving it its common name of "branched horsetail". Scale-like leaves form a whorled sheath above each node along the aerial stem. These leaves are narrowly lance-olate with a single vein and are often shiny-black in color (Hyde et al., 2018; Roux, 2003).

3. Distribution

E. ramosissimum is widely distributed across South Africa (Eastern Cape, Free State, Gauteng, KwaZulu-Natal, Limpopo, Mpumalanga, Northern Cape, and North West), occurring mostly in terrestrial areas along perennial rivers or streams and areas that are seasonally flooded (wetlands) (Roux, 2003).

4. Ethnobotanical usage

E. ramosissimum is a sweet yet slightly bitter tasting plant that is traditionally used in South Africa for a variety of ailments. Infertile women drink a decoction made from the rhizome to aid in fertilization while a paste made from the branches is applied to areas to treat fractured or dislocated bones. *E. ramosissimum* is also known to possess diuretic, haemostatic, antifungal, and antiviral properties. The Zulu communities have been reported to use the sap from the plant to reduce the pain of toothaches and heal wounds of tooth extractions (Banjamin and Manickam, 2007; Gerstner, 1939).

5. Phytochemical constituents

There have been 17 compounds that were previously isolated from the whole plant of *E. ramosissimum*: 5α,6α-expoxy-β-ionone-3-O-β-D-gluco-pyranoside (1), loliolide (2), cycloart-24(30)-ene-3β-ol (3), cycloart-22(23)-ene-3β-ol (4), ergost-6,22-diene-3β,5α,8α-triol (5), friedelinol (6), apigene (7), genkwanin (8), genkwanin-5-O-β-D-glucopyranoside (9), apigene-5-O-β-D-glucopyranoside (10), luteolin (11), quercentin-3-O-β-D-glucopyranoside (12), kaempferol-3-β-D-glucopyranoside (13), kaempferol-3-O-β-D-glucose-7-O-β-D-glucopyranoside (14), adenine (15), β-sitosterol (16), and β-daucosterol (17) (Wang and Jia, 2005).

6. TLC fingerprinting of plant extract

To observe the separation on *E. ramosissimum*, 2 mg of an ethanolic extract was weighed out and dissolved in 200 μL ethanol. For the thin layer chromatography (TLC) analysis of *E. ramosissimum* crude extract, silica gel 60 F254 TLC plates were used to observe the separation of the compounds present within the extract. Plate markings were made with a soft pencil and glass capillaries were used to spot the samples onto the TLC plate. The spots were left to dry before it was placed in a TLC tank, which contained a 10 mL eluent 9.5:0.5 methanol: DCM solvent system. The samples were allowed to separate until the solvent system reached 1 cm from the top of the TLC plate. The plate was observed under ultraviolet (UV light) (long and short wavelength), followed by spraying with freshly prepared vanillin to detect the bands on the TLC plate.

7. Pharmacological properties

E. ramosissimum has been relatively understudied for its in vitro medicinal properties. Considering the number of constituents available in the plant, there is an opportunity for exploring its medicinal value.

7.1 Antibacterial activity

The whole plant of *E. ramosissimum* was collected in Pietermaritzburg, South Africa, and three extracts were prepared thereafter (aqueous, methanol, and ethyl acetate). The extracts were then tested in a disc diffusion assay against seven bacterial species (*Bacillus subtilis, Escherichia coli, Klebsiella pneumoniae, Micrococcus luteus, Pseudomonas aeruginosa, Staphylococcus aureus*, and *Staphylococcus epidermidis*). From the results of this report, neither the aqueous, methanol or ethyl acetate extracts of *E. ramosissimum* showed any bacterial inhibitory potential against the seven strains of bacteria (Kelmanson et al., 2000).

7.2 Antioxidant and anticancer activity

The antioxidant and free radical scavenging activities of the aerial parts of *E. ramosissimum* were previously reported. The aerial portions of the plant were collected from Vojvodina, Serbia, and phosphate buffer (pH 7) extracts were prepared. The extract was tested for its antioxidant activity through the determination of antioxidant enzyme activities of superoxide dismutase (SOD), glutathione peroxidase (GSH-Px), guaiacol peroxidase (GPx), and catalase (CAT) as well as the total antioxidant activity using the ferric reducing ability of plasma (FRAP) assay. The phosphate buffer extracts of the aerial portions of *E. ramosissimum* results indicated the following for the antioxidant enzyme activities: 118.5 ± 1.74 U/mg protein (SOD), 0.945 ± 0.030 U/mg protein (GSH-Px), 231.5 ± 1.23 U/mg protein (GPx), and 325.6 ± 6.56 U/mg protein (CAT). These results indicate that the phosphate buffer extracts of *E. ramosissimum* contain a high level of catalase activity although a very low activity of 5.44 ± 0.72 FRAP units (1 unit equals 100 μM Fe (II)) (Stajner et al., 2009).

In another report, the methanol extracts of *E. ramosissimum* were tested for its antioxidant activity using the 2,2′-azinobis-3-ethylbenzothiazoline-6-sulfonic acid (ABTS) and diphenylpicrylhydrazyl (DPPH) radical scavenging assays. The whole plant of *E. ramosissimum* was collected in the Salem district of Tamil Nadu (India), thereafter 100% methanol extracts were prepared using soxhlet extraction methods. At 250 μg/mL, the methanol extract of *E. ramosissimum* showed a $73.46 \pm 0.14\%$ inhibition of DPPH free radical while the ABTS radical scavenging assay indicated a total antioxidant activity of 1946.36 ± 2.12 μmol/g. The high-radical scavenging activities of these methanol extracts against DPPH and ABTS suggested that *E. ramosissimum* could be a promising natural source of antioxidants (Paulsamy et al., 2013).

A recent publication found that consuming medicinal plants, such as *Equisetum* species, containing kaempferol and kaempferol glycosides has a positive effect on reducing the risk of developing chronic diseases including cancer. Kaempferol has been found to exhibit a wide range of pharmacological activities, including antioxidant, antiinflammatory, antimicrobial, anticancer, cardioprotective, neuroprotective, antidiabetic, antiosteoporotic, estrogenic/antiestrogenic, anxiolytic, analgesic, and antiallergic (Calderon-Montano et al., 2011). In addition to these activities, kaempferol has been reported to induce anticancer activity on a molecular level by modulating numerous key factors within the cell signaling pathways involved in apoptosis, angiogenesis, inflammation and metastasis by inhibiting angiogenesis and the growth of cancerous cells, while protecting the viability of normal cells yet inducing the apoptosis of cancer cells (Chen and Chen, 2013).

7.3 Antityrosinase activity

The mushroom tyrosinase inhibition of various extracts of *E. ramosissimum* was determined. The whole plant of *E. ramosissimum* was collected and ethyl acetate, dichloromethane, hexane, methanol, and aqueous extracts were prepared. According to the results, the percentage inhibition of mushroom tyrosinase for each extract at 100 μg/mL was reported as follows: 23.79 ± 3.84% (dichloromethane), 23.82 ± 4.25% (hexane), 23.27 ± 1.67% (methanol), and 23.82 ± 1.24% (aqueous) all had similar inhibitory potential while the ethyl acetate extract was recorded to have the strongest inhibiting effect with 38.93 ± 3.09% at 100 μg/mL (Li et al., 2016).

8. Additional information

8.1 Therapeutic (proposed) usage

Anticancer and antityrosinase

8.2 Safety data

The ethyl acetate, dichloromethane, hexane, methanol, and aqueous extracts of *E. ramosissimum* showed no toxic effects on human epidermal keratinocytes (HaCaT) and dermal fibroblasts as after a 24 h treatment, the cell viabilities at various concentrations (0–100 μg/mL) exceeded 65% (Li et al., 2016).

8.3 Trade information

Not threatened, not endangered, and abundant

8.4 Dosage

Not available

References

Adrian, 2012. Estróbilo de *Equisetum ramosissimum*. Moncofar, Castellón, España. Available online: https://commons.wikimedia.org/wiki/File:Equisetum_ramosissimum_CS1.jpg. The copyright holder of this work, release this work into the public domain. This applies worldwide.

Banjamin, A., Manickam, V.S., 2007. Medicinal pteridophytes from the Western Ghats. Indian Journal of Traditional Knowledge 6, 611—618.

Calderon-Montano, J.M., Burgos-Morón, E., Pérez-Guerrero, C., López-Lázaro, M., 2011. A review on the dietary flavonoid kaempferol. Mini Reviews in Medicinal Chemistry 11 (4), 298—344.

Chen, A.Y., Chen, Y.C., 2013. A review of the dietary flavonoid, kaempferol on human health and cancer chemoprevention. Food Chemistry 138 (4), 2099—2107.

Filippov, P., 2005. *Equisetum ramosissimum* slavičín, Czech Republic. Available online: https://commons.wikimedia.org/wiki/File:Equisetum_ramosissimum,_Slavi%C4%8D%C3%ADn,_Czech_Republic.jpg (CC BY-SA 3.0).

GBIF, 2018. *Equisetum Ramosissimum* Desf. In GBIF Secretariat. GBIF Backbone Taxonomy. Checklist dataset. https://doi.org/10.15468/39omei.

Gerstner, J., 1939. A preliminary checklist of Zulu names and plants with short notes. Bantu Studies 13, 46—64.

Hyde, M.A., Wursten, B.T., Ballings, P., Coates Palgrave, M., 2018. Flora of Zimbabwe: *Equisetum Ramosissimum*. https://www.zimbabweflora.co.zw/speciesdata/species.php?species_id=100210v.

Kelmanson, J.E., Jäger, A.K., van Staden, J., 2000. Zulu medicinal plants with antibacterial activity. Journal of Ethnopharmacology 69 (3), 241—246.

Li, P.H., Chiu, Y.P., Shih, C.C., Wen, Z.H., Ibeto, L.K., Huang, S.H., Chiu, C.C., Ma, D.L., Leung, C.H., Chang, Y.N., Wang, H.M., 2016. Biofunctional activities of *Equisetum ramosissimum* extract: protective effects against oxidation, melanoma, and melanogenesis. Oxidative Medicine and Cellular Longevity 9. Article ID 2853543.

Martin, J., 2010. *Equisetum ramosissimum* close up, in Sierra de Alfacar y Víznar. Granada, Spain. Available online: https://commons.wikimedia.org/wiki/File:Equisetum_ramosissimum_Enfoque_2010-7-17_SierradeAlfacar.jpg. The copyright holder of this work, release this work into the public domain. This applies worldwide.

Paulsamy, S., Moorthy, D., Nandakumar, K., Saradha, M., 2013. Evaluation of *in vitro* antioxidant potential of methanolic extracts of the ferns, *Actiniopteris radiata* (Sw) Link. and *Equisetum ramosissimum* Desf. International Journal of Pharmaceutical Sciences and Research 2 (3), 451—455.

Roux, J.P., 2003. Swaziland Ferns and Fern Allies. http://plants.jstor.org/stable/10.5555/al.ap.flora.sffa001370184100001.

Štajner, D., Popović, B.M., Čanadanović-Brunet, J., Anačkov, G., 2009. Exploring *Equisetum arvense* L., *Equisetum ramosissimum* L. and *Equisetum telmateia* L. as sources of natural antioxidants. Phytotherapy Research 23 (4), 546—550.

Wang, X., Jia, Z., 2005. Chemical constituents of *Equisetum ramosissimum*. Acta Botanica Boreali-Occidentalia Sinica 25 (12), 2524—2528.

C H A P T E R
14

Eriosema kraussianum

Riana Kleynhans, Ivy Masefako Makena, Babalwa Matsiliza-Mlathi

Tshwane University of Technology, Pretoria, Gauteng, South Africa

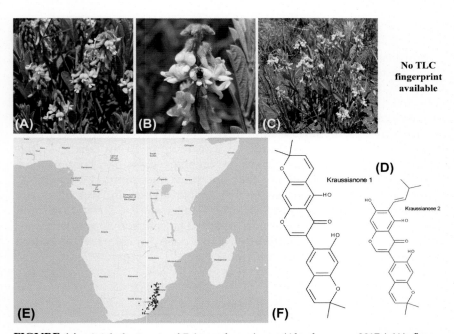

FIGURE 14 Arial plant parts of *Eriosema kraussianum* (Alandmanson, 2017a) (A), flower of *E. kraussianum* (Alandmanson, 2017b) (B), arial plant parts of *E. kraussianum* (Alandmanson, 2017c) (C), no TLC fingerprint available (D), distribution of *E. kraussianum* in Sub-Saharan Africa (GBIF, 2018) (E), chemical structures of kraussianone 1 and 2 (F).

Underexplored Medicinal Plants from Sub-Saharan Africa
https://doi.org/10.1016/B978-0-12-816814-1.00014-4
99

1. General description

1.1 Botanical nomenclature

Eriosema kraussianum Meisn

1.2 Botanical family

Fabaceae

1.3 Vernacular names

Pale yellow eriosema (English)
uBangalala (Zulu)

2. Botanical description

Eriosema kraussianum is a dwarf, erect, fairly small perennial, herb from the Fabaceae family. The specific species epithet *kraussianum* refers to Christian Ferdinand Friedrich von Krauss, a German scientist who collected this plant for the first time from the Natal (now KwaZulu-Natal) province of South Africa (Ngalo, 2015). The species can be classified as a small shrublet with several unbranched, stems covered in silvery silky hairs. The branches form clumps and grow up to 15 cm tall. The alternately arranged, evergreen leaves are on short stalks and contain three conspicuously veined leaflets that are silky and mottled beneath. *E. kraussianum* flowers from September to November. Inflorescences are about 35 mm tall and arranged as terminal racemes. The flowers are 7 mm long and are creamy white or pale yellow. The species has gnarled roots, which produce an oil (rapidly turning to a deep red color) when injured (Drewes et al., 2013; Ngalo, 2015).

3. Distribution

Eriosema kraussianum naturally occurs among rocky areas of grassland and woodland, throughout eastern South Africa (Eastern Cape, Free State, Kwa Zulu Natal, and Mpumalanga provinces) and Swaziland (Ngalo, 2015; Von Staden and Dayaram, 2011).

4. Ethnobotanical usage

The roots of *E. kraussianum* are traditionally chewed by Zulu warriors and are used as an aphrodisiac (Bryant, 1966; Hutchings et al., 1996). The Zulu traditional health practitioners believe that the roots of *E. kraussianum* and other *Eriosema* species are effective remedies for the treatment of erectile dysfunction or impotence (Malviya et al., 2011). The roots are the mostly used morphological part of *E. kraussianum*, either as hot milk infusions or pounded boiled roots (Bryant, 1966; Hulme, 1954).

5. Phytochemical constituents

Seven pyrano-isoflavones have been isolated from *E. kraussianum* roots (Drewes et al., 2002, 2004). These pyrano-isoflavones were named Kraussianone 1, 2, 3, 4, 5, 6, and 7. The kraussianones were isolated from finely milled roots with dichloromethane subsequently followed by dichloromethane/methanol (50:50). Leaves and stems have not been studied, and information on other chemical constituents is still limited.

6. TLC fingerprinting of plant extract

Thin layer chromatography (TLC) fingerprint is not available for this plant.

7. Pharmacological properties

Although known for its use in traditional medicine in South Africa, *E. kraussianum* remains one of the understudied *Eriosema* species, with potential to be investigated further.

7.1 Erectile dysfunction activity

The traditional use of *E. kraussianum* for the treatment of erectile dysfunction and/or impotence by Zulu health practitioners was validated by Drewes et al. (2002). Drewes et al. (2002) screened the five pyrano-isoflavones (kraussianones 1—5) from the rootstock of *E. kraussianum* for smooth muscle relaxation of rabbit penile muscle.

The most active compounds (kraussionaone 1 and 2) had an activity of 85% and 65% respectively of that found in Viagra at a dose of 78 ng/mL (Drewes et al., 2002). *E. kraussianum* is therefore one of the promising plant species of South Africa with potential for development as a remedy in the treatment of impotence and/or erectile dysfunction (Pavan et al., 2015).

7.2 Vasodilatory and hypoglycaemic activity

Ojewole et al. (2006) investigated the vasodilatory and hypoglycaemic properties of kraussianone 1 and 2 in experimental rat models. The two constituents (20–80 mg/kg p.o.) caused dose-dependent and significant hypoglycemia in rats and also showed secondary, vasorelaxant effects. Ojewole and Drewes (2007) furthermore obtained experimental evidence, which showed that the hydro-alcohol extract of *E. kraussianum* resulted in a dose-dependent and significant reduction of blood glucose levels in healthy normoglycaemic and Streptozotocin-treated diabetic rats.

7.3 Preeclampsia

A study by Ramesar et al. (2012) reported that kraussianone 2 (Kr2) has a potential benefit in improving fetal mortality during compromised pregnancies. The authors investigated the effect of Kr2 application in a preeclampsia induced (L-NAME) rat model. The application of Kr2 significantly decreased fetal mortality and demonstrated a trend toward increasing birth and placental weights. Kr2 administration also significantly reduced blood pressure amplification as compared to the pre-eclampsia induced group (Ramesar et al., 2012).

8. Additional informtion

8.1 Therapeutic (proposed) usage

Erectile dysfunction, preeclampsia, and antidiabetic

8.2 Safety data

No cytotoxicity data could be found related to *E. kraussianum*

8.3 Trade information

Widespread, common, and not threatened with a stable population trend and least concern status (Von Staden and Dayaram, 2011).

8.4 Dosage

Not available

References

Alandmanson, 2017a. *Eriosema Kraussianum* in Grassland on Cedara Research Farm. KwaZulu-Natal. Available online: https://commons.wikimedia.org/wiki/File: Eriosema_2017_10_25_2204.jpg (CC BY 4.0).

Alandmanson, 2017b. *Eriosema Kraussianum* in Grassland on Cedara Research Farm. KwaZulu-Natal. Available online: https://commons.wikimedia.org/wiki/File: Eriosema_2017_10_25_2212.jpg (CC BY 4.0).

Alandmanson, 2017c. *Eriosema Kraussianum* in Grassland on Cedara Research Farm. KwaZulu-Natal. Available online: https://commons.wikimedia.org/wiki/File: Eriosema_2017_10_25_2245.jpg (CC BY 4.0).

Bryant, A.T., 1966. Zulu Medicine and Medicine-Men. Centaur Struik, Cape Town.

Drewes, S.E., Horn, M.M., Munro, O.Q., Dhlamini, J.T.B., Meyer, J.J.M., Rakuambo, N.C., 2002. Pyrano-isdflavones with erectile-dysfunction activity from *Eriosema kraussianum*. Phytochemistry 59 (7), 739—747.

Drewes, S.E., Horn, M.M., Khan, F., Munro, O.Q., Dhlamini, J.T.B., Rakuambo, N.C., Meyer, J.J.M., 2004. Minor pryano-isoflavones from *Eriosema kraussianum*: activity-structure and chemical reaction studies. Phytochemistry 65, 1955—1961.

Drewes, S.E., Selepe, M.A., Van Heerden, F.R., Archer, R.H., Mitchell, D., 2013. Unraveling the names, origins and chemistry of "muthis" used for male sexual disorder in KwaZulu Natal, South Africa. South African Journal of Botany 88, 310—316. https://doi.org/10.1016/j.sajb.2013.08.010.

GBIF, 2018. *Eriosema kraussianum* Meisn. In: GBIF Secretariat (2017). GBIF Backbone Taxonomy. Checklist dataset. https://doi.org/10.15468/39omei.

Hulme, M.M., 1954. Wild Flowers of Natal. Shuter & Shooter, Pietermaritzburg.

Hutchings, A., Scott, A.H., Lewis, G., Cunningham, A., 1996. Zulu Medicinal Plants: An Inventory. University of Natal Press, Pietermaritzburg.

Malviya, N., Jain, S., Gupta, B.V., Vyas, S., 2011. Recent studies on aphrodisiac herbs for the management of male sexual dysfunction — a review. Drug Research 68 (1), 3—8.

Ngalo, S., 2015. *Eriosema Kraussianum* Meisn. PlantZAfrica. Online. Available from: http://pza.sanbi.org/eriosema-krassianum.

Ojewole, J.A.O., Drewes, S.E., Khan, F., 2006. Vasodilatory and hypoglycaemic effects of two pyrano-isoflavone extractives from *Eriosema kraussianum* N.E.Br. [Fabaceae] rootstock in experimental rat models. Phytochemistry 67, 610—617. https://doi.org/10.1016/j.phytochem.2005.11.019.

Ojewole, J.A.O., Drewes, S.E., 2007. Hypoglycaemic effect of *Eriosema kraussianum* N.E.Br [Fabaceae] rootstock hydro-alcohol extract in rats. Journal of Natural Medicines 61, 244—250. https://doi.org/10.1007/s11418-006-0129-0.

Pavan, V., Mucignat-Caretta, C., Redaelli, M., Ribaudo, G., Zagotto, G., 2015. The old made new: natural compounds against erectile dysfunction. Arch Parm Chememistry of Life Science. 348, 607—614. https://doi.org/10.1002/ardp.201500075.

Ramesar, S.V., Drewes, S.E., Gathiram, P., Moodley, J., Mackraj, I., 2012. The effect of Kraussianone-2 (Kr2) a natural pyrano-isoflavones from *Eriosema kraussianum*, in an L-Name-induced Pre-eclamptic rat model. Phytotherapy Research 26, 1375—1380. https://doi.org/10.1002/ptr.3697.

Von Staden, L., Dayaram, A., 2011. *Eriosema Kraussianum* Meisn. National Assessment: Red List of South African Plants Version 2017 1. http://redlist.sanbi.org/species.php?species=451-24.

Further Reading

Selepe, M.A., 2011. Synthesis and Analysis of *Eriosema* Isoflavonids and Derivatives Thereof. PhD study. University of KwaZulu-Natal, Pietermartisburg.

Erythrophleum lasianthum

Sipho H. Chauke, Quenton Kritzinger

Department of Plant and Soil Sciences, University of Pretoria, Pretoria, Gauteng, South Africa

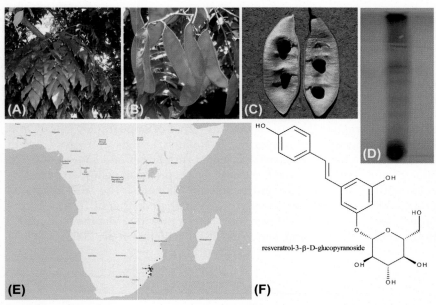

FIGURE 15 Aerial parts of *Erythrophleum lasianthum* (JMK, 2015a) (A), seeds of *E. lasianthum* (JMK, 2016) (B), open seed pod of *E. lasianthum* (JMK, 2015b) (C), TLC chromatogram, fingerprint of *E. lasianthum* (D), distribution of *E. lasianthum* in sub-Saharan Africa (GBIF, 2017) (E), chemical structure of resveratrol-glucopyranoside (F).

Underexplored Medicinal Plants from Sub-Saharan Africa
https://doi.org/10.1016/B978-0-12-816814-1.00015-6   **105**

1. General description

1.1 Botanical nomenclature

Erythrophleum lasianthum Corbishley

1.2 Botanical family

Fabaceae

1.3 Vernacular names

Maputaland ordeal tree (English)
Maputaland oordeelboom (Afrikaans)
Umbhemesi (Zulu)

2. Botanical description

Erythrophleum lasianthum is a medium to large tree with canopy heights ranging between 12 and 17 m. The bark of *E. lasianthum* is grayish-brown in color with a rough surface. The leaves are hairless with a narrowly tapered tip and alternating leaflets. The leaves of *E. lasianthum* are similar to those of *Erythrophleum suavoelens* in terms of appearance, shape, and leaflet arrangement. However, *E. lasianthum* leaflets can grow up to 40 × 20 mm, whereas *E. suavoelens* leaflets are larger and can grow up to 50 × 25 mm. The flowers of *E. lasianthum* are greenish yellow to a creamy color with wool-like hairs on the stamen filaments. The fruit occurs as pods, which are often thin woody, brown, flat, and straight. The seeds are brown, lens-shaped, 12−15 mm long, 4−6 mm wide (Mucina et al., 2017; Roux, 2003; Van Wyk and Van Wyk, 2013; Williams et al., 2008).

3. Distribution

E. lasianthum is commonly distributed in the KwaZulu Natal province of South Africa, Mozambique, and eSwatini (formerly known as Swaziland). It occurs naturally in hot and dry bushvelds or sandy forests (Van Wyk and Van Wyk, 2013).

4. Ethnobotanical usage

In KwaZulu Natal, the powdered bark of *E. lasianthum* is snuffed for the treatment of headaches and migraines. It is also taken internally as a potent purgative for the relief of abdominal pains. Furthermore, infusions made from the bark are used as enemas and emetics. In southern Africa, the powder form of the bark is snuffed to treat colds and lung diseases in cattle. The bark and the leaves of *E. lasianthum* are also taken as decoctions for the treatment of heart problems, fever, and as an anthelmintic (Johnson, 1999; Neuwinger, 1996; Nielsen et al., 2012; Palmer and Pittman, 1972; Watt and Beyer-Brandwijk, 1962).

5. Phytochemical constituents

The chemical constituents present in *E. lasianthum* bark, flowers, and leaves have not been studied. However, three compounds have been isolated from *E. lasianthum* seeds. The isolated compounds are 3-β-hydroxynoerythrosuamine, 3-O-β-D-glucopyranoside, and resveratrol-3-β-D-glucopyranoside (Orsini et al., 1997).

Alkaloids were found to be present in the extracts prepared from the seeds of *E. lasianthum* collected from the dry sand forests of KwaZulu Natal in South Africa (Verrota et al., 1995).

6. TLC fingerprinting of plant extract

The separation of constituents present in the leaf extract of *E. lasianthum* was observed by weighing out 2 mg of the dried ethanolic extract, which was dissolved in 200 µL of ethanol. For the analysis of the *E. lasianthum* leaf extract, silica gel 60 F254 thin layer chromatography (TLC) plates were used to observe the separation of the compounds present within the extract. Two lines, 1 cm from the bottom and 1 cm from the top of the TLC plate, were drawn with a soft pencil. The extract was then spotted using a glass capillary on the line at the bottom of the TLC plate. The spot was allowed to dry completely before placing the TLC plate in a chromatography tank containing a 10 mL eluent of 9:1 chloroform: methanol solvent system. When the solvent system reached 1 cm from the top of the TLC plate, the developed plate was allowed to dry and then sprayed with freshly prepared vanillin/sulfuric acid (2%), for detecting the bands on the TLC plate as well as for the observation of the bands under ultraviolet (UV) light (short and long wavelength).

7. Pharmacological properties

The medicinal properties of *E. lasianthum* have not been extensively studied both in vivo and in vitro.

7.1 Antibacterial activity

In a study by Nielsen et al. (2012), the leaves and stem of *E. lasianthum* collected in August 2007 (winter), from the Manie van Schijff Botanical Garden, University of Pretoria, Pretoria, South Africa, were prepared into crude extracts using methanol as an extractant. The crude extract was then tested against *Mycobacterium smegmatis* ATCC 70084, *Mycobacterium tuberculosis* H37Rv ATCC 27294, Methicillin-resistant *Staphylococcus aureus* (MRSA, LMP805), *Escherichia coli* (βL^{+} EC, LMP701), Chloramphenicol-resistant *Citrobacter* (CRCF, LMP802) and Ampicillin-resistant *Klebsiella pneumoniae* (ARKP, LMP803). The crude methanol extracts showed no activity against *M. smegmatis* and *M. tuberculosis*. However, moderate activity (minimum inhibitory concentration of 625 µg/mL) of the *E. lasianthum* leaves and stem extract was observed against CRCF, ARKP, and MRSA (Nielsen et al., 2012).

7.2 Antioxidant activity

In a study by Twilley et al. (2017), an ethanolic leaf extract of *E. lasianthum* was prepared and investigated for its antioxidant activity using the diphenylpicrylhydrazyl (DPPH) radical scavenging bioassay. The leaf extract showed antioxidant activity with a 50% inhibitory concentration (IC_{50}) value of 5.25 ± 0.08 µg/mL when compared to that of the positive control, ascorbic acid (1.98 ± 0.01 µg/mL).

8. Additional information

8.1 Therapeutic (proposed) usage

Antibacterial and antioxidant

8.2 Safety data

The bark and roots are toxic (Watt and Breyer-Brandwijk, 1962)

8.3 Trade information

Threatened (Williams et al., 2008)

8.4 Dosage

Not available

References

GBIF, 2017. *Erythrophleum Lasianthum* Corbishley in GBIF Secretariat (2017).GBIF Backbone Taxonomy. Checklist dataset. https://doi.org/10.15468/39omeiaccessed via GBIF.org on 2018-07-03.

JMK, 2015a. Foliage of a Maputaland Ordeal Tree at the Manie van der Schijff Botanical Garden at the University of Pretoria. Available online: https://commons.wikimedia. org/wiki/File:Erythrophleum_lasianthum,_loof,_Manie_van_der_Schijff_BT,_b.jpg. (CC BY-SA 3.0).

JMK, 2015b. Open seed pod of a Maputaland Ordeal Tree at the Manie van der Schijff Botanical Garden at the University of Pretoria. https://commons.wikimedia.org/wiki/File: Erythrophleum_lasianthum,_oop_peul,_Manie_van_der_Schijff_BT,_a.jpg.

JMK, 2016. Green seed pods of a Maputaland Ordeal Tree at the Manie van der Schijff Botanical Garden at the University of Pretoria. Available at: https://commons.wikimedia.org/ wiki/File:Erythrophleum_lasianthum,_groen_peule,_Manie_vd_Schijff_BT,_a.jpg.

Johnson, T., 1999. CRC Ethnobotany Desk Reference. CRC Press Inc., Florida, p. 1213.

Mucina, L., Lötter, M.C., Tichy, L., Siebert, S.J., Scott-Shaw, C.R., 2017. Classification of the Eastern Scarp forests. In: Mucina, L. (Ed.), Vegetation Survey and Classification of Subtropical Forests of Southern Africa. Springer, Switzerland, p. 170.

Neuwinger, H.D., 1996. African Ethnobotany— Poison and Drugs. Chapman and Hall, London, pp. 295–314.

Nielsen, T.R., Kuete, V., Jager, A.K., Meyer, J.J.M., Lall, N., 2012. Antimicrobial activity of selected South African medicinal plants. BMC Complementary and Alternative Medicine 12, 1–6.

Orsini, F., Pelizzoni, F., Verotta, L., Aburjai, T., Ragers, C.B., 1997. Isolation, synthesis and antiplatelet aggregation activity of resveratrol 3-O-β-D-glucopyranoside and related compounds. Journal of Natural Products 60, 1082–1087.

Palmer, E., Pitman, N., 1972. Trees of Southern Africa, vol. 2. Balkema, Cape town, pp. 833–835.

Roux, J.P., 2003. Flora of South Africa. In: Flora of Southern Africa. South African Biodiversity Institute (SANBI), Cape Town. Available at: https://www.aluka.org/collection/FLOSA? si=851&scope=plants.

Twilley, D., Langhansova, L., Palaniswamy, D., Lall, N., 2017. Evaluation of traditionally used medicinal plants for anticancer, antioxidant, anti-inflammatory and antiviral (HPV-1) activity. South African Journal of Botany 112, 494–500.

Van Wyk, B., Van Wyk, P., 2013. Field Guide of Trees of Southern Africa. Struik Nature, Cape Town, p. 600.

Verotta, L., Aburjai, T., Rogers, C.B., Dorigo, P., Marango, I., Fraccallo, D., Santostasi, G., Gaion, R.M., Floreani, M., Carpenedo, F., 1995. Chemical and pharmacological characterization of *Erythrophleum lasianthum* alkaloids. Planta Medica 61, 271–274.

Watt, J.M., Breyer-Brandwijk, M.G., 1962. The Medicinal and Poisonous Plants of Southern and Eastern Africa. E and S Livingstone Ltd, Edinburg, pp. 66–67.

Williams, V.L., Raimondo, D., Crouch, N.R., Cunningham, A.B., Scott-Shaw, C.R., Lötter, M., Ngwenya, A.M., 2008. Erythrophleum Lasianthum Corbishley. National Assessment Red List of South Africa. Available at: http://redlist.sanbi.org/species.php?species=455-4.

Euclea natalensis

Carel B. Oosthuizen, Namrita Lall

Department of Plant and Soil Sciences, University of Pretoria, Pretoria, Gauteng, South Africa

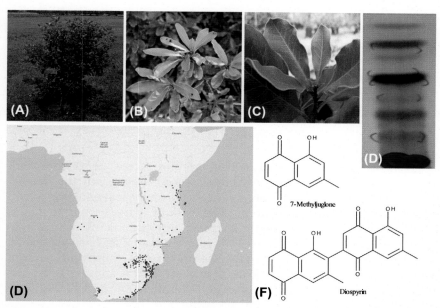

FIGURE 16   Juvenile specimen of *Euclea natalensis* (A), leaves of *E. natalensis* (B), shoot and leaves of *E. natalensis* (C) (Oosthuizen, 2017), TLC chromatogram, fingerprint of *E. natalensis* (D), distribution map of *E. natalensis* in sub-Saharan Africa (GBIF, 2017) (E), chemical structures of 7-methyljuglone and diospyrin (F).

Underexplored Medicinal Plants from Sub-Saharan Africa
https://doi.org/10.1016/B978-0-12-816814-1.00016-8   **111**

1. General description

1.1 Botanical nomenclature

Euclea natalensis A.DC.

1.2 Botanical family

Ebenaceae

1.3 Vernacular names

Natal guarri, Natal ebony, large-leaved guarri (English)
Natalghwarrie, berggwarrie, swartbasboom (African)
umTshekisani, umKhasa (Xhosa)
iDungamuzi, iChitamuzi, isiZimane, umTshikisane, inKunzane,
inKunzi-emnyama, umHlalanyamazane, umAnyathi (Zulu)
umHlangula (Tsonga)
nhlangulane (Chopi)
motlhakola (Ngwaketse)
nhlangulane (Shangana)

2. Botanical description

Euclea natalensis is a small to medium shrub/tree. Leaves are dark green on both sides, with wavy edges. *Euclea natalensis* is the hairiest species of the family. Small glands can be seen on the leave surfaces when magnified at 10× magnification. The bark is dark brown to black. *E. natalensis* is found growing under many different conditions in a wide variety of habitats, from arid rocky scrub to dune bush, open grassveld, woodland, forest, forest margin, riverine fringes, bushveld, and in swamps, from sea level to 1200 m. In arid scrub, it is stunted, often less than a meter tall, whereas in a forest or under favorable conditions, it can become about 12−18 m tall with spreading branches.

3. Distribution

Euclea natalensis is widespread, from Clanwilliam in the Western Cape, southward and eastward along the coast through the Eastern Cape to KwaZulu-Natal, Mpumalanga, Limpopo, Gauteng, and further north in

South Africa. It is also distributed from Swaziland, Mozambique, to tropical east Africa to Ethiopia.

4. Ethnobotanical usage

Zulus frequently use roots of these plant species as a purgative. It is also used to treat abdominal pains usually in the form of an infusion (Watt and Breyer-Brandwijk, 1962). The root is also applied to the skin lesions in leprosy and taken internally for ancylostomiasis. The Tsonga apply the powdered root for the relief of toothache and headache. An infusion of the shoots and bark is taken as an emetic in certain chest diseases to treat complications such as chest pains, bronchitis, pleurisy, and asthma. A decoction of the root is used as a remedy for syphilis. The roots are also famed to produce a distinctive black dye.

Communities involved include Zulus, Tsongas, and Xhosas.

5. Phytochemical constituents

A range of different chemical compounds have been isolated from *E. natalensis*, most of these belong to the naphthoquinone class. Diospyrin and closely related compounds, 8-hydroxydiospyrin isodiospyrin and neodiospyrin, have been isolated from the roots. Other quinones isolated from the plant include 7-methyljuglone, euclanone, galpinone, mamegakinone, natalenone, and shinanolone. Some pentacyclic terpenoids have also been isolated, these include β-sitosterol, botulin, and lupeol (Lall et al., 2006; Lopes and Paul, 1973; Maroyi, 2017; Tannock, 1973; van der Kooy et al., 2006; Weigenand et al., 2004).

6. TLC fingerprinting of plant extract

The plant material was crushed and ground after an air drying process. The dried material was ground into a fine powder and ethanol was added in a 1:10 (weight:volume) ratio. The extract was shaken for 48 h, filtered, and dried using rotary evaporation. The dried extract was collected and stored at 4°C. To observe the separation of the phytochemicals of *E. natalensis*, thin layer chromatography (TLC) was used. Two milligrams of the ethanolic extract was weighed out and dissolved in 200 μL of ethanol. The extract was spotted on the plate. The TLC plate was developed up to 8 cm from the bottom of the plate using the mobile phase ethyl acetate: hexane (3:1). The plate was air dried and examined under ultraviolet light and sprayed with vanillin/sulfuric acid (2%) solution.

7. Pharmacological properties

Due to the traditional usage of *E. natalensis*, the extract has been proposed to be used as a possible adjuvant for patients suffering from tuberculosis.

7.1 Antibacterial activity

Extracts produced from different parts of *E. natalensis* have shown a broad spectrum of antibacterial properties. In a study by Lall and Meyer (2000), the water and acetone extracts of the roots of *E. natalensis* were evaluated for their antimicrobial properties against *Bacillus cereus, Bacillus pumilus, Bacillus subtilis, Enterobacter aerogenes, Enterobacter cloacae, Escherichia coli, Klebsiella pneumoniae, Micrococcus kristinae, Pseudomonas aeruginosa, Serratia marcescens*, and *Staphylococcus aureus*. It was found that both extracts inhibited the growth of the *Bacillus* spp. *M. kristinae* and *S. aureus* at concentrations ranging between 0.1 and 6.0 mg/mL. In another study, the ethanolic and dichloromethane extracts of the leaves were evaluated against bacterial pathogens associated with sexually transmitted infections (*Gardnerella vaginalis, Neisseria gonorrhoeae, Oligella ureolytica*, and *Ureaplasma urealyticum*). The extracts showed to be active with the minimum inhibitory concentration (MIC) values ranging between 1.5 and 2.0 mg/mL (Van Vuuren and Naidoo, 2010).

The antimycobacterial activity of the acetone and water root extract showed to be active with an MIC of 0.5 mg/mL (Lall and Meyer, 1999). In a study conducted by Lall et al. (2016), the ethanolic shoot extract exhibited an antimycobacterial activity with an MIC of 125 µg/mL (Lall et al., 2016). It was further confirmed in an in vivo mice model, where the same extract was able to reduce the bacterial load in mice infected with *Mycobacterium tuberculosis* H37Rv (Lall et al., 2016).

7.2 Antiplasmodial activity

In a study conducted by Clarkson et al. (2004), the dichloromethane and methanol (1:1) root and leaf extracts showed promising activities with 50% inhibition concentration (IC_{50}) values of 5.1 and 5.3 µg/mL, respectively, against *Plasmodium falciparum* using the parasite lactate dehydrogenase assay.

7.3 Hepatoprotective activity

The hepatoprotective property of the ethanolic shoot extract of *E. natalensis* was evaluated on acetaminophen-induced toxic liver cells (HepG2). It was found that the extract was able to have a 50% protective effect at a concentration of 12.5 µg/mL (Lall et al., 2016). Similarly, in an in vivo mice preclinical study, the same extract exhibited a protective effect by reducing the levels of toxic lever marker, alanine aminotransferase (ALT) (Lall et al., 2016).

8. Additional information

8.1 Therapeutic (proposed) usage

Antimycobacterial, immunostimulatory, and hepatoprotective

8.2 Safety data

The cellular toxicity of *E. natalensis* has been assessed on different cell lines and was found to have low to no observable toxicity. The toxicity of the ethanolic extract was evaluated in an acute and subacute in vivo mice trial. It was found that the median lethal dose (LD_{50}) was higher than 2000 mg/mL.

8.3 Trade information

Not threatened, not endangered, and abundant

8.4 Dosage

Not available

References

Clarkson, C., Maharaj, V.J., Crouch, N.R., Grace, O.M., Pillay, P., Matsabisa, M.G., Bhagwandin, N., Smith, P.J., Folb, P.I., 2004. In vitro antiplasmodial activity of medicinal plants native to or naturalised in South Africa. Journal of Ethnopharmacology 92 (2-3), 177–191.

GBIF, 2017. *Euclea natalensis* A.DC. In: GBIF Secretariat.

Lall, N., Kumar, V., Meyer, D., Gasa, N., Hamilton, C., Matsabisa, M., Oosthuizen, C.B., 2016. In vitro and in vivo antimycobacterial, hepatoprotective and immunomodulatory activity of *Euclea natalensis* and its mode of action. Journal of Ethnopharmacology 194, 740–748. https://doi.org/10.1016/j.jep.2016.10.060.

Lall, N., Meyer, J.J.M., 1999. In vitro inhibition of drug-resistant and drug-sensitive strains of Mycobacterium tuberculosis by ethnobotanically selected South African plants. Journal of Ethnopharmacology 66 (3), 347—354.

Lall, N., Meyer, J.J.M., 2000. Antibacterial activity of water and acetone extracts of the roots of *Euclea natalensis*. Journal of Ethnopharmacology 72, 313—316. https://doi.org/10.1016/S0378-8741(00)00231-2.

Lall, N., Weiganand, O., Hussein, A.A., Meyer, J.J.M., 2006. Antifungal activity of naphthoquinones and triterpenes isolated from the root bark of *Euclea natalensis*. South African Journal of Botany 72, 579—583.

Lopes, M.H., Paul, I.M., 1973. Triterpenóides pentac'clicos de *Euclea natalensis* e *Euclea divinorum*. Revista Portuguesa de Química 15, 213—217.

Maroyi, A., 2017. Review of ethnomedicinal uses, phytochemistry and pharmacological properties of *Euclea natalensis* A. DC. Molecules 22, 2128.

Oosthuizen, C., 2017. Photos of *Euclea natalensis* A.DC.

Tannock, J., 1973. Naphthaquinones from *Diospyros* and *Euclea* species. Phytochemistry 12, 2066—2067. https://doi.org/10.1016/S0031-9422(00)91546-2.

van der Kooy, F., Meyer, J.J.M., Lall, N., 2006. Antimycobacterial activity and possible mode of action of newly isolated neodiospyrin and other naphthoquinones from *Euclea natalensis*. South African Journal of Botany 72, 349—352. https://doi.org/10.1016/j.sajb.2005.09.009.

Van Vuuren, S.F., Naidoo, D., 2010. An antimicrobial investigation of plants used traditionally in southern Africa to treat sexually transmitted infections. Journal of Ethnopharmacology 130, 552—558. https://doi.org/10.1016/j.jep.2010.05.045.

Watt, J.M., Breyer-Brandwijk, M.G., 1962. The Medicinal and Poisonous Plants of Southern Africa and Eastern Africa: Being an Account of Their Medicinal and Other Uses, Chemical Composition, Pharmacological Effects and Toxicology in Man and Animal. Livingstone.

Weigenand, O., Hussein, A.A., Lall, N., Meyer, J.J.M., 2004. Antibacterial activity of naphthoquinones and triterpenoids from *Euclea natalensis* root bark. Journal of Natural Products 67, 1936—1938.

CHAPTER

17

Eugenia crassipetala

Mala Ranghoo Sanmukhiya,
Joyce Govinden Soulange, Jean-Claude Sevastian,
Avinash Budloo, Rachel Brunchault,
Srutee Ramprosand

Faculty of Agriculture, University of Mauritius, Reduit, Mauritius

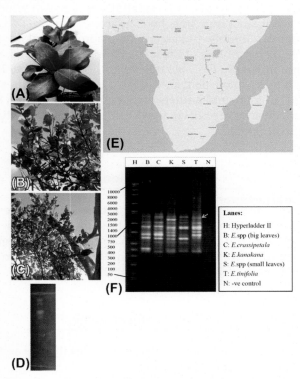

FIGURE 17   *Eugenia crassipetala* (**A**), (**B, C**) TLC of Eugenia crassipetala crude methanolic extract (**D**), distribution of *E. crassipetala* in sub-Saharan Africa (GBIF, 2018) (**E**), ISSR profile of Eugenia crassipetala in comparison with other Eugenia species (**F**).

Underexplored Medicinal Plants from Sub-Saharan Africa
https://doi.org/10.1016/B978-0-12-816814-1.00017-X

117

1. General description

1.1 Botanical nomenclature

Eugenia crassipetala J.Guého & A.J.Scott.

1.2 Botanical family

Myrtaceae.

1.3 Vernacular names

None (Surinam cherry — *E. uniflora*).

2. Botanical description

Eugenia crassipetala is a shrub which reaches 5 m in height, with smooth bark, pale pink detaching slowly in small flakes, beneath which the new bark is pale greenish orange in color. The leaves have petioles reaching 3 mm in length, minutely pubescent or glabrous, oval or ellipsoidal 1.2—3.5 × 0.9—2.2 cm, obtuse at the apex. Flowers are scented, sometimes sessile, 1.5 mm in length. Flower buds are piriform in shape, 10 × 7 mm. Petals are white in color, oboval, 17—20 × 15—18 mm. The stamen are numerous (200 in total) and anthers are globulous of 1 mm in length and cream colored, Ovaries are bilocular, with 20 ovules and the style is white 10—12 mm (Scott, 1990).

3. Distribution

Eugenia crassipetala is endemic to Mauritius Islands. The species is typically found in mountain ranges but is considered rare and endangered. It normally flowers in March and May. It has been reported in Mont du Lion, Creve Coeur near Grand Peak which is in the Moka mountain range near Pieter Both (Scott, 1990).

4. Ethnobotanical usage

The only reference to traditional usage includes the use as an antibacterial agent in Mauritian folk medicine.

5. Phytochemical constituents

Crude extracts of *E. crassipetala* have been reported to contain tannins, phenols, flavonoids, alkaloids, terpenes, traces of coumarins and saponins (Brunchault et al., 2014). The phytochemicals present in *E. crassipetala* are terpenes, phenols, flavonoids, tannins, leucoanthocyanins, anthraquinones and traces of alkaloids (Brunchault et al., 2014). *Eugenia crassipetala* is rich in total flavonoids and total phenolics as compared to other *Eugenia* species endemic to Mauritius.

6. TLC fingerprinting of plant extract

Thin layer chromatography (TLC) fingerprint is shown in Figure 17 (D).

7. Pharmacological properties

7.1 Antibacterial properties

It has been reported that *E. crassipetala* displayed antimicrobial properties. In a comparative study of *Eugenia* species, *E. crassipetala* was found to be amongst the species with highest antibacterial activity against *E. coli, P. mirabilis* and *S. aureus* with minimum inhibitory concentrations (MIC) even lower than the positive control chloramphenicol (Brunchault et al., 2014).

7.2 Antioxidant properties

The diphenylpicrylhydrazyl (DPPH) assay was used to ascertain the antioxidant property of *E. crassipetala*. Antioxidant activity was found to be the highest in polar extracts which inhibited the radical scavenging between 95.50 and 91.88 ± 0.02% at 100 μg/mL of extract. The free radical scavenging activity correlated with the high phenolic content of the extract.

8. Additional information

8.1 Therapeutic (proposed) usage

Antibacterial and antioxidant.

8.2 Safety data

Not available.

8.3 Trade information

Endangered.

8.4 Dosage

Not available.

References

Brunchault, R., Govinden-Soulange, J., Ranghoo-Sanmukhiya, V.M., Sevastian, J.C., 2014. Molecular and bioactive profiling of selected *Eugenia* species from Mauritius Island. International Journal of Plant Biology 5, 1—6.

GBIF, 2018. *Eugenia crassipetala* J.Gueho & A.J.Scott in GBIF Secretariat (2017). GBIF Backbone Taxonomy. Checklist dataset. https://doi.org/10.15468/39omeiaccessed via GBIF.org on 2019-02-24.

Scott, A.J., 1990. 92. Myrtacées. In: Bosser, J., Cadet, T., Guého, J., Marais, W. (Eds.), Flore des Mascareignes: La Réunion, Maurice, Rodrigues. 90. Rhizophoracées - 106. Araliacées. Institut de Recherche pour le Développement, Paris; Mauritius Sugar Industry Research Institute, Ile Maurice. The Royal Botanic Gardens, Kew, 70 pp.

18

Eugenia tinifolia

Nawraj Rummun[1,2], Cláudia Baider[3],
Theeshan Bahorun[1],
Vidushi S. Neergheen-Bhujun[1,2]

[1] ANDI Centre of Excellence for Biomedical and Biomaterials Research, University of Mauritius, Réduit, Republic of Mauritius; [2] Department of Health Sciences, Faculty of Science, University of Mauritius, Réduit, Republic of Mauritius; [3] The Mauritius Herbarium, Agricultural Services, Ministry of Agro-Industry and Food Security, Réduit, Republic of Mauritius

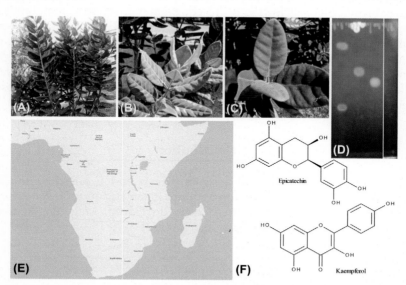

FIGURE 18 Aerial parts of *Eugenia tinifolia* (Molteno, 2014) (A), stem of *E. tinifolia* (Shawka, 2012) (B), leaves of *E. tinifolia* (C), TLC chromatogram, Lane 1 bottom; rutin, top; quercitrin; Lane 2 bottom; hyperoside, top; quercetin; Lane 3; chlorogenic acid; Lane 4; *E. tinifolia* leaf extract (D), distribution of *E. tinifolia* in sub-Saharan Africa (GBIF, 2017) (E), chemical structures of epicatechin and kaempferol (F). *(B) Picture courtesy: N. Rummun.*

1. General description

1.1 Botanical nomenclature

Eugenia tinifolia Lam.

1.2 Botanical family

Myrtaceae

1.3 Vernacular names

Mauritius: Bois de nèfles à feuilles coriaces

2. Botanical description

Tree up to 7 m tall, reaching 20—30 cm in diameter, bark pale brown, flaking. Leaves with 1—2.5 cm petiole, tomentose; blade elliptical or oval, 6—11.5 × 2.8—7 cm, tip acute or obtuse; base cunated or obtuse; coriaceous, tomentose to glabrous, margins strongly revoluted, dark green above, brown below. Flowers 3—3.5 cm diameter, solitary, sometimes a raceme of 2—3 pairs on branchlets, central flower sessile, lateral flowers with peduncle; calice lobes oblong, obtuse or acute, 4 × 6—8 mm, tomentose; petals subcircular, 8—9 mm long, white to beige, margin tomentose, many stamens, 7—11 mm, anthers globose. Ovary bilocular, style 5 mm long. Fruit globose or ellipsoid, 10—20 mm long, tomentose. Seeds 1—3, 10 mm long (Adapted from Scott, 1990).

3. Distribution

This endemic tree is found in drier forests and exposed mountain summits, where it can be rare to common. It can be found in the native remnants of Le Pouce, Mt Ory, Corps de Garde, Magenta, Yemen, Chamarel, and Le Morne, among other sites.

4. Ethnobotanical usage

The leaves of *E. tinifolia* are used as depurative and to treat dermatological diseases (Rummun et al., 2018).

5. Phytochemical constituents

The reported phytochemical profile of *E. tinifolia* leaf comprises tannins, anthraquinones, leucoanthocyanidins, flavonoids, saponins, alkaloids, terpenes, and phenols (Brunchault et al., 2014). The aqueous extract of its leaf is reported to contain (per gram of fresh leaf) (+)-catechin (3855 ± 16 µg), (−)-epicatechin (7636 ± 25 µg), (−)-epigallocatechin gallate (2447 ± 2 µg), (−)-epigallocatechin (1057 ± 2 µg), procyanidin B1 (2327 ± 3 µg), procyanidin B2 (731 ± 1 µg), and gallic acid (478 ± 6 µg) (Neergheen et al., 2006). Furthermore, the leaf extract also contained kaempferol and quercetin (Ramhit et al., 2018).

6. TLC fingerprinting of plant extract

The air-dried leaf was exhaustively extracted with aqueous methanol (80%, v/v) and partitioned with dichloromethane. The aqueous phase was lyophilized, and 5 mg of the powdered extract was dissolved in 1 mL of aqueous methanol (80%, v/v). For the reference standards, quercitrin, quercetin, rutin, hyperoside, and chlorogenic acid were purchased from Extrasynthèse (France), and 1 mg of each standard was dissolved in 1 mL methanol. For the chromatographic separation, 10 µL of extract and 5 µL of reference standard were spotted on a silica gel 60 F254 thin layer chromatography (TLC) plate (20×20 cm). The spots were left to dry and the plate was placed in a TLC tank, presaturated with 100 mL mobile phase. The mobile phase comprises ethyl acetate, formic acid, and water in ratio 8:1:1 (v/v). The samples were allowed to separate until the solvent front reached about 15 cm from the baseline. The plate was dried and sprayed with 1% methanolic diphenyl boric acid aminoethyl ester and examined under ultraviolet light at 365 nm to detect the bands on the TLC plates.

7. Pharmacological properties

The pharmacological activities of *E. tinifolia* remain underexplored as only a few reports in relation to its in vitro antioxidant, antimicrobial, and cancer cell inhibitory activities have been documented.

7.1 Antioxidant activity

The in vitro antioxidant activity of *E. tinifolia* leaf extracts were reported against a battery of antioxidant models including the ferric reducing antioxidant assay, 2,2'-azino-bis(3-ethylbenzothiazoline-6-sulfonic acid), hypochlorous (HOCl), hydroxyl (OH⁻), diphenylpicrylhydrazyl (DPPH), nitric oxide (NO·), and superoxide anion (O_2^-) free radical scavenging assays (Brunchault et al., 2014; Neergheen et al., 2006; Ramhit et al., 2018). The extract further attenuated both 2,2'-azobis (2-amidinopropane) hydrochloride induced and iron ascorbate—mediated in vitro lipid peroxidation of beef liver microsomes (Neergheen et al., 2006).

7.2 Antibacterial activity

Eugenia tinifolia leaf extract exhibited potent antibacterial activity against *Escherichia coli* (American type culture collection [ATCC] 25922), *Proteus mirabilis* (ATCC 12453), and *Staphylococcus aureus* (ATCC 29213) having a minimum inhibitory concentration (MIC) lower than that of chloramphenicol, a clinically used antibiotic (Brunchault et al., 2014). Along similar lines, Ramhit et al. (2018) reported the broad spectrum antibacterial activity of *E. tinifolia* hydroalcoholic leaf extract against *E. coli* (ATCC 25922), *Klebsiella oxytoca* (ATCC 43086), *Salmonella enterica* (ATCC 14028), *Pseudomonas aeruginosa* (ATCC 27853), *Pseudomonas fluorescens* (ATCC 13525), *Serratia marcescens* (ATCC 13880), and *Bacillus cereus* (ATCC 11778) with MIC values ranging from 9.7 to 78.1 µg fresh weight/mL.

7.3 Anticancer activity

Eugenia tinifolia hydro-alcoholic leaf extracts inhibited the cellular proliferation of MDAMB 231 human breast cancer cells, in a dose-dependent manner, as evaluated by 1-(4,5-Dimethylthiazol-2-yl)-3,5-diphenylformazan (MTT) viability assay (Neergheen et al., 2011). Similar dose-dependent antiproliferative effect was reported against Hs578T human breast cancer cells (ATCC HTB-126) (Ramhit et al., 2018).

8. Additional information

8.1 Therapeutic (proposed) usage

Antibacterial and anticancer

8.2 Safety data

Eugenia tinifolia hydro-alcoholic leaf extract showed low cytotoxicity against normal breast cell line, Hs578BsT (ATCCHTB-125), whereby at concentration of 1 mg fresh weight/mL, the extract showed less than 50%

growth inhibition of the nonmalignant Hs578BsT cells (Ramhit et al., 2018).

8.3 Trade information

This species has been classified as rare (Walter and Gillet, 1998) in the 1997 International Union for Conservation of Nature (IUCN) Red List. No update was done since. However, giving its distribution, global population size, and threats, the species would probably be classified under Vulnerable following the Red List of the IUCN category (IUCN, 2001).

8.4 Dosage

Not available

References

Brunchault, R.V., Soulange, J.G., Sanmukhiya, V.M.R., Sevathian, J.C., 2014. Molecular and bioactive profiling of selected *Eugenia* species from Mauritius island. International Journal of Plant Biology 5, 1—7. https://doi.org/10.4081/pb.2014.4728.

GBIF Secretariat, 2017. Eugenia tinifolia in GBIF Backbone Taxonomy. Checklist dataset. https://doi.org/10.15468/39omei.

IUCN, 2001. IUCN Red List Categories and Criteria, Version 3.1. IUCN Species Survival Commission, Gland, Switzerland and Cambridge, United Kingdom.

Molteno, S., 2014. *Eugenia tinifolia* — Bois de Nefles — Monvert Arboretum— Mauritius. Available online: https://commons.wikimedia.org/wiki/File:Eugenia_tiniifolia_-_bois_de_nefles_-_Monvert_arboretum_-_Mauritius.jpg. (CC0).

Neergheen, V., Bahorun, T., Aruoma, O.I., 2011. In vitro antiproliferative and apoptotic screening of Mauritian endemic plants. University of Mauritius Research Journal 17, 240—255.

Neergheen, V.S., Soobrattee, M.A., Bahorun, T., Aruoma, O.I., 2006. Characterization of the phenolic constituents in Mauritian endemic plants as determinants of their antioxidant activities in vitro. Journal of Plant Physiology 163, 787—799. https://doi.org/10.1016/j.jplph.2005.09.009.

Ramhit, P., Ragoo, L., Bahorun, T., Neergheen-Bhujun, V.S., 2018. Multi-targeted effects of untapped resources from the Mauritian endemic flora. South African Journal of Botany 115, 208—216. https://doi.org/10.1016/j.sajb.2018.01.020.

Rummun, N., Neergheen-Bhujun, V.S., Pynee, K.B., Baider, C., Bahorun, T., 2018. The role of endemic plants in Mauritian traditional medicine — potential therapeutic benefits or placebo effect? Journal of Ethnopharmacology 213, 111—117. https://doi.org/10.1016/j.jep.2017.10.006.

Shawka, A., 2012. *Eugenia tinifolia* — Bois de Nefle — Mauritius Endemic Tree. Available online: https://commons.wikimedia.org/wiki/File:Eugenia_tinifolia_-_bois_de_nefle_-_Mauritius_endemic_tree_2.jpg. (CC0).

Scott, A.J., 1990. 92. Myrtacées. In: Bosser, J., Cadet, T., Guého, J., Marais, W. (Eds.), Flore des Mascareignes — La Réunion, Maurice, Rodrigues. MSIRI/ORSTOM/KEW. Imprimerie de Montligeon, France.

Walter, K.S., Gillett, H.J., 1998. 1997 IUCN Red List of Threatened Plants. IUCN Species Survival Commission, Gland, Switzerland and Cambridge, United Kingdom.

Ficus glumosa

Analike Blom van Staden, Namrita Lall

Department of Plant and Soil Sciences, University of Pretoria, Pretoria,
Gauteng, South Africa

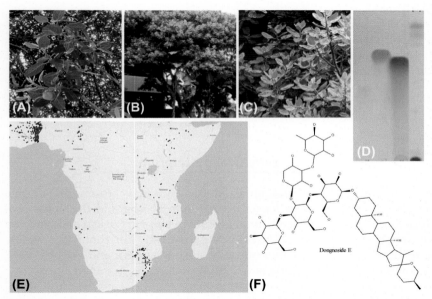

FIGURE 19 Leaves of *Ficus glumosa* (JMK, 2013a) (A), large specimen of *F. glumosa* (JMK, 2013b) (B), shoots and leaves of *F. glumosa* (JMK, 2013c) (C), TLC chromatogram, Lane 1; myricetin, Lane 2; quercetin, Lane 3; catechin, Lane 4; *F. glumosa* extract (D), distribution of *F. glumosa* in sub-Saharan Africa (GBIF, 2017) (E), chemical structure of dongnoside (F).

Underexplored Medicinal Plants from Sub-Saharan Africa
https://doi.org/10.1016/B978-0-12-816814-1.00019-3

1. General description

1.1 Botanical nomenclature

Ficus glumosa Delile

1.2 Botanical family

Moraceae

1.3 Vernacular names

African Rock-Fig, Goldenhair Fig, Hairy Rock Fig, Mountain Fig, Mountain Rock Fig (English)

Berg-Rotsvy, Bergvy, Bergvyeboom, Harige Rotsvy, Rots-Vyeboom (Afrikaans)

Inkokhokho, Magnyea (Siswati)

Lelothwane (South Sotho)

Inkokhokho, Omnyama, Umdenda, Umdenda Omnyama, Umdende, Umnyaxa (Zulu)

Mphaya (North Sotho)

Tshikululu (Venda)

Umthombe (Xhosa)

2. Botanical description

Ficus glumosa is a medium-sized tree but may become a tall tree reaching 20 m. The hairy leaves are ovate to oblong and the stems produce a white latex. The fig fruits are found in pairs in the leaf axils and can be smooth to puberulous. The branches are mostly horizontal and widely spread, which are often supported by stilt roots (Berg and Wiebes, 1992; Nana et al., 2012; Ntchapda et al., 2014).

3. Distribution

Ficus glumosa is not endemic to South Africa but is found in the Eastern Cape, Kwazulu-Natal, Limpopo, and Mpumalanga, stretching toward Senegal and the Arabian Peninsula (Sanbi, 2016; Van Noort and Rasplus, 2014).

4. Ethnobotanical usage

The fruits of *F. glumosa* are traditionally used for skin diseases, chest pain, and lung problems, such as cough, pneumonia, and bronchitis. *F. glumosa* is used in Cameroon, East Africa, and Senegal for hypertension, hemorrhoids, stomatitis, edema, diabetes, and rheumatism. The aqueous extract is used as an oral rinse for toothaches, caries, and gingivitis in the Central African Republic (Arbonnier, 2000; Boulesteix and Guinko, 1979; Koné and Atindehou, 2008; Nana et al., 2012; Ntchapda et al., 2014; Olaokun et al., 2013; Sultana et al., 2014).

5. Phytochemical constituents

Compounds and phytochemical groups previously identified from *F. glumosa* are tannins, flavonoids, furanocoumarins, and two new ceramides, namely compound 1, (2R,7E)-2-hydroxy-N-[(2S,3S,4R)-1,3, 4-trihydroxyhexadecan-2-yl] hexacos-7-enamide, and compound 2, (2R)-N-{(2S,3S,4R,9Z)-1-O-[(β-D-glucopyranosyl]-3,4-dihydroxyheptadec-9-en-2-yl}-2-hydroxypentacosanamide. Twenty-one known compounds have been isolated from *F. glumosa*, namely chiricanine A, lanosta-7,24-dien-3-one, lanosta-8,24-dien-3-one, alpinumisoflavone, β-amyrine, catechin, lupeol, 3,4-dihydroxybenzoic acid, 6-prenylpinocembrin, bergapten, genistein, luteolin, wighteone, polystachyol, 6-prenylapigenin, 2,4,5-trihydroxybenzoic acid, lyoniresinol-2a-O-β-D-xylopyranoside, 4'-O-methylalpinumisoflavone, β-sitosterol-3-O-(6'-O-heptadecanoyl)-β-D-glucopyranosyl, β-sitosterol-3-O-β-D-glucopyranoside, and dongnoside E (Compound 23) (Nana et al., 2012; Ntchapda et al., 2014; Sultana et al., 2014).

6. TLC fingerprinting of plant extract

For the separation of the compounds from *F. glumosa*, 2 mg of the ethanolic extract was weighed out and dissolved in 200 µL ethanol. For the standards, myricetin, quercetin, and catechin (Sigma—Aldrich Co. St Louis, MO, USA) were weighed out in the same manner as the extract and dissolved in 600 µL of ethanol. For the thin layer chromatography (TLC) analysis of *F. glumosa* crude extract, silica gel 60 F254 TLC plates were used to observe the separation of the compounds present in the extract. Plate markings were made with a soft pencil and glass capillaries were used to spot the samples on the TLC plate. Reference standards, myricetin, quercetin, and catechin, were spotted to determine whether it was present in the extract. The spots were left to dry completely before placing the plate in a TLC tank, which contained 10 mL eluent 9:1 dichloro-methane:methanol solvent system. The plate was observed under ultra-violet (UV light) (long and short wavelength), followed by spraying with freshly prepared vanillin/sulfuric acid (2%) to detect the bands on the TLC plate.

7. Pharmacological properties

Ficus glumosa has not been extensively researched for its in vitro and in vivo medicinal properties. Although it is a widely distributed and well-known plant in South Africa, there is still an opportunity for research and development regarding this plant.

7.1 Antibacterial activity

In a study done earlier, the leaves and stems of *F. glumosa* were collected (February to March 2015) from the Manie van der Schijff botanical garden of the University of Pretoria. An ethanol extract was prepared. The ethanolic crude extract showed growth inhibitory activity against *Propionibacterium acnes*, American type culture collection (ATCC) 6919 and ATCC 11827 strains, with a minimum inhibitory concentration (MIC) of 500 µg/mL. No bactericidal effect was observed for *F. glumosa* (Blom van Staden and Lall, 2018). When the extract of *F. glumosa* was combined with the known antibiotic, tetracycline, the synergistic effect, at a ratio of 9:1, resulted in the MIC for the extract to reduce to 56.25 µg/mL, whereas the MIC of the drug reduced to 0.625 µg/mL for the ATCC 11827 strain (Blom van Staden and Lall, 2018). The synergistic effect, at a ratio of 5:5 for the ATCC 6919 strain, resulted in the MIC for the extract to reduce to 3.91 µg/mL, while the MIC of the drug reduced to 0.391 µg/mL. A study done by Kwazo in 2015 showed that the water extract of *F. glumosa* showed antibacterial activity toward *Salmonella typhi* and *Salmonella paratyphi*. The bacterial growth inhibition was observed by utilizing the agar diffusion method (Kwazo et al., 2015).

7.2 Antidiabetic activity

The potential antidiabetic activity of the *Ficus* species has previously been investigated. The antidiabetic activity was determined by evaluating the digestive enzymes regarding the antioxidant activity, polyphenol content, and glucose uptake in muscle, fat, and liver. Antidiabetic studies included the investigation of insulin secretion and the effect on cells through cytotoxicity assays. The acetone extract of *F. glumosa* inhibited the α-amylase, with 65.1%, and α-glucosidase enzymes, with 38.7%. The methanol extract of the stems and bark of *F. glumosa* has shown glucose-lowering potential in vivo at the effective dose of 65 mg/kg (Olaokun, 2012; Olaokun et al., 2013).

7.3 Phytochemical content and antioxidants

The leaves and stems ethanol extracts of *F. glumosa*, obtained from the University of Pretoria, were collected and screened for its phytochemical constituents. The extract was tested for total tannins, saponins, alkaloids, cardiac glycosides, terpenes, flavonoids, and total phenolics. The ethanol extracts of *F. glumosa* showed the presence of tannins, alkaloids, saponins, and cardiac glycosides. *F. glumosa* showed its optimum antioxidant activity in diphenylpicrylhydrazyl (DPPH) spectrophotometric assay at the concentration of 100 μg/mL. The ferric-reducing antioxidant power showed a significant concentration dependent increase in the total antioxidant power (Madubunyi et al., 2012).

8. Additional information

8.1 Therapeutic (proposed) usage

Antibacterial, antidiabetic, and antioxidant

8.2 Safety data

Not available

8.3 Trade information

Least concern

8.4 Dosage

Not available

References

Arbonnier, M., 2000. Arbres, arbustes et lianes des zones sèches d'Afrique de l'Ouest Trees, shrubs and lianas of West Africa dry zones, Mali, Ouagadougou: centre de Coopération Internationale en Recherche Agronomique pour le développement/Muséum national d'histoire naturelle/Union mondiale pour la nature. In: CIRAD/MNHN/UICN.

Berg, C.C., Wiebes, 1992. *Ficus glumosa*. http://www.figweb.org/Ficus/Subgenus_Urostigma/Section_Galoglychia/Subsection_Platyphyllae/Ficus_glumosa.htm. Accessed 30 July 2018.

Blom van Staden, A., Lall, N., 2018. Medicinal plants as alternative treatments for progressive macular hypomelanosis. In: Medicinal Plants for Holistic Health and Well-Being, pp. 145–182.

Boulesteix, M., Guinko, S., 1979. Plantes médicinales utilisées par les Gbayas dans la région de Bouar (Empire Centrafricain). In: Quatrième colloque du Conseil africain de Malgache pour l'enseignement supérieur (CAMES), Libreville, Gabon.

GBIF, 2017. *Ficus glumosa* Delile in GBIF Secretariat (2017). GBIF Backbone Taxonomy. Checklist dataset. https://doi.org/10.15468/39omei. accessed via GBIF.org on 2018-08-01.

JMK, 2013a. Sub-canopy foliage and fruit of a Mountain fig growing near the Manie van der Schijff Botanical Garden at the University of Pretoria, South Africa. Available online: https://commons.wikimedia.org/wiki/File:Ficus_glumosa,_loof_en_vrugte,_b,_Tuks.jpg.

JMK, 2013b. Mountain fig growing near the Manie van der Schijff Botanical Garden at the University of Pretoria, South Africa. Available online: https://commons.wikimedia.org/wiki/File:Ficus_glumosa,_habitus,_Tuks.jpg.

JMK, 2013c. Foliage and fruit of a Mountain fig growing near the Manie van der Schijff Botanical Garden at the University of Pretoria, South Africa. Available online: https://commons.wikimedia.org/wiki/File:Ficus_glumosa,_loof_en_vrugte,_a,_Tuks.jpg.

Koné, W., Atindehou, K.K., 2008. Ethnobotanical inventory of medicinal plants used in traditional veterinary medicine in Northern Côte d'Ivoire (West Africa). South African Journal of Botany 74 (1), 76–84.

Kwazo, H., Faruq, U., Dangoggo, S., Malami, B., Moronkola, D., 2015. Antimicrobial activity and phytochemical screening of crude water extract of the stem bark of *Ficus glumosa*. Scientific Research and Essays 10 (5), 177–183.

Madubunyi, I.I., Onoja, S.O., Asuzu, I.U., 2012. In vitro antioxidant and in vivo antidiabetic potential of the methanol extract of *Ficus glumosa* Del (Moraceae) stem bark in alloxan-induced diabetic mice. Comparative Clinical Pathology 21 (4), 389–394.

Nana, F., Sandjo, L.P., Keumedjio, F., Ambassa, P., Malik, R., Kuete, V., Rincheval, V., Choudhary, M.I., Ngadjui, B.T., 2012. Ceramides and cytotoxic constituents from *Ficus glumosa* Del.(Moraceae). Journal of the Brazilian Chemical Society 23 (3), 482–487.

Ntchapda, F., Abakar, D., Kom, B., Nana, P., Bonabe, C., Kakesse, M., Talla, E., Dimo, T., 2014. Diuretic activity of the aqueous extract leaves of *Ficus glumosa* del.(moraceae) in rats. Science World Journal 2014.

Olaokun, O.O., 2012. The value of extracts of *Ficus lutea* (Moraceae) in the management of Type II diabetes in a mouse obesity model. University of Pretoria.

Olaokun, O.O., McGaw, L.J., Eloff, J.N., Naidoo, V., 2013. Evaluation of the inhibition of carbohydrate hydrolysing enzymes, antioxidant activity and polyphenolic content of extracts of ten African *Ficus* species (Moraceae) used traditionally to treat diabetes. BMC Complementary and Alternative Medicine 13 (1), 1.

SANBI, 2016. *Ficus glumosa* Delile. SANBI red data list. http://redlist.sanbi.org/species.php?species=1906-18. Accessed 30 July 2018.

Sultana, S., Nandi, J.K., Rahman, S., Jahan, R., Rahmatullah, M., 2014. Preliminary antihyperglycemic and analgesic activity studies with Angiopteris evecta leaves in Swiss albino mice. World Journal of Pharmacy and Pharmaceutical Sciences 3 (10), 1–12.

Van Noort, S., Rasplus, J.Y., 2014. Ficus glumosa. Figweb. http://www.figweb.org/Ficus/Subgenus_Urostigma/Section_Galoglychia/Subsection_Platyphyllae/Ficus_glumosa.htm. Accessed 30 July 2018.

Ficus lutea

Analike Blom van Staden, Namrita Lall

Department of Plant and Soil Sciences, University of Pretoria, Pretoria, Gauteng, South Africa

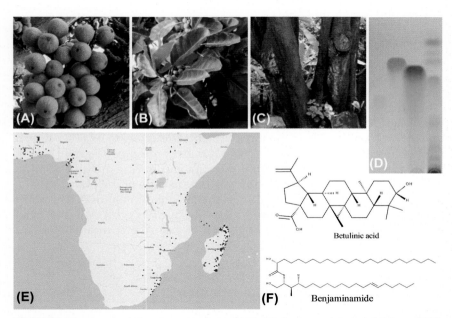

FIGURE 20   Fruits of *Ficus lutea* (Atamari, 2007) (A), leaves and fruits of *F. lutea* (JMK, 2013a) (B), bark of *F. lutea* (JMK, 2013b) (C), TLC chromatogram, Lane 1; myricetin, Lane 2; quercetin, Lane 3; catechin, Lane 4; *F. lutea* extract (D), distribution of *F. lutea* in sub-Saharan Africa (GBIF, 2018) (E), chemical structures of betulinic acid and benjaminamide (F).

133

1. General description

1.1 Botanical nomenclature

Ficus lutea Vahl

1.2 Botanical family

Moraceae

1.3 Vernacular names

Giant-leaved fig (English)
Reuseblaarvy (Afrikaans)
Umthombe, uluzi (Xhosa)
Umvubu, omkhulu (Zulu)

2. Botanical description

Ficus lutea is a large fig tree that grows 25 m in height, and its branches can span 30–45 m in width. It is a deciduous tree. However, the surroundings affect its dimensions; in open areas the tree has a short buttressed trunk and in forest environments it is likely to be taller with a narrower spread. The tree is known for its large glossy ovate leaves, varying between 130 and 430 mm in length and having a width of up to 200 mm. The leaves are positioned toward the ends of the branches. The bark is dark gray to brown and is relatively smooth-textured. The hairy fruits (syconia) are mostly found in spring but has been detected from June to October. The fruits vary between 15 and 30 mm in diameter and are stalkless (Burring, 2004).

3. Distribution

Ficus lutea is native to the tropical areas of Africa but has been planted all over South Africa. *F. lutea* has also been spotted in Madagascar, the Seychelles, and Comores. The natural habitat ranges from riverine forests and coastal areas to woodlands and evergreen forests (Burrows and Burrows, 2003; Van Noort and Rasplus, 2004: Ware and Compton, 1992).

4. Ethnobotanical usage

The fruits of *F. lutea* are traditionally used for wound healing and the treatment of sores and boils in Oman and consumed by people in West Africa. The bark is used in the clothing industry in Mozambique. The wood of the tree is used for creating bowls, and the latex is used for bird-lime (Burrows and Burrows, 2003; Marwah et al., 2007; Pooley, 1993).

5. Phytochemical constituents

Compounds and phytochemical groups previously identified from *F. lutea* are triterpenoids, phytol, lupeol, β-amyrin, β-amyrin acetate, betulinic acid, Coumarins, α-tocopherol, flavonoids, acorenone, ceramide glycoside (lutaoside), flavonoids, epiafzelechin, β-sitosterol glucoside (Marwah et al., 2007; Ogunwande et al., 2008; Olaokun et al., 2014; Poumale et al., 2011).

6. TLC fingerprinting of plant extract

For the separation of compounds from *F. lutea*, 2 mg of the ethanolic extract was weighed out and dissolved in 200 μL ethanol. For the standards, myricetin, quercetin, and catechin (Sigma—Aldrich Co. St Louis, MO, USA) were weighed out in the same manner as the extract and dissolved in 600 μL of ethanol. For the thin layer chromatography (TLC) analysis of *F. lutea* crude extract, silica gel 60 F254 TLC plates were used to observe the separation of the compounds present within the extract. Plate markings were made with a soft pencil, and glass capillaries were used to spot the samples onto the TLC plate. Reference standards, myricetin, quercetin, and catechin, were spotted to determine whether it was present in the extract. The spots were left to dry completely before placing the plate in a TLC tank, which contained 10 mL eluent 9:1 dichloromethane: methanol solvent system. The plate was observed under ultraviolet (UV light) (long and short wavelength), followed by spraying with freshly prepared vanillin/sulfuric acid (2%) to detect the bands on the TLC plate.

7. Pharmacological properties

Ficus lutea has not been extensively researched for its in vitro and in vivo medicinal properties. Although it is a widely distributed and is a well-known plant in South Africa, there is still an opportunity for research and development regarding this plant.

7.1 Antibacterial activity

In one study, the leaves and stems of *F. lutea* were collected. An ethanolic extract was prepared and the ethanolic crude extract was found to show growth inhibitory activity against *Propionibacterium acnes*, American type culture collection (ATCC) 6919 and ATCC 11827 strains, with a minimum inhibitory concentration (MIC) of 500 μg/mL (Blom van Staden and Lall, 2018). When the extract of *F. lutea* was combined with the known antibiotic, tetracycline, the synergistic effect, at a ratio of 4:6, it resulted in the MIC of the extract to reduce to 9.83 μg/mL, whereas the MIC of the drug reduced to 0.625 μg/mL for the ATCC 11827 strain. The synergistic effect, at a ratio of 5:5 for the ATCC 6919 strain, resulted in the MIC for the extract to reduce to 3.91 μg/mL, whereas the MIC of the drug reduced to 0.391 μg/mL. No bactericidal effect was observed for *F. lutea* (Blom van Staden and Lall, 2018). In another study, the antifungal and antibacterial activity of compounds isolated from the wood of *F. lutea* were determined using the agar diffusion method. Lutaoside showed growth inhibition toward *Chlorella vulgaris*, *Scenedesmus subspicatus*, *Chlorella sorokiniana*, *Mucor miehei*, *Bacillus subtilis* and *Candida albicans*. Benjaminamide showed growth inhibition toward *S. subspicatus*, *C. sorokiniana*, *M. miehei*, *Bacillus subtilis*, and *C. albicans* (Poumale et al., 2011).

7.2 Antidiabetic activity

The potential antidiabetic activity of the *Ficus* species has previously been investigated. The antidiabetic activity can be determined by evaluating the digestive enzymes regarding the antioxidant activity, polyphenol content, and glucose uptake in muscle, fat, and liver. Antidiabetic studies include the investigation of insulin secretion and the effect on cells through cytotoxicity assays. The acetone extracts of *F. lutea* inhibited the α-amylase and α-glucosidase enzymes and stimulated glucose uptake in the primary and established muscle and fat cell cultures. The extract of *F. lutea* enhanced the insulin secretion in RIN-m5F pancreatic cell line. The crude extract of *F. lutea* was fractioned into six fractions. The ethyl acetate fraction was found to be the most active in inhibiting sucrase activity and in enhancing glucose uptake in C_2C_{12} muscle and H-4-II-E liver in the absence of insulin. Five compounds were isolated from the ethyl acetate fraction of *F. lutea*, namely stigmasterol, α-amyrin acetate, lupeol, epicatechin, and epiafzelechin. Four compounds isolated are known to possess antidiabetic activity. It may be concluded that the antidiabetic activity of *F. lutea* is due to the inhibition of the enzymes responsible for the breakdown of carbohydrate and the increase in glucose uptake in the fat, muscle, and liver and the secretion of insulin (Olaokun, 2012).

7.3 Phytochemical content and antioxidant

The leaves and stems ethanol extracts of *F. lutea*, obtained from the University of Pretoria, were collected and screened for its phytochemical constituents. The extract was tested for total tannins, saponins, alkaloids, cardiac glycosides, terpenes, flavonoids, and total phenolics. The ethanol extracts of *F. lutea* showed the presence of tannins, alkaloids, saponins, cardiac glucosides, and phenolics. Plants were collected by Marwah et al. in October 2001 and September 2002 from Royal Botanic Gardens, Kew, Richmond, UK. The plant material was initially extracted with chloroform for 2 weeks and later extracted with 20% aqueous ethanol for another 2 weeks. *F. lutea* was tested for its antioxidant activity using the diphenylpicrylhydrazyl (DPPH) radical scavenging assays and exhibited a 50 % inhibitory concentration (IC_{50}) value of $11.9 \pm 0.3\,\mu g/mL$ against the DPPH free radical (Marwah et al., 2007).

8. Additional information

8.1 Therapeutic (proposed) usage

Antibacterial, antidiabetic, antioxidant, and wound healing

8.2 Safety data

Not available

8.3 Trade information

Not threatened, not endangered and abundant

8.4 Dosage

Not available

References

Atamari, 2007. Ficus lutea. Available online: https://commons.wikimedia.org/wiki/File: Ficus_lutea_0004.jpg. (CC BY-SA 3.0). Accessed June 2018.

Blom van Staden, A., Lall, N., 2018. Medicinal plants as alternative treatments for progressive macular hypomelanosis. In: Medicinal Plants for Holistic Health and Well-Being, pp. 145–182.

Burring, J.H., 2004. *Ficus Lutea*. Plantzafrica. http://www.plantzafrica.com/plantefg/ficuslutea.htm. Accessed 30 July 2018.

Burrows, J., Burrows, S., 2003. Figs of Southern and South-Central Africa. Umdaus Press, Hatfield, South Africa viii, 379pp.-illus., col. illus. ISBN, 1919766243.

GBIF, 2018. *Ficus Lutea* Vahl in GBIF Secretariat (2017). GBIF Backbone Taxonomy. Checklist dataset. https://doi.org/10.15468/39omei. accessed via GBIF.org on 2018-08-01.

JMK, 2013a. Foliage and Fruit of a Giant-leaved Fig in the Manie van der Schijff Botanical Garden. University of Pretoria, South Africa. Available online: https://commons. wikimedia.org/wiki/File:Ficus_lutea,_loof_en_vrugte,_b,_Manie_van_der_Schijff_BT. jpg. (CC BY-SA 3.0). Accessed June 2018.

JMK, 2013b. Main Trunks of a Giant-leaved Fig in the Manie van der Schijff Botanical Garden. University of Pretoria, South Africa. Available online: https://commons.wikimedia.org/ wiki/File:Ficus_lutea,_hoofstamme,_Manie_van_der_Schijff_BT.jpg (CC BY-SA 3.0). Accessed June 2018.

Marwah, R.G., Fatope, M.O., Al Mahrooqi, R., Varma, G.B., Al Abadi, H., Al-Burtamani, S.K.S., 2007. Antioxidant capacity of some edible and wound healing plants in Oman. Food Chemistry 101 (2), 465–470.

Ogunwande, I.A., Sonibare, M.A., Thang, T.D., Dung, N.X., Soladoye, M.O., Morohunfolu, O.O., 2008. Comparative analysis of the oils of three *Ficus* species from Nigeria. Journal of Essential Oil Research 20 (5), 386–389.

Olaokun, O.O., 2012. The Value of Extracts of *Ficus Lutea* (Moraceae) in the Management of Type II Diabetes in a Mouse Obesity Model. University of Pretoria.

Olaokun, O.O., McGaw, L.J., Awouafack, M.D., Eloff, J.N., Naidoo, V., 2014. The potential role of GLUT4 transporters and insulin receptors in the hypoglycaemic activity of *Ficus lutea* acetone leaf extract. BMC Complementary and Alternative Medicine 14 (1), 269.

Pooley, E., 1993. Complete Field Guide to Trees of Natal. Natal Flora Publications Trust, Zululand & Transkei.

Poumale, H.M.P., Djoumessi, A.V.B.S., Ngameni, B., Sandjo, L.P., Ngadjui, B.T., Shiono, Y., 2011. A new ceramide isolated from *Ficus lutea* Vahl (moraceae). Acta Chimica Slovenica 58, 81–86.

Van Noort, S., Rasplus, J.Y., 2004. Ficus Lutea Vahl 1805. Figweb. http://www.figweb.org/ Ficus/Subgenus_Urostigma/Section_Galoglychia/Subsection_Galoglychia/Ficus_lutea. htm.

Ware, A.B., Compton, S.G., 1992. Breakdown of pollinator specificity in an African fig tree. Biotropica 544–549.

Ficus sur

Analike Blom van Staden, Namrita Lall

Department of Plant and Soil Sciences, University of Pretoria, Pretoria, Gauteng, South Africa

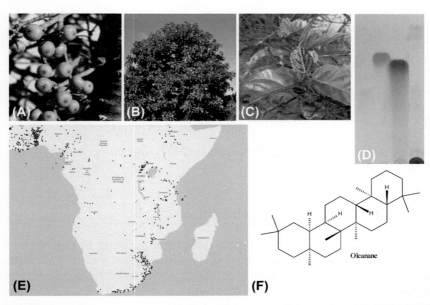

FIGURE 21 Fruits of *Ficus sur* (JMK, 2012a) (A), large specimen of *F. sur* (Wiebe, 2012) (B), leaves of *F. sur* (JMK, 2012b) (C), TLC chromatogram, Lane 1; myricetin, Lane 2; quercetin, Lane 3; catechin, Lane 4; *F. sur* extract (D), distribution of *F. sur* in sub-Saharan Africa (GBIF, 2017) (E), chemical structure of oleanane (F).

1. General description

1.1 Botanical nomenclature

Ficus sur Forssk

1.2 Botanical family

Moraceae

1.3 Vernacular names

Broom cluster fig (English)
Besem-trosvy (Afrikaans)
Mogo-tshetlo (North Sotho)
Umkhiwane (Xhosa)
Umkhiwane (Zulu)

2. Botanical description

Ficus sur is an evergreen tree that can grow up to 35 m in height. It has elliptic to ovate-shaped leaves that are very hairy. The fruits, figs, are produced in clusters and can be found in the spring and summer months, from September to March (Plantzafrica, 2007; Van Noort and Rasplus, 2014).

3. Distribution

Ficus sur is not endemic to South Africa but is found in the Western Cape, up to North Africa stretching toward Senegal and the Arabian Peninsula. It is found mostly in woodlands and moist forests, although it has been seen on river banks and drier woodlands (Plantzafrica, 2007; Van Noort and Rasplus, 2014).

4. Ethnobotanical usage

The fruit of *F. sur* is eaten by the indigenous people. The fruits are also mixed with other plants, such as *Terminalia macroptera* to treat snake bites. *Ficus sur* fruit is ground into flour and included in meals or drinks with red potassium and some amount of water, together with sugar or honey and is taken for up to 4 weeks to treat thyroid fever. The bark, on the other hand, is used as a compress for boils (Faleyimu et al., 2010; Inngjerdingen et al., 2004; Mabona et al., 2013).

5. Phytochemical constituents

Compounds and phytochemical groups previously identified from *F. sur* are saponins, saponin glycosides, oleanane, ursine, tannins, flavonoids, anthracenosides, anthocyanins, coumarins, and steroids (Eldeen et al., 2005; Eldeen and Van Staden, 2007; Feleke and Brehane, 2005; Kunle et al., 1999; Ramde-Tiendrebeogo et al., 2012; Solomon—Wisdom et al., 2011).

6. TLC fingerprinting of plant extract

To observe the separation of the compounds of *F. sur*, 2 mg of the ethanolic extract was weighed out and dissolved in 200 µL ethanol. For the standards, myricetin, quercetin, and catechin (Sigma—Aldrich Co. St Louis, MO, USA) were weighed out in the same manner as the extract and dissolved in 600 µL of ethanol. For the thin layer chromatography (TLC) analysis of *F. sur* crude extract, silica gel 60 F254 TLC plates were used to observe the separation of the compounds present within the extract. Plate markings were made with a soft pencil and glass capillaries were used to spot the samples onto the TLC plate. Reference standards, myricetin, quercetin, and catechin, were spotted to determine whether it was present in the extract. The spots were left to dry completely before placing the plate in a TLC tank, which contained 10 mL eluent 9:1 dichloromethane: methanol solvent system. The plate was observed under ultraviolet (UV light) (long and short wavelength), followed by spraying with freshly prepared vanillin/sulfuric acid (2%) to detect the bands on the TLC plate.

7. Pharmacological properties

Ficus sur has not been extensively researched for its in vitro and in vivo medicinal properties. Although it is a widely distributed and well-known plant in South Africa, there is still an opportunity for research and development regarding this plant.

7.1 Antibacterial activity

In one the leaves and stems of *F. sur* were collected and an ethanolic extract was prepared. The ethanol crude extract showed growth inhibitory activity against *Propionibacterium acnes*, American type culture collection (ATCC) 6919 and ATCC 11827 strains, with a minimum inhibitory concentration (MIC) of 500 µg/mL (Blom van Staden and Lall, 2018). No bactericidal effect was observed for *F. sur*. When the extract of *F. sur* was combined with the known antibiotic, tetracycline, the synergistic effect, at a ratio of 7:3, resulted in the MIC for the extract to reduce to 2.34 µg/mL, whereas the MIC of the drug reduced to 0.547 µg/mL for the ATCC 11827 strain. The synergistic effect, at a ratio of 5:5 for the ATCC 6919 strain, resulted in the MIC for the extract to reduce to 7.81 µg/mL, whereas the MIC of the drug reduced to 0.781 µg/mL (Blom van Staden and Lall, 2018).

The MIC values recorded for the bark aqueous extract of *F. sur* for the different skin pathogens, namely *Staphylococcus aureus* ATCC 25923, methicillin-resistant *S. aureus*, gentamycin methicillin-resistant *S. aureus*, *Staphylococcus epidermidis* ATCC 2223, *Pseudomonas aeruginosa* ATCC 27858, *Candida albicans* ATCC 10231, *Microsporum canis* ATCC 3629, and *Brevibacillus agri* ATCC 51663, were >16.00 mg/mL. However, the MICs for the dichloromethane: methanol extracts were as follows; 0.75 mg/mL for *S. aureus*, 1.00 mg/mL for *S. epidermidis* ATCC 2223, 1.25 mg/mL for *P. aeruginosa* ATCC 27858, 2.00 mg/mL for *C. albicans* ATCC 10,231, >16.00 mg/mL for *M. canis* ATCC 3629, and 8.00 mg/mL for *B. agri* ATCC 51663.

The MIC values recorded for the leaf aqueous extract of *F. sur* for the different skin pathogens, namely *S. aureus* ATCC 25923, methicillin-resistant *S. aureus*, gentamycin methicillin-resistant *S. aureus*, *S. epidermidis* ATCC 2223, *P. aeruginosa* ATCC 27858, *M. canis* ATCC 3629, and *B. agri* ATCC 51663 were >16.00 mg/mL, except for *C. albicans* ATCC 10231 and *M. canis* ATCC 3629, which were found to be 4.00 mg/mL. However, the MICs for the dichloromethane: methanol leaf extracts were as follows; 4.00 mg/mL for *S. aureus*, 2.00 mg/mL for *S. epidermidis* ATCC 2223, 4.00 mg/mL for *P. aeruginosa* ATCC 27858, 1.00 mg/mL for *C. albicans* ATCC 10231, 1.00 mg/mL for *M. canis* ATCC 3629, and 2.00 mg/mL for *B. agri* ATCC 51663. Another study found that *F. sur* had a MIC of 2.5 for *S. aureus* and *E. coli* (Mabona et al., 2013; Ramde-Tiendrebeogo et al., 2012).

7.2 Antidiabetic activity

The potential antidiabetic activity of the *Ficus* species has previously been investigated. The antidiabetic activity was determined by evaluating the digestive enzymes regarding the antioxidant activity, polyphenol content, and glucose uptake by the muscle, fat, and liver cells. Antidiabetic studies included the investigation of insulin secretion and the effect on cells through cytotoxicity assays. The acetone extract of *F. sur* inhibited the α-amylase and α-glucosidase enzymes (Olaokun, 2012; Olaokun et al., 2013).

7.3 Phytochemical content and antioxidant

The leaf and stem ethanolic extracts of *F. sur*, obtained from the University of Pretoria, were collected and screened for its phytochemical constituents. The extract was tested for total tannins, saponins, alkaloids, cardiac glycosides, terpenes, flavonoids, and total phenolics. The ethanol extracts of *F. sur* showed the presence of tannins, saponins, alkaloids, cardiac glycosides, terpenes, flavonoids, and phenolics. Phenolic compounds are vital plant components, as they are mostly responsible for a plant's antioxidant activity, via the interaction with free radicals and the prevention of the breakdown of hydro-peroxides. The flavonol content in *F. sur* was determined as 0.27 ± 0.01 mg/g and the 50 % inhibitory concentration (IC_{50}) value for the antioxidant activity against diphenylpicrylhydrazyl (DPPH) was found to be 31.83 ± 0.55 µg/mL (Ramde-Tiendrebeogo et al., 2012).

8. Additional information

8.1 Therapeutic (proposed) usage

Antibacterial, antimicrobial, and antidiabetic

8.2 Safety data

Not available

8.3 Trade information

Not threatened, not endangered and abundant

8.4 Dosage

Not available

References

Solomon—Wisdom, G., Shittu, G., Agboola, Y., 2011. Antimicrobial and phytochemical screening activities of Ficus sur (Forssk). New York Science Journal 4 (1), 15—18.

Blom van Staden, A., Lall, N., 2018. Medicinal plants as alternative treatments for progressive macular hypomelanosis. In: Medicinal Plants for Holistic Health and Well-Being, pp. 145—182.

Eldeen, I., Van Staden, J., 2007. Antimycobacterial activity of some trees used in South African traditional medicine. South African Journal of Botany 73 (2), 248—251.

Eldeen, I., Elgorashi, E., Van Staden, J., 2005. Antibacterial, anti-inflammatory, anticholinesterase and mutagenic effects of extracts obtained from some trees used in South African traditional medicine. Journal of Ethnopharmacology 102 (3), 457—464.

Faleyimu, O., Akinyemi, O., Idris, Y., 2010. Survey of forest plants used in traditional treatment of typhoid fever in Chikun Local Government Area of Kaduna State, Nigeria. International Journal of Biomedicine and Health Sceinces 6, 2.

Feleke, S., Brehane, A., 2005. Triterpene compounds from the latex of Ficus sur I. Bulletin of the Chemical Society of Ethiopia 19 (2), 307—310.

GBIF, 2017. Ficus sur Forssk. In: GBIF Secretariat (2017). GBIF Backbone Taxonomy. Checklist dataset. https://doi.org/10.15468/39omei. accessed via GBIF.org on 2018-08-01.

Inngjerdingen, K., Nergård, C.S., Diallo, D., Mounkoro, P.P., Paulsen, B.S., 2004. An ethnopharmacological survey of plants used for wound healing in Dogonland, Mali, West Africa. Journal of Ethnopharmacology 92 (2), 233—244.

JMK, 2012a. Fig cluster on a Cape fig, near Louwsburg, KwaZulu-Natal. Available online: https://commons.wikimedia.org/wiki/File:Ficus_sur,_vyetros_b,_Louwsburg.jpg (CC BY-SA 3.0). Accessed June 2018.

JMK, 2012b. Fresh winter leaves of a Cape fig, near Louwsburg, KwaZulu-Natal. Argentine ants are patrolling the leaves. Available online: https://commons.wikimedia.org/wiki/File:Ficus_sur,_vars_winterblare,_Louwsburg.jpg (CC BY-SA 3.0). Accessed June 2018.

Kunle, O., Shittu, A., Nasipuri, R., Kunle, O., Wambebe, C., Akah, P., 1999. Gastrointestinal activity of Ficus sur. Fitoterapia 70 (6), 542—547.

Mabona, U., Viljoen, A., Shikanga, E., Marston, A., Van Vuuren, S., 2013. Antimicrobial activity of southern African medicinal plants with dermatological relevance: from an ethnopharmacological screening approach, to combination studies and the isolation of a bioactive compound. Journal of Ethnopharmacology 148 (1), 45—55.

Olaokun, O.O., 2012. The Value of Extracts of Ficus Lutea (Moraceae) in the Management of Type II Diabetes in a Mouse Obesity Model. University of Pretoria.

Olaokun, O.O., McGaw, L.J., Eloff, J.N., Naidoo, V., 2013. Evaluation of the inhibition of carbohydrate hydrolysing enzymes, antioxidant activity and polyphenolic content of extracts of ten African Ficus species (Moraceae) used traditionally to treat diabetes. BMC Complementary and Alternative Medicine 13 (1), 1.

Plantzafrica, 2007. Marcini Govender. http://www.plantzafrica.com/plantab. Accessed 30 July 2018.

Ramde-Tiendrebeogo, A., Tibiri, A., Hilou, A., Lompo, M., Millogo-Kone, H., Nacoulma, O.G., Guissou, I.P., 2012. Antioxidative and antibacterial activities of phenolic compounds from Ficus sur Forssk. and Ficus sycomorus L.(Moraceae): potential for sickle cell disease treatment in Burkina Faso. International Journal of Brain and Cognitive Sciences 6 (1), 328—336.

Wiebe, K., 2012. Cape fig in a garden in Kaapsehoop, Mpumalanga. Available online: https://commons.wikimedia.org/wiki/File:Ficus_sur,_Kaapsehoop.jpg (CC BY-SA 3.0). Accessed June 2018.

Van Noort, S., Rasplus, J.Y., 2014. Ficus Glumosa. Figweb. http://www.figweb.org/Ficus/Subgenus_Urostigma/Section_Galoglychia/Subsection_Platyphyllae/Ficus_glumosa.htm. Accessed 30 July 2018.

22

Greyia radlkoferi

Marco Nuno De Canha, Namrita Lall

Department of Plant and Soil Sciences, University of Pretoria, Pretoria, Gauteng, South Africa

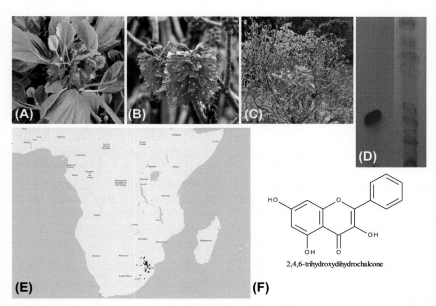

2,4,6-trihydroxydihydrochalcone

(A) (B) (C) (D) (E) (F)

FIGURE 22   Aerial plant parts of *Greyia radlkoferi* (Shebs, 2005) (A), flower of *G. radlkoferi* (Shebs, 2006a) (B), view of *G. radlkoferi* in autumn (Shebs, 2006b) (C), TLC chromatogram, Lane 1; 2,4,6-trihydroxydihydrochalcone, Lane 2; *G. radlkoferi* extract (D), distribution of *G. radlkoferi* in sub-Saharan Africa (GBIF, 2017) (E), chemical structure of 2,4,6-trihydroxydihydrochalcone (F).

Underexplored Medicinal Plants from Sub-Saharan Africa
https://doi.org/10.1016/B978-0-12-816814-1.00022-3

1. General description

1.1 Botanical nomenclature

Greyia radlkoferi Szyszyl

1.2 Botanical family

Greyiaceae

1.3 Vernacular names

Woolly Bottlebrush, Wild Bottlebrush, Transvaal Bottlebrush, Natal bottlebrush, Bottlebrush and
Bottlebrush Tree (English)
Transvaalse Baakhout, Wollerige Baakhout, Glase-waaierbos, and Baakhout (Afrikaans)
inHlazane (Siswati)
inDlebelembila (Swazi)

2. Botanical description

The Greyiaceae family is endemic to South Africa and consists of three species, including *Greyia radlkoferi*. It is an attractive ornamental species with snarled branches and scarlet flowers. It is a shrub or small tree that can grow up to 5 m in length, with a yellowish bark that turns gray as the tree ages. The leaves are oval, lobed at the base, and very woolly on the petioles and the underside of the leaves. This characteristic is a distinguishing feature of its closely related cousin *Greyia sutherlandii*. The red flowers are funnel-shaped and form clusters as a raceme inflorescence (Bohm and Chan, 1992; De la Cruz, 2016).

3. Distribution

In South Africa, *G. radlkoferi* occurs mainly in the mist-belt mountains of Mpumalanga and in KwaZulu-Natal close to Ngome. This species can also be found in Swaziland. It is also distributed in areas including deep channels along misty streambanks, the borders of evergreen forest, and among rocks (De La Cruz, 2016).

4. Ethnobotanical usage

There is minimal information related to this species and its medicinal and economic importance, apart from the use as an ornamental plant.

5. Phytochemical constituents

This species is rich in flavonoid compounds. Compounds isolated from this species include 2,4,6-trihydroxydihydrochalcone; 3,5,7-trihydroxyflavone; 4',5,7-trihydroxyisoflavone; 5,7-dihydroxyflavanone; and 2',6'-dihydroxy- 4' − methoxydihydrochalcone (Lall et al., 2016).

6. TLC fingerprinting of plant extract

To observe the separation of *G. radlkoferi*, 2 mg of the ethanolic extract was weighed out and dissolved in 200 µL ethanol. For the standard, 2, 4, 6-trihydroxydihydrochalcone was weighed off in the same manner as the extract and dissolved in 600 µL of ethanol. For the thin layer chromatography (TLC) analysis of *G. radlkoferi* crude extract, silica gel 60 F_{254} TLC plates were used to observe the separation of the compounds present within the extract. Plate markings were made with a soft pencil, and glass capillaries were used to spot the samples onto the TLC plate. Reference standard 2, 4, 6-trihydroxydihydrochalcone was spotted to determine whether it was present in the extract. The spots were left to dry completely, before placing the plate in a TLC tank, which contained 10 mL eluent 9:1 chloroform: methanol solvent system. The samples were allowed to separate until the solvent system reached 1 cm from the top of the TLC plate. The plate was observed under ultraviolet (UV light) (long and short wavelength), followed by spraying with freshly prepared vanillin/sulfuric acid (2%) to detect the bands on the TLC plate.

7. Pharmacological properties

Greyia radlkoferi has not been extensively researched for its in vitro and in vivo medicinal properties. Although it is a widely distributed and well-known plant in South Africa, there is still an opportunity for research and development with regard to this plant.

7.1 Effects on tyrosinase activity and melanin production

The ethanol extract of *G. radlkoferi* was able to inhibit tyrosinase enzyme activity by 50% (IC_{50}) at a concentration of 17.96 µg/mL. There were five compounds isolated from this extract. Compound 1 (2′, 4′, 6′-trihydroxydihydrochalcone) was the most active with an inhibitory concentration of 17.70 µg/mL (68.48 µM). Compound 2 (3, 5, 7-trihydroxyflavone) showed inhibitory activity at a concentration of 113.60 µg/mL (420.37 µM). The tyrosinase inhibitory activity of Compound 1 was explained by molecular docking of this molecule to the active site of the enzyme, which showed the highest GOLD score of 55.58 as compared to that of the known inhibitor kojic acid, which showed a docking score of 47.95. The extract of *G. radlkoferi* was able to decrease melanin content in melanocytes by 50% at a concentration of 12.50 µg/mL. Compound 1 was able to reduce melanin content by 25% at the same concentration, while Compound 2 inhibited 30% of melanin content (De Canha et al., 2013; Lall et al., 2016).

8. Additional information

8.1 Therapeutic (proposed) usage

Even skin tone

8.2 Safety data

To determine the effect on melanin production, the cytotoxicity of the extract and compounds was tested on B16–F10 mouse melanocytes. The extract inhibited cell viability by 50% at a concentration of 40.89 µg/mL, whereas Compound 1 showed the same effect at a concentration of 56.59 µg/mL (218.95 µM). Compound 2 did not affect cell viability at the highest concentration tested (200 µg/mL) (De Canha et al., 2013).

8.3 Trade information

Least concern

8.4 Dosage

Formulated cream

References

Bohm, B.A., Chan, J., 1992. Flavonoids and affinities of Greyiaceae with a discussion of the occurrence of B-ring deoxyflavonoids in dicotyledonous families. Systematic Botany 17, 272–281.

De Canha, M.N., Lall, N., Hussein, A., Mogapi, E., Moodley, I., 2013. The Extract of *Greyia radlkoferi* and Use Thereof. WO/2013/171720.

De La Cruz, P., 2016. *Greyia radlkoferi* Szyszyl. http://www.plantzafrica.com/plantefg/greyrad.htm.

GBIF, 2017. *Greyia radlkoferi* Szyszył. https://doi.org/10.15468/39omei.

Lall, N., Mogapi, E., De Canha, M.N., Crampton, B., Nqephe, M., Hussein, A.A., Kumar, V., 2016. Insights into tyrosinase inhibition by compounds isolated from *Greyia radlkoferi* Szyszyl using biological activity, molecular docking and gene expression analysis. Bioorganic & Medicinal Chemistry 24, 5953–5959.

Shebs, S., 2005. Photo of *Greyia radlkoferi* at the San Francisco Botanical Garden. Available online: https://commons.wikimedia.org/wiki/File:Greyia_radlkoferi_1.jpg. (CC BY-SA 3.0).

Shebs, S., 2006a. Photo of *Greyia radlkoferi* at the University of California Botanical Garden. Available online: https://commons.wikimedia.org/wiki/File:Greyia_radlkoferi_5.jpg. (CC BY-SA 3.0).

Shebs, S., 2006b. Photo of *Greyia radlkoferi* at the University of California Botanical Garden. Available online: https://commons.wikimedia.org/wiki/File:Greyia_radlkoferi_4.jpg. (CC BY-SA 3.0).

Haemanthus albiflos

Balungile Madikizela[1,2], Lyndy Joy McGaw[1]

[1] Phytomedicine Programme, Department of Paraclinical Sciences, Faculty of Veterinary Sciences, University of Pretoria, Pretoria, Gauteng, South Africa; [2] University of KwaZulu-Natal, Durban, KwaZulu-Natal, South Africa

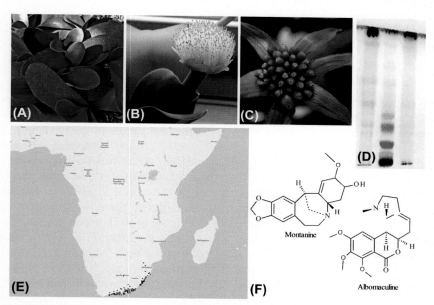

FIGURE 23 Aerial parts of *Haemanthus albiflos* (Zell, 2009) (A), flower of *H. albiflos* (Wolf, 2006) (B), fruit of *H. albiflos* (Raasgat, 2004) (C), TLC chromatogram, Lane 1; *H. albiflos* bulb acetone extract, Lane 2; *H. albiflos* bulb ethanol extract, Lane 3; *H. albiflos* leaf acetone extract (D), distribution of *H. albiflos* in sub-Saharan Africa (GBIF, 2017) (E), chemical structures of montanine and albomaculine (F).

Underexplored Medicinal Plants from Sub-Saharan Africa
https://doi.org/10.1016/B978-0-12-816814-1.00023-5

1. General description

1.1 Botanical nomenclature

Haemanthus albiflos Jacq.

1.2 Botanical family

Amaryllidaceae

1.3 Vernacular names

White paint brush or dappled snowbrush or white April fool or powder puff, white bloody lily, shaving brush, Elephant's tongue (English)
   Gevlekte poeierkwas or witpoeierkwas (Afrikaans)
   Licishamlilo (Siswati)
   Umathunga or isithithibala (Xhosa)
   Uzeneke (Zulu)

2. Botanical description

Haemanthus albiflos is an evergreen bulbous plant of the Amaryllidaceae family, and the most commonly known of the three *Haemanthus* species. The genus *Haemanthus* was created by Linnaeus in 1753 and is derived from Greek words "haima" and "anthos," meaning "blood flower" The species *"albiflos,"* which means "white flower" in English, was given its name due to the color of the flowers of this plant. *Haemanthus albiflos* is variable, growing up to about 250 mm in height when flowering. It has variable leaves; oblong, usually smooth and sometimes shiny with varying colors from pale to dark green or grayish-green. The leaves may be covered with short, soft hairs, or have yellowish spots on the upper surface. The upper half of the bulb is bright green and is usually exposed above ground. This plant has a long flowering period that extends from early April to July (autumn and winter) in the wild. However, when cultivated, sporadic blooms may appear at any time of the year. The flower head (botanically known as an umbel) consists of numerous erect, narrow white flowers, and enclosed greenish-white bracts. The fruit is a bright orange or red fleshy berry, producing a distinctive musty odor when ripe (PlantZAfrica, 2018).

3. Distribution

Haemanthus albiflos, native to southern Africa, varies considerably throughout its distribution range along the eastern coastal belt and inland Cape region of southern Africa. In South Africa, it is found in the Western

Cape, Eastern Cape, and KwaZulu-Natal Provinces, in deep shade on forest floors, on rocky seashores exposed to salt spray, in coastal dune forest, on cliff faces in river valleys, and in shady places on inland mountain ranges (PlantZAfrica, 2018).

4. Ethnobotanical usage

This plant finds usage in traditional medicine for the treatment of various diseases and ailments. The Xhosa people in the Eastern Cape drink a bulb infusion to assist with healing broken bones or they apply roots as a poultice over fractured bones to assist healing. The bulb infusion is also used by Xhosas in the eastern region of the OR Tambo district for treating tuberculosis, whereas the people in the Amathole district use the leaf concoction prepared in alcohol for the same purpose (Lawal et al., 2014; Madikizela et al., 2017). The bulb decoction prepared together with *Scadoxus puniceus* L. and *Crinum macowanii* Baker is reported for traditional use against amenorrhea and pregnancy-related conditions. The Zulus use the bulb as an emetic, whereas the Xhosas use it as an infusion for the treatment of chronic coughs (Hutchings et al., 1996). A bulb decoction is administered orally for the treatment of skin-related diseases and wounds (Thibane et al., 2019). The whole plant is reported for use against sexually transmitted infections, as a blood purifier, body cleanser, for pains and arthritis. The bulb is reported for traditional use in the Western Cape in Rasta bush medicine for treating internal bruises, broken bones, ulcers, and asthma, and the leaves are applied topically to draw out water from swelling ankles and to relieve water retention (Philander, 2011). The plant is also used as a purgative and diuretic (Philander, 2011). Leaves are used topically for skin ulcers, sores, wounds, and burns (Hutchings et al., 1996; Afolayan et al., 2014). The fleshy bulb is applied to aching skin and is also used to ward off lightning (Pooley, 1998).

5. Phytochemical constituents

Fresh bulbs (2 kg) and leaves (1 kg) of the plant collected from Zulu-land are macerated and extracted in 2 L of ethanol at room temperature with continuous agitation for approximately 4 days (Crouch et al., 2005). A gumlike residue was obtained for both plant parts, and this was partitioned in dichloromethane: methanol (1:1). The compounds were then separated using various ratios of dichloromethane: methanol using column chromatography with silica gel as solid phase. Three isoquinoline alkaloids were isolated from both the leaves and the bulbs of *H. albiflos*, and they included homolycorine (1), albomaculine (2) and the O-methyl-lycorenium salt (3) (Crouch et al., 2005).

To determine alkaloid diversity of the bulb, the pulverized plant material (300 mg) was macerated in 400 μL methanol for 5 min, and then 3 mL of 0.1% H_2SO_4 was added. The material was then extracted for 45 min under ultrasonication, shaken for 2 h, and centrifuged for 10 min at 4000 rpm. The supernatant was removed. Extraction was repeated twice and during the second extraction, the sample was left overnight. The extract was retained on an ion-exchange solid phase extraction column (Isolute SCX, 500 mg, 3 mL) preconditioned with 2 mL methanol and 2 mL 0.1% H_2SO_4. The column was washed with 2 mL 0.1% H_2SO_4 and 4 mL methanol after alkaloid extract addition. The alkaloid extracts were then eluted three times with 2 mL 25% NH_4OH in methanol, pH 11–12, concentrated under vacuum until dryness and redissolved to a concentration of 5 mg/mL in methanol. The sample was centrifuged for 10 min at 4000 rpm, and the supernatant was removed. The alkaloid profiles were obtained by gas chromatography–mass spectrometry (GC-MS), and they included homolycorine and montanine (Bay-Smidt et al., 2011). According to our knowledge, which is based on literature search, there are no phytochemical investigations that have been reported on the flowers and fruits of this plant yet.

6. TLC fingerprinting of plant extract

For the separation of compounds present within the crude extracts of *H. albiflos*, 10 mg of bulb acetone and ethanolic extracts were dissolved in 1 mL ethanol. The leaf acetone extract of this plant was prepared the same way as that of a bulb. Silica gel $60F_{254}$ thin layer chromatography (TLC) plates (Merk, Germany) were used to observe the separation of the compounds of *H. albiflos*. Exactly 10 μL of each extract was spotted in a line of 1 cm wide on a TLC plate using capillaries, allowed to dry completely and developed by placing the plate in a saturated TLC tank, which contained 100 mL eluent 8:2:1 ethyl acetate: methanol: formic acid solvent system. The TLC plate was removed from the tank when the solvent system reached 1 cm from the top and dried under a stream of air to evaporate the solvent. An observation under ultraviolet (UV) light (at 254 nm wavelength) was made, and freshly prepared vanillin/sulfuric acid (2%) was sprayed to detect the bands on the TLC plate.

7. Pharmacological properties

This plant has been studied in vitro for pharmacological properties. However there are no existing reports of in vivo pharmacological activities or extensive toxicity studies done. Therefore further research is required.

7.1 Antimicrobial activity

In a study done by Motsei et al. (2003), investigating the antifungal activity of several plants including *H. albiflos*, the leaf and bulb of the plant were collected in Pietermaritzburg Botanical Garden and extracts were prepared by extracting 1 g of dried plant material separately in 10 mL of water, ethanol, ethyl acetate, and hexane. However, all the extracts showed no activity against *Candida albicans* (clinical isolates from human baby and adult, and the American type culture collection [ATCC] 10231 strain) with minimum inhibitory concentration (MIC) values ranging from 2.09 to 25 mg/mL.

In another study, the bulb was used to determine the antimicrobial potential of the plant against infectious skin microorganisms and skin dermatophytes: *Bacillus subtilis*, *Staphylococcus aureus*, *S. epidermidis*, *Escherichia coli*, *Klebsiella pneumoniae*, *Brevibacillus agri*, *C. albicans*, *Trichophyton mentagrophytes*, *Trichophyton tonsurans*, and *Micrococcus canis*. Different solvents of varying polarities were used to extract plant material at a ratio of 20 mL/g (v/w), and they included petroleum ether, dichloromethane, 70% aqueous ethanol (v/v), and water. The petroleum ether and dichloromethane extracts from the bulb showed antibacterial activity only against *K. pneumoniae*, whereas the ethanol and water extract of the bulb showed activity against *E. coli* with MIC values of 0.78 and 0.098 mg/mL, respectively. All the extracts were inactive against the fungal strains tested with MIC values ranging between 1.56 and 12.5 mg/mL (Thibane et al., 2019).

When tested for antimycobacterial activity, the leaf and bulb acetone extracts had some activity against *Mycobacterium fortuitum* and *Mycobacterium smegmatis* (leaf extract), *Mycobacterium bovis* BCG, and *Mycobacterium gordonae* (bulb extract) with an MIC of 0.63 mg/mL in all cases. Water and ethanol extracts showed no activity against all tested strains: *M. smegmatis*, *M. fortuitum*, *M. bovis* BCG, *M. aurum*, and *M. gordonae*, with MIC values ranging from 1.25 to 2.50 mg/mL (Madikizela and McGaw, 2018).

7.2 Antioxidant activity

The 50% aqueous methanol extract from the bulb was tested for antioxidant activity in the diphenylpicrylhydrazyl (DPPH) radical scavenging assay and ferric reducing antioxidant power (FRAP) assay and also for their ability to delay the oxidation of β-carotene in the β-carotene linoleic acid model. The bulb extract showed a 50% inhibition concentration (IC_{50}) value of 2.45 µg/mL in the DPPH assay and a 50% effective concentration (EC_{50}) of 1.12 µg/mL in the FRAP assay, ORR_{60min}; 0.22 and ORR_{90min}; 0.19 in the β-carotene linoleic acid model (Thibane et al., 2019).

7.3 Photoprotective effect

The aqueous ethanol bulb extract prepared from 1 g of powdered plant material in 20 mL of 70% ethanol was tested for photoprotective (measure sun protective factor, SPF) effect in a study by Thibane et al. (2019). The SPF result, which is the ratio of ultraviolet (UV) radiation required to produce a minimal erythema dose in protected skin to unprotected skin, confirmed the ability of the plant extract to provide minimal protection (SPF <12).

7.4 Antityrosinase activity

In an antityrosinase activity study, a 20 mL/g (v/w) ratio was used to prepare the 70% aqueous ethanol leaf extract of the powdered plant material. Inhibition of tyrosinase was determined using the dopachrome method with 3,4-dihydroxy-L-phenylalanine (L-DOPA) as a substrate. The leaf ethanol extract was reported to have insignificant antityrosinase activity with an IC_{50} value of 79.58 µg/mL (Thibane et al., 2019).

7.5 Acetylcholinesterase inhibitory activity

The acetylcholinesterase inhibitory activity of the methanolic extract from the bulb was reported to be insignificant with a 50% inhibitory concentration (IC_{50}) of 50 µg/mL (Bay-Smidt et al., 2011).

7.6 Affinity to the serotonin reuptake transport protein

The affinity to serotonin reuptake transport of the methanolic extract from the bulb was reported as insignificant with a 50% inhibitory concentration (IC_{50}) of 50 µg/mL (Bay-Smidt et al., 2011).

7.7 Antiinflammatory activity

Acetone and aqueous bulb extracts were screened to determine their inhibitory effect against phospholipase A2 activity using the secretory phospholipase A2 (sPLA2) inhibitor screening assay kit. The acetone extract was reported to have significantly inhibited sPLA2 with a 50 % inhibition concentration (IC_{50}) of 0.9835 µg/mL, which was comparable to that of the positive control, thioether amide PC, with an IC_{50} of 0.9556 µg/mL (Thibane et al., 2018).

7.8 Antiviral activity

The hydroethanolic extract of the bulb was prepared from plant material collected in the garden of the Faculty of Pharmacy, Paris, in early autumn. The bulb was dried at 25°C, ground by crushing in a Culatti grinder, extracted with 70% ethanol (28 g in 400 mL) and evaporated under vacuum, leaving the aqueous solution, which was then filtered through a 0.22 μM filter and frozen at −70°C in 1 mL fractions. Poliovirus type I propagated on HeLa cells was used to determine the antiviral activity of the extract (Husson et al., 1993). For each experiment, 1 mL of the frozen aqueous solution was thawed and incorporated into the culture medium at appropriate concentrations. In that study, the bulb extract was reported to inhibit RNA synthesis at concentrations of 0.1, 0.2, and 0.3 μL/mL by 17%, 44%, and 58%, respectively. The same extract also inhibited kinetics of cellular DNA synthesis by 44% and 40% at concentrations of 0.1 and 0.2 μL/mL, respectively. The hydroethanolic extract of the bulb also showed inhibition of the rate of viral RNA synthesis up to 210 min by 90% at 0.2, 0.5, and 1 μL/mL, and higher concentrations were reported to have blocked RNA viral synthesis. The mechanism of action of antiviral activity of the bulb hydroethanolic extract at a concentration of 0.2 μL/mL was studied on poliovirus, and the rates of cellular RNA, DNA, and protein synthesis were inhibited at 44%, 40%, and 52%, respectively, with a 95% decrease of viral RNA synthesis over 210 min (Husson et al., 1993).

The hydroethanolic extract of the bulb had antiviral activity against moloney murine leukemia virus derived from SVX shuttle with resistance to G418 antimitotic and human immunodeficiency virus (HIV). The extract inhibited the formation of G418 resistant 3T3 clones by 88% and showed an IC_{50} value of 4 μL/mL on HIV-infected lymphocytic cells (Husson et al., 1997). In a study by Husson et al. (1991), a hydroethanolic leaf extract had antiviral activity against herpes simplex virus type I, poliovirus type I, vesicular stomatitis virus, and simian rotavirus SA 11. In another study, the hydroethanolic extract (7 μL/mL) of the leaves inhibited replication of poliovirus type I and protein viral synthesis by 4.5 log units and 97%, respectively (Husson et al., 1994).

8. Additional information

8.1 Therapeutic (proposed) usage

Antiviral, antibacterial, antiinflammatory, photoprotective, and antioxidant.

8.2 Safety data

The 7 µL/mL concentration of the aqueous ethanol leaf extract showed 20% inhibition of monkey kidney cells (Husson et al., 1994). Cytotoxicity with 32%, 50%, 63%, and 70% inhibition was reported with 2, 7, 14, and 28 µL of extract, respectively in a calorimetric assay of NIH 3T3 (fibroblast mouse) cells fixed with crystal violet (Husson et al., 1997). Albomaculine, a compound isolated from this plant, was not found to be cytotoxic when tested against hepatoma and fibroblast cells at a concentration of 4 µM (Gasparini et al., 2017).

8.3 Trade information

Haemanthus albiflos is one of the species mentioned in the Redlist of South East Africa and Redlist of South African plants in the least concern category (Ifrim and Zaharia, 2015).

8.4 Dosage

Not available

References

Afolayan, A.J., Grierson, D.S., Mbeng, W.O., 2014. Ethnobotanical survey of medicinal plants used in the management of skin disorders among the Xhosa communities of the Amathole District, Eastern Cape, South Africa. Journal of Ethnopharmacology 153, 220–232.

Bay-Smidt, M.G.K., Jäger, A.K., Krydsfeldt, K., Meerow, A.W., Stafford, G.I., Van Staden, J., Rønsted, N., 2011. Phylogenetic selection of target species in Amaryllidaceae tribe Haemantheae for acetylcholinesterase inhibition and affinity to the serotonin reuptake transport protein. South African Journal of Botany 77, 175–183.

Crouch, N.R., Pohl, T.L., Mulholland, D.A., Ndlovu, E., 2005. Alkaloids from three ethnomedicinal *Haemanthus* species: *H. albiflos*, *H. deformis* and *H. pauculifolius* (Amaryllidaceae). South African Journal of Botany 71, 49–52.

Gasparini, L.S., Macedo, N.D., Pimentel, E.F., Fronza, M., Junior, V.L.J., Borges, W.S., Cole, E.R., Andrade, T.U., Endringer, D.C., Lenz, D., 2017. In vitro cell viability by CellProfiler® software as equivalent to MTT assay. Pharmacognosy Magazine 13, S365–S369.

GBIF, 2017. *Haemanthus albiflos* Jacq, GBIF Secretariat, GBIF Backbone Taxonomy. Checklist dataset. https://doi.org/10.15468/39omei. Accessed via GBIF.org on 2018-08-28.

Hutchings, A., Scott, A.H., Lewis, G., Cunningham, A., 1996. Zulu Medicinal Plants. An Inventory. University of Natal Press, Pietermaritzburg. ISBN 0869809237.

Husson, G.P., Subra, F., Lai-Kuen, R., Vilagines, R., 1997. Antiviral activity of hydroalcoholic extract from *Haemanthus albiflos* on the moloney murine leukemia virus and the human immunodeficiency virus. Comptes Rendus des Seances de la Societe de Biologie et de Ses Filiales 191, 473–485.

Husson, G.P., Vilagines, P., Sarrette, B., Vilagines, R., 1991. Antiviral effect of *Haemanthus albiflos* leaves extract on herpes virus, adenovirus, vesicular stomatitis virus, rotavirus and poliovirus. Annales Pharmaceutiques Françaises 49, 40–48.

Husson, G.P., Sarrette, B., Vilagines, P., Vilagines, R., 1993. Investigations on antiviral action of *Haemanthus albiflos* natural extract. Phytotherapy Research 7, 348—351.

Husson, G.P., Vilagines, P., Sarrette, B., Vilagines, R., 1994. Antiviral effect of the alkaloid extract isolated from *Haemanthus albiflos*. Annales Pharmaceutiques Françaises 52, 311—322.

Ifrim, C., Zaharia, G., 2015. Indoor plants cultivated in botanical garden Iassy used in traditional medicine. Analele Ştiinţifice ale Universităţii "Al. I. Cuza" Iaşis. II a. Biologie vegetală 61, 75—87.

Lawal, I.O., Grierson, D.S., Afolayan, A.J., 2014. Phytotherapeutic information on plants used for the treatment of tuberculosis in Eastern Cape Province, South Africa. Evidence-based Complementary and Alternative Medicine 2014. Article ID 735423, 11 pages.

Madikizela, B., Kambizi, L., McGaw, L.J., 2017. An ethnobotanical survey of plants used traditionally to treat tuberculosis in the eastern region of O.R. Tambo district, South Africa. South African Journal of Botany 109, 231—236.

Madikizela, B., McGaw, L.J., 2018. Scientific rationale for traditional use of plants to treat tuberculosis in the eastern region of the OR Tambo district, South Africa. Journal of Ethnopharmacology 224, 250—260.

Motsei, M.L., Lindsey, K.L., Van Staden, J., Jäger, A.K., 2003. Screening of traditionally used South African plants for antifungal activity against Candida albicans. Journal of Ethnopharmacology 86 (2—3), 235—241.

Philander, L.A., 2011. An ethnobotany of Western Cape Rasta bush medicine. Journal of Ethnopharmacology 138, 578—594.

PlantZAfrica, 2018. *Haemanthus albiflos*. Online. Available at: http://pza.sanbi.org/haemanthus-albiflos.

Pooley, E., 1998. A Field Guide to Wildflowers: KwaZulu-Natal and the Eastern Region. Natal Flora Publications Trust, Durban.

Raasgat, 2004. *Haemanthus Albiflos* Jacq. Fruits. Available online: https://commons.wikimedia.org/wiki/File:Haemanthus_albiflos01.jpg (The copyright holder of this work, release this work into the public domain. This applies worldwide).

Thibane, V.S., Ndhlala, A.R., Abdelgadir, H.A., Finnie, J.F., Van Staden, J., 2019. The cosmetic potential of plants from the Eastern Cape Province traditionally used for skincare and beauty. South African Journal of Botany 122, 475—483. https://doi.org/10.1016/j.sajb.2018.05.003.

Thibane, V.S., Ndhlala, A.R., Abdelgadir, H.A., Finnie, J.F., Van Staden, J., 2018. Plants as natural inhibitors of enzymes involved in skin inflammation. South African Journal of Botany 115, 311.

Wolf, M., 2006. *Haemanthus Albiflos* in Blüte. Available online: https://commons.wikimedia.org/wiki/File:Haemanthus_albiflos.jpg. (CC BY-SA 3.0).

Zell, H., 2009. *Haemanthus Albiflos*, Amaryllidaceae, Elephant's Tongue, Shaving-Brush Plant, Habitus. Botanical Garden KIT, Karlsruhe, Germany. Available online: https://commons.wikimedia.org/wiki/File:Haemanthus_albiflos_001.JPG. (CC BY-SA 3.0).

24

Heteropyxis canescens

Dikonketso Bodiba, Namrita Lall

Department of Plant and Soil Sciences, University of Pretoria, Pretoria, Gauteng, South Africa

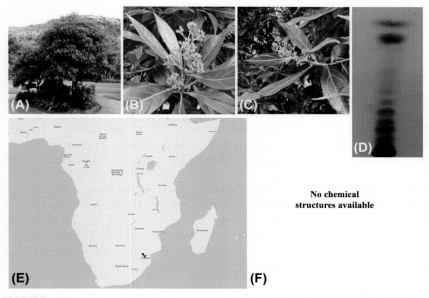

No chemical
structures available

FIGURE 24   Aerial plant parts of *Heteropyxis canescens* (JMK, 2013a) (A), flower of *H. canescens* (JMK, 2013b) (B), stem of *H. canescens* (JMK, 2013c) (C), TLC chromatogram, fingerprint of *H. canescens* extract (D), distribution of *H. canescens* in sub-Saharan Africa (GBIF, 2018) (E), no chemical compounds have been reported (F).

1. General description

1.1 Botanical nomenclature

Heteropyxis canescens Oliv.

1.2 Botanical family

Heteropyxidaceae

1.3 Vernacular names

Bastard Lavender tree (English)
Forest Lavender tree (English)
Inkunzana (Swati)
Basterlaventelboom (Afrikaans)

2. Botanical description

Heteropyxis canescens is an evergreen, semideciduous tree that is rare and hardy and typically grows up to heights of 3—5 meters. It has a sparkling beige bark that flakes off in patches revealing blotches. The leaves are relatively large and decorative, with fascinating venation. The leaves produce a lavender smell when crushed. The leaves turn a magnificent red, purple, and maroon in autumn, holding up almost all winter. In the summer they are glossy dark green and paler underneath. The flowers are small and yellow-green, occurring in clusters at the end of their branches from September to March. The flowers attract birds, butterflies, and other small insects. The fruit is a spherical pale brown capsule 3 mm in diameter. These trees grow best in moist conditions but can tolerate garden-like environments (Boon, 2010; Hilton-Taylor, 1996; Raimondo et al., 2009; Victor, 2005).

3. Distribution

Heteropyxis canescens occurs in forested ravines and riverine forests in a restricted area of Mpumalanga and Swaziland (Victor, 2005).

4. Ethnobotanical usage

Heteropyxis canescens has no reported traditional/ethnobotanical uses.

5. Phytochemical constituents

There no reports on isolated compounds/major constituents or essential oils from *H. canescens*.

6. TLC fingerprinting of plant extract

A thin layer chromatography (TLC) fingerprint of the *H. canescens* was prepared with the ethanolic extract. The separation of the compounds was observed by weighing out 2 mg of the extract dissolved in 500 μL of ethanol. For examining the crude extract of *H. canescens*, TLC was used. Silica gel 60 F254 TLC plates were used to examine the separation of compounds that were present in the crude extract. The plates were marked with a soft pencil and 100 μL tips were used to spot the samples onto the TLC plate. The spots were allowed to dry completely and the plate was placed in a tank, containing 20 mL of the eluent, 8:2 dichloromethane:hexane as the solvent system. The samples were allowed to separate until the solvent system reached 0.5 cm from the top of the TLC plate. Vanillin/sulfuric acid (2%) was freshly prepared and used for detection of bands on the plate, whereas some bands were observed under ultraviolet (UV) light (long and short wavelength).

7. Biological activities

There are no published reported studies that have been conducted on *H. canescens* in literature. A study with unpublished results was conducted at the University of Pretoria, evaluating the possible biological activity of the ethanolic extracts of this plant.

7.1 Antibacterial activity

In a previous study, the leaves and twigs of *H. canescens* were collected in the late summer time (January–February) at the University of Pretoria Hatfield campus and were used to prepare an ethanolic extract. The extract showed good activity against gram-positive *Streptococcus mutans* American type culture collection (ATCC) 25175 (minimum inhibitory concentration [MIC] of 0.29 mg/mL) and moderate activity against *Candida albicans* ATCC 25175 (MIC of 3.125 mg/mL), using the microdilution method (Bodiba, 2016)

7.2 Combinational studies

A study was conducted to determine the possibility of synergism between ethanolic extracts of *H. canescens* as well as another member of the Heteropyxidaceae family, *Heteropyxis dehniae*. The plant extracts of *H. canescens* and *H. dehniae* were combined and used to determine antimicrobial activity. The two plant extracts were also combined with two other samples: Peppermint essential oil (PEO) and TEAVIGO, which are known for its antiplaque/anticaries, antigingivitis activities, and combating bad breath. These compounds are common in formulations for oral products. A combination of the checkerboard and ratio methods was used to determine the effect of combining these two plant samples and the selected compounds (Moody, 1992: Orhan et al., 2005).

7.3 Antioxidant capacity

The diphenylpicrylhydrazyl (DPPH) was used for testing antioxidant activity (Du Toit et al., 2001). Nitric oxide (NO) and superoxide are stable free radicals that can be used to determine the general and specific antioxidant potential of a sample. Nitric oxide is important in vasodilatation, regulation of mineralized tissue function, neurotransmission, etc. In periodontal tissue, NO and saliva are part of a nonspecific natural defense mechanism against pathogenic bacteria. However, under pathological conditions, NO has damaging effects, particularly involving tissue damage. NO inhibitors are, therefore, of interest when looking for treatments of oral diseases.

The ethanolic extract of *H. canescens* had good overall antioxidant activity, exhibiting specific activity against nitric oxide and superoxide. This suggested that *H. canescens* was able to not only directly affect the bacterial growth itself but could also have an indirect mechanism that targets bacterial metabolic processes such as oxidation, thereby also exhibiting inhibition. This antioxidant capacity alludes to the value of *H. canescens* not only as antibacterial agents but also antioxidant agents that could help minimize the damage that may result from bacteria's metabolic processes (Kuete et al., 2015)

8. Additional information

8.1 Therapeutic (proposed) usage

Antibacterial and antioxidant

8.2 Safety data

There is currently no data available on the possible toxicity of *H. canescens* essential oils, major constituents or leaf extracts.

8.3 Trade information

Falls under the least concern category, not endangered, abundant in countries such as Swaziland and Mpumalanga province.

8.4 Dosage

Not available

References

Bodiba, D.C., 2016. Biological Activity of *Heteropyxis Canescens* and *Heteropyxis Dehniae* and Their Mechanisms against *Streptococcus Mutans*. University of Pretoria, South Africa (Dissertation).

Boon, R., 2010. Pooley's Trees of Eastern South Africa. Flora and Fauna Publications Trust, Durban.

Du-Toit, R., Volsteedt, Y., Apostolides, Z., 2001. Comparison of the antioxidant content of fruits, vegetables and teas measured as vitamin C equivalent. Toxicology 166, 63—69.

GBIF, 2018. *Heteropyxis Canescens* Oliv. In GBIF Secretariat (2018). GBIF Backbone Taxonomy. Checklist dataset. https://doi.org/10.15468/39omei. accessed via GBIF.org on 2018-09-25.

Hilton-Taylor, C., 1996. Red Data List of Southern African Plants. Strelitzia 4. South African National Botanical Institute, Pretoria.

JMK, 2013a. Forest Lavender at the Walter Sisulu National Botanical Garden in Western Roodepoort. South Africa. This threatened species is endemic to Mpumalanga and Swaziland. Available online: https://commons.wikimedia.org/wiki/File:Heteropyxis_canescens,_habitus,_a,_Walter_Sisulu_NBT.jpg. (CC BY-SA 3.0).

JMK, 2013b. Fruit and Foliage of a Forest Lavender at the Walter Sisulu National Botanical Garden in Western Roodepoort. South Africa. This threatened species is endemic to Mpumalanga and Swaziland. Available online: https://commons.wikimedia.org/wiki/File: Heteropyxis_canescens,_loof_en_vrugte,_b,_Walter_Sisulu_NBT.jpg. (CC BY-SA 3.0).

JMK, 2013c. Foliage of a Forest Lavender at the Walter Sisulu National Botanical Garden in Western Roodepoort. South Africa. This threatened species is endemic to Mpumalanga and Swaziland. Available online: https://commons.wikimedia.org/wiki/File: Heteropyxis_canescens,_lower,_a,_Walter_Sisulu_NBT.jpg. (CC BY-SA 3.0).

Kuete, V., Sandjo, L., Seukep, J., Maen, Z., Ngadjui, B., Efferth, T., 2015. Cytotoxic compounds from the fruits of Uapacatogoensis towards multi-factorial drug-resistant cancer cells. Planta Medica 81, 32—38.

Moody, J.A., 1992. Synergy testing: broth microdilution checkerboard and broth macrodilution methods. In: Eisenberg, H.D. (Ed.), Clinical Microbiology Procedures Handbook. American Society for Microbiology, Washington, DC.

Orhan, G., Bayram, A., Zer, Y., Balci, I., 2005. Synergy tests by E test and checkerboard methods of antimicrobial combinations against *Brucella melitensis*. Journal of Clinical Microbiology 43 (1), 140−143.

Raimondo, D., von Staden, L., Foden, W., Victor, J.E., Helme, N.A., Turner, R.C., Kamundi, D.A., Manyama, P.A., 2009. Red List of South African Plants. Strelitzia 25. South African National Biodiversity Institute, Pretoria.

Victor, J.E., 2005. Heteropyxis Canescens Oliv. National Assessment: Red List of South African Plants Version 2017.1.

Further reading

Bodiba, D.C., 2013. Mechanism of Action of *Heteropyxis* against Oral Pathogens. University of Pretoria, South Africa. Dissertation.

Heteropyxis dehniae

Dikonketso Bodiba, Namrita Lall

Department of Plant and Soil Sciences, University of Pretoria, Pretoria, Gauteng, South Africa

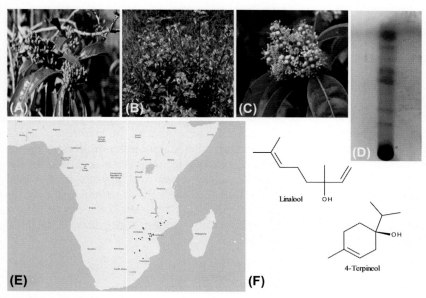

FIGURE 25 Flower buds of *Heteropyxis dehniae* (A), aerial parts of *H. dehniae* (B), flowers of *H dehniae* (Baumann, 2016) (C), TLC chromatogram, fingerprint of *H. dehniae* extract (D), distribution of *H. dehniae* in sub-Saharan Africa (GBIF, 2018) (E), chemical structures of 4-terpineol and linalool (F).

167

1. General description

1.1 Botanical nomenclature

Heteropyxis dehniae Seuss

1.2 Botanical family

Heteropyxidaceae

1.3 Vernacular names

Chisurudza (Shona)
Inkiza ye ntaba (Ndebele)
Lavender tree (English)
Mubanda (Shona)
Mutandavarombo (Shona)
Nyakanebve (Shona)

2. Botanical description

Heteropyxis dehniae is medium in height, with pale gray bark. This tree closely resembles *H. natalensis*, another member of the Heteropyxidaceae family. The leaves are alternate, with a hairy light green undersurface and a smooth upper surface. The leaves go from pinkish to green as they mature. The flowers are light yellow-green and appear in the early summer (October–December), whereas the fruits are small and oval that first appear in late October. The fruit bears a number of seeds in three to five valves that split open when ready (Foden and Potter, 2005; Hyde et al., 2018; Sibanda et al., 2004).

3. Distribution

Heteropyxis dehniae is commonly found in bushveld and rocky places. It is distributed across the Southern African region covering countries such as Mozambique, Zimbabwe, Swaziland, and several regions of the Limpopo province (Foden and Potter, 2005).

4. Ethnobotanical usage

The leaves and roots of *H. dehniae* are traditionally used for the treatment of several ailments. Some medicinal uses include the preparation of medicinal teas used as blood purifiers and as a perfume. In addition to this, dried fresh leaves can be smoked to relieve headaches. The steam from a decoction of the roots is used to treat nosebleeds. The roots are also used for the treatment of mental disorders as well as menorrhagia (Arnold and Gulumian, 1984; Foden and Potter, 2005; Hyde et al., 2018; Raimondo et al., 2009; Sibanda et al., 2004)

5. Phytochemical constituents

The only phytochemical constituents that have been isolated from this species are their essential oils from the leaves. Gas chromatography—mass spectrometry (GC-MS) revealed that these oils mainly contain 78.2% oxygenated monoterpenoids, 9.5% sesquiterpene hydrocarbons, and 6.7% oxygenated sesquiterpenoids. Linalool (58.3%), 4-terpineol (9.8%), terpineol (3.6%), and caryophyllene oxide (3.1%) are the most abundant essential oil components (Sibanda et al., 2004).

6. TLC fingerprinting of plant extract

A thin layer chromatography (TLC) fingerprint of the *H. dehniae* was prepared with the ethanolic extract. The separation was observed by weighing out 2 mg of the extract dissolved it in 500 μL of ethanol. For examining the crude extract of *H. dehniae* silica gel 60 F254 TLC plates were used to analyze the separation of compounds present. The plates were marked with a soft pencil, and capillaries were used to spot the samples onto the TLC plate. The spots were allowed to dry completely, and the plate was placed in a tank, containing 20 mL of the eluent, 9:1 chloroform: methanol as the solvent system. The samples were allowed to separate until the solvent system reached 0.5 cm from the top of the TLC plate. Acidic Vanillin/sulfuric acid (2%) was freshly prepared and used for detection of bands on the plate, whereas some bands were observed under ultraviolet (UV) light (long and short wavelength).

7. Biological activities

Limited studies have been conducted using the ethanolic extracts of *H. dehniae*, but the leaf oils were studied in more biological assays.

7.1 Antibacterial activity

The leaf oils isolated from *H. dehniae* showed good activity against several microorganisms including *Staphylococcus aureus, Pseudomonas aeruginosa*, *Escherichia coli*, and *Candida albicans* using the disc diffusion method. The leaf oils exhibited a minimum inhibitory concentration (MIC) value of 0.625 mg/mL against *C. albicans* (Sibanda et al., 2004).

In another study, the leaves and twigs of *H. dehniae* were collected in the late summer time (January–February) at the University of Pretoria experimental farm and were used to prepare an ethanolic extract. The extract showed moderate activity against gram-positive *Streptococcus mutans* American type culture collection (ATCC) 25175 (MIC: 1.56 mg/mL) and *C. albicans* ATCC 25175 (MIC: 2 mg/mL), using the microdilution method (Bodiba, 2013)

7.2 Combination studies

A study was conducted to determine the possibility of synergism between ethanolic extracts of *H. dehniae* as well as another member of the Heteropyxidaceae family, *H. canescens*. The plant extracts of *H. canescens* and *H. dehniae* were combined and were used to determine antimicrobial activity against oral pathogens. The two plant extracts were added in combination with two samples: peppermint essential oil and TEAVIGO, which are known for its antiplaque/anticaries, antigingivitis, and combating bad breath. These compounds are common in formulations for oral products. A combination of the checkerboard and ratio methods was used to determine the effect of combining the two plant samples and the selected compounds (Moody, 1992; Orhan et al., 2005). In combination, it was shown that the MIC values of the plant extract were reduced at least twofold, indicating a positive effect of the combination of the extracts (Bodiba, 2013).

8. Additional information

8.1 Therapeutic (proposed) usage

Antibacterial and anticancer

8.2 Safety data

A study was conducted using the leaf oils and purified major constituents of *H. dehniae*, where the samples were screened for possible cytotoxic activity against PC-3 (human prostatic adenocarcinoma).

MDA-MB-231 (human mammary adenocarcinoma), Hs 578T (human mammary ductal carcinoma), MCF7 (human mammary adenocarcinoma), SK-MEL-28 (human melanoma), and 5637 (human primary bladder carcinoma). The leaf oils showed in vitro cytotoxic activity against human melanoma (SK-MEL-28) and human bladder carcinoma (5637) cells. Caryophyllene oxide, which forms part of the major components of the leaf oils, may be responsible for the observed cytotoxic activity of the *H. dehniae* leaf essential oil (Sibanda et al., 2004).

8.3 Trade information

Falls under the least concern category, not endangered, and abundant in countries such as Zimbabwe

8.4 Dosage

Not available

References

Arnold, H.J., Gulumian, M., 1984. Pharmacopoeia of traditional medicine in Venda. Journal of Ethnopharmacology 12, 1. https://doi.org/10.1016/0378-8741(84)90086-2.

Baumann, G., 2016. PhotoID: 55249. Species: *Heteropyxis Dehniae* Suess. Available online: http://www.africanplants.senckenberg.de/root/index.php?page_id=78&id=7205#image=55249.

Bodiba, D.C., 2013. Mechanism of Action of *Heteropyxis* against Oral Pathogens. University of Pretoria, South Africa. Dissertation.

Foden, W., Potter, L., 2005. *Heteropyxis Dehniae* Suess. National Assessment: Red List of South African Plants Version 2017.1.

GBIF, 2018. *Heteropyxis Dehniae* Suess. In GBIF Secretariat (2017). GBIF Backbone Taxonomy. Checklist dataset. https://doi.org/10.15468/39omei. accessed via GBIF.org on 2019-02-24.

Hyde, M.A., Wursten, B.T., Ballings, P., Coates Palgrave, M., 2018. Flora of Zimbabwe: Species information.Heteropyxisdehniae. https://www.zimbabweflora.co.zw/speciesdata/species.php?species_id=142480. retrieved 21 September 2018.

Moody, J., 1992. Synergism testing: broth microdilution checkerboard and broth macrodilution methods. In: Clinical Microbiology Procedures Handbook, vol. 5. American Society for Microbiology, Washington, DC, p. 22.

Orhan, G., Bayram, A., Zer, Y., Balci, I., 2005. Synergy tests by E test and checkerboard methods of antimicrobial combinations against Brucella melitensis. Journal of Clinical Microbiology 43, 140–143.

Raimondo, D., von Staden, L., Foden, W., Victor, J.E., Helme, N.A., Turner, R.C., Kamundi, D.A., Manyama, P.A., 2009. Red List of South African Plants. Strelitzia, vol. 25. South African National Biodiversity Institute, Pretoria.

Sibanda, S., Chigwada, G., Poole, M., Gwebu, E.T., Noletto, J.A., Schmidt, J.M., Rea, A.I., Setzer, W.N., 2004. Composition and bioactivity of the leaf essential oil of *Heteropyxis dehniae* from Zimbabwe. Journal of Ethnopharmacology 92, 107–111.

Hypericum revolutum subsp. revolutum

Analike Blom van Staden, Namrita Lall

Department of Plant and Soil Sciences, University of Pretoria, Pretoria, Gauteng, South Africa

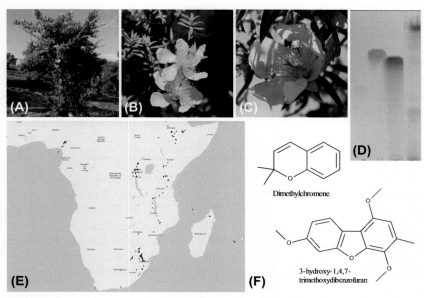

FIGURE 26 Aerial plant parts of *Hypericum revolutum* (Rae, 2010) (A), flower of *H. revolutum* in the sun (Knobel, 2010) (B), flower of *H. revolutum* in the shade (Dwergen-paartje, 2017) (C), TLC chromatogram, Lane 1; myricetin, Lane 2; quercetin, Lane 3; catechin, Lane 4; *H. revolutum* extract (D), distribution of *H. revolutum* in sub-Saharan Africa (GBIF, 2017) (E), chemical structures of dimethylchromene and 3-hydroxy-1,4,7-trimethoxydibenzofuran (F).

Underexplored Medicinal Plants from Sub-Saharan Africa
https://doi.org/10.1016/B978-0-12-816814-1.00026-0   173

1. General description

1.1 Botanical nomenclature

Hypericum revolutum Vahl subsp. *revolutum*

1.2 Botanical family

Hypericaceae

1.3 Vernacular names

Curry bush, Forest Primrose (English)
Kerriebos (Afrikaans)
Ruhurukuru (Shona)
Mudyanongo (Venda)

2. Botanical description

Hypericum revolutum is a multistemmed shrub or small tree (3 m high). It is fast-growing and evergreen. The branches are drooping reddish brown and have scaly bark stems. It has bright yellow flowers, and its fruit is a reddish-brown capsule present from June to November (Hyde et al., 2002).

3. Distribution

H. revolutum is native to South Africa and Zimbabwe. Although it is primarily found in sub-Saharan Africa, it has been identified in Southwest Arabia, Fernando, Comoro Island, Indian Ocean islands, and Cameroon. *H. revolutum* grows in damp areas, at the edges of forests and next to stream banks. In South Africa it can mainly be found in Gauteng, the Eastern Cape, Mpumalanga, KwaZulu-Natal and along the Cape coastal area (Hyde et al., 2002: Viljoen and Velembo, 2014).

4. Ethnobotanical usage

H. revolutum is medicinally used to treat stomach ache and rheumatism. Traditional medical practitioners in Uganda use *H. revolutum* for the treatment of tuberculosis. In Cameroon, *H. revolutum* is used as a medicine against protozoal diseases such as malaria (Orhan et al., 2013; Tabuti et al., 2010; Viljoen and Velembo, 2014; Yineger et al., 2013).

5. Phytochemical constituents

Compounds and phytochemical groups previously identified from *H. revolutum* are acylphloro-glucinols, xanthones, flavonoids, tannins, benzopyrans coumarins, hyperforin, 8-isobutyryl-5,7-dihydroxy-6-methyl-2,2 dimethylchromene, 3-hydroxy-1,4,7-trimethoxydibenzofuran, 4-(3-O-3″)-3″-methylbutenyl-6-phenyl-pyran-2-one, and pyranols (Abdollahi et al., 2012; Bennett and Lee, 1989; Crockett et al., 2005; Dall'agnol et al., 2003; Decosterd et al., 1986a; Decosterd et al., 1986b; Decosterd et al., 1989; Décostered et al., 1987; Dulger and Dulger, 2014; Ploss et al., 2001; Shiu and Gibbons, 2009).

6. TLC fingerprinting of plant extract

For observing the separation on *H. revolutum*, 2 mg of the ethanolic extract was weighed out and dissolved in 200 μL of ethanol. For the standards, myricetin, quercetin, and catechin (Sigma—Aldrich Co. St Louis, MO, USA) were weighed out in the same manner as the extract and dissolved in 600 μL of ethanol. For the thin layer chromatography (TLC) analysis of *H. revolutum* crude extract, silica gel 60 F254 TLC plates were used to observe the separation of the compounds present within the extract. Plate markings were made with a soft pencil, and glass capillaries were used to spot the samples onto the TLC plate. Reference standards: myricetin, quercetin, and catechin were spotted to determine whether it was present in the extract. The spots were left to dry completely before placing the plate in a TLC tank, which contains 10 mL eluent 9:1 dichloromethane:methanol as the solvent system. The plate was observed under ultraviolet (UV light) (long and short wavelength), followed by spraying with freshly prepared vanillin/sulfuric acid (2%) to detect the bands on the TLC plate.

7. Pharmacological properties

The *Hypericum* species has been thoroughly investigated, except the well-known South African species, namely *H. revolutum*. *H. revolutum* has not been extensively researched for its in vitro and in vivo medicinal properties; therefore, there is a lot of opportunity for research and development regarding this plant.

7.1 Antibacterial activity

In one study, the leaves and stems of *H. revolutum* were collected (February to March 2015) from the Manie van der Schijff botanical garden of the University of Pretoria. An ethanol extract was prepared. The ethanol crude extract showed growth inhibitory activity against *Propionibacterium acnes*, American type culture collection (ATCC) 6919 and ATCC 11827 strains, with a minimum inhibitory concentration (MIC) of 500 μg/mL (Blom van Staden and Lall, 2018). No bactericidal effect was observed for *H. revolutum*. When the extract of *H. revolutum* was combined with the known antibiotic, tetracycline, the synergistic effect, at a ratio of 9:1, resulted in an MIC of 56.25 μg/mL for the extract (10-fold reduction), whereas the MIC of the drug was found to be 0.625 μg/mL for the ATCC 11827 strain. The synergistic effect, at a ratio of 5:5 for the ATCC 6919 strain, resulted in the MIC for the extract to be 3.91 μg/mL (approximately 100-fold reduction), whereas the MIC of the drug was found to be 0.391 μg/mL (Blom van Staden and Lall, 2018).

In a study conducted by Adugna et al. (2014) it was found that the methanol extract of *H. revolutum* exhibited a growth inhibition zone, through the disc diffusion method, of 11.3 and 5.6 mm against *Escherichia coli* and *Salmonella typhi*, respectively, but no inhibition was observed for *Salmonella typhimurium* and *Salmonella paratyphi*. The methanol extract of *H. revolutum* exhibited a growth inhibition zone of 9 and 12 mm against *Shigella* spp and *Pseudomonas aeruginosa*, respectively. The MIC of *H. revolutum* against *Shigella* spp and *P. aeruginosa* were found to be 125 mg/mL and 250 mg/mL respectively (Adugna et al., 2014; Andualem et al., 2014).

7.2 Antimalarial activity

A study conducted by Zofou et al., in 2011 showed that the ethylacetate subextract of *H. revolutum* exhibited a good activity (50 % inhibitory concentration (IC_{50}) lower than 10 μg/mL) against the W2mef strain of *Plasmodium falciparum*. The fractionation of the ethylacetate extract into five major fractions, produced one active fraction against the W2mef strain. Three fractions showed good antiplasmodial activity with IC_{50} values lower than 5 μg/mL (Zofou et al., 2011).

7.3 Phytochemical content

The leaf and stem ethanolic extracts of *H. revolutum*, obtained from the University of Pretoria, were collected and screened for its phytochemical constituents. The extract was tested for total tannins, saponins, alkaloids, cardiac glycosides, terpenes, flavonoids and total phenolics. The ethanol extracts of *H. revolutum* showed the presence of saponins (Blom van Staden and Lall, 2018). A study conducted by Andualem et al., in 2014, identified terpenoids, flavonoids, and tannins in the crude extract of *H. revolutum* (Andualem et al., 2014).

8. Additional information

8.1 Therapeutic (proposed) usage

Antiinflammatory, antimalarial, and wound healing

8.2 Safety data

Not available

8.3 Trade information

Least concern

8.4 Dosage

Not available

References

Abdollahi, F., Shafaghat, A., Salimi, F., 2012. Biological activity and a biflavonoid from *Hypericum scabrum* extracts. Journal of Medicinal Plants Research 6 (11), 2131–2135.

Adugna, B., Terefe, G., Kebede, N., 2014. Potential in vitro antibacterial action of selected medicinal plants against *Escherichia coli* and three *Salmonella* species. International Journal of Microbiological Research 5, 85–89.

Andualem, G., Umar, S., Getnet, F., Tekewe, A., Alemayehu, H., Kebede, N., 2014. Antimicrobial and phytochemical screening of methanol extracts of three medicinal plants in Ethiopia. Advances in Biological Research 8 (3), 101–106.

Blom van Staden, A., Lall, N., 2018. Medicinal plants as alternative treatments for progressive macular hypomelanosis. In: Medicinal Plants for Holistic Health and Well-Being, pp. 145–182.

Bennett, G.J., Lee, H.-H., 1989. Xanthones from guttiferae. Phytochemistry 28 (4), 967–998.

Crockett, S.L., Schaneberg, B., Khan, I.A., 2005. Phytochemical profiling of new and old world *Hypericum* (St. John's Wort) species. Phytochemical Analysis 16 (6), 479–485.

Dall'Agnol, R., Ferraz, A., Bernardi, A., Albring, D., Nör, C., Sarmento, L., Lamb, L., Hass, M., Von Poser, G., Schapoval, E., 2003. Antimicrobial activity of some *Hypericum*species. Phytomedicine 10 (6), 511–516.

Decosterd, L., Stoeckli-Evans, H., Msonthi, J., Hostettmann, K., 1986a. A new antifungal chromene and a related di-chromene from *Hypericum revolutum*. Planta Medica 5, 429.

Decosterd, L., Stoeckli-Evans, H., Msonthi, J., Hostettmann, K., 1986b. A new antifungal chromene and a related di-chromene from *Hypericum revolutum*. Planta Medica 52 (5), 429.

Decosterd, L.A., Stoeckli-Evans, H., Chapuis, J.C., Msonthi, J.D., Sordat, B., Hostettmann, K., 1989. New hyperforin derivatives from *Hypericum revolutum* Vahl with growth inhibitory activity against a human colon carcinoma cell line. Helvetica Chimica Acta 72 (3), 464–471.

Décostered, L.A., Hostettmann, K., Stoeckli-Evans, H., Msonthi, J.D., 1987. New antifungal chromenyl ketones and their pentacyclic dimers from *Hypericum revolutum* Vahl. Helvetica Chimica Acta 70 (7), 1694–1702.

Dulger, G., Dulger, B., 2014. Antifungal activity of *Hypericum havvae* against some medical Candida yeast and cryptococcus species. Tropical Journal of Pharmaceutical Research 13 (3), 405–408.

Dwergenpaartje, 2017. The Arabo-African Species of St. John's-Wort *Hypericum Revolutum*, Photographed along the Chogoria Route, Mount Kenya, at Approximately 3000 M Altitude. Available online: https://commons.wikimedia.org/wiki/File:Hypericum_revolutum_mtkenya.jpg (CC BY-SA 4.0). Accessed 30 July 2018.

GBIF, 2017. *Hypericum Revolutum* Vahl in GBIF Secretariat (2017). GBIF Backbone Taxonomy. Checklist dataset. https://doi.org/10.15468/39omei. accessed via GBIF.org on 2018-08-01.

Hyde, M., Wursten, B., Ballings, P., Palgrave, M.C., 2002. *Hypericum Revolutum*. Flora of Zimbabwe.   http://www.zimbabweflora.co.zw/speciesdata/species.php?species_id=140380. Accessed 30 July 2018.

Knobel, J.C., 2010. Spring Flowers of a Curry Bush, Jan Celliers Park, Pretoria. Available online: https://commons.wikimedia.org/wiki/File:Hypericum_revolutum,_blomme,_Jan_Celliers_Park.jpg (CC BY-SA 3.0). Accessed 30 July 2018.

Orhan, I.E., Kartal, M., Gülpinar, A.R., Cos, P., Matheeussen, A., Maes, L., Tasdemir, D., 2013. Assessment of antimicrobial and antiprotozoal activity of the olive oil macerate samples of *Hypericum perforatum* and their LC−DAD−MS analyses. Food Chemistry 138 (2), 870−875.

Ploss, O., Petereit, F., Nahrstedt, A., 2001. Procyanidins from the herb of *Hypericum perforatum*. Die Pharmazie 56 (6), 509−511.

Rae, A., 2010. *Hypericum Revolutum* I Know that Some Species of St John's Wort Can be a Little Woody but I Didn't Realise They Could be Shrubs Several Metres High. This is in the Semien Mountains at C 3300m. Available online: https://commons.wikimedia.org/wiki/File:Hypericum_revolutum_1.jpg (CC BY-SA 2.0). Accessed 30 July 2018.

Shiu, W.K.P., Gibbons, S., 2009. Dibenzofuran and pyranone metabolites from *Hypericum revolutum* ssp. *revolutum* and Hypericum choisianum. Phytochemistry 70 (3), 403−406.

Tabuti, J.R., Kukunda, C.B., Waako, P.J., 2010. Medicinal plants used by traditional medicine practitioners in the treatment of tuberculosis and related ailments in Uganda. Journal of Ethnopharmacology 127 (1), 130−136.

Viljoen, C., Velembo, S., 2014. *Hypericum Revolutum* Vahl. Plantzafrica. http://www.plantzafrica.com/planthij/hypericumrevol.htm. Accessed 30 July 2018.

Yineger, H., Kelbessa, E., Bekele, T., Lulekal, E., 2013. Plants used in traditional management of human ailments at Bale Mountains National Park, Southeastern Ethiopia. Journal of Medicinal Plants Research 2 (6), 132−153.

Zofou, D., Kowa, T.K., Wabo, H.K., Ngemenya, M.N., Tane, P., Titanji, V.P., 2011. *Hypericum lanceolatum* (Hypericaceae) as a potential source of new anti-malarial agents: a bioassay-guided fractionation of the stem bark. Malaria Journal 10 (1), 1.

Juncus effusus

Carel B. Oosthuizen, Matthew Fisher, Namrita Lall

Department of Plant and Soil Sciences, University of Pretoria, Pretoria, Gauteng, South Africa

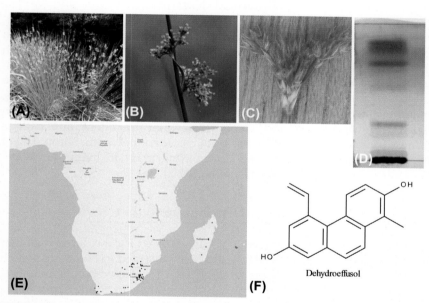

Dehydroeffusol

FIGURE 27   Aerial plant parts of *Juncus effusus* (Meggar, 2005) (A), flower of *J. effusus* (Peigimccann, 2008) (B), close-up of inflorescence (Rasbak, 2006) (C), TLC chromatogram, fingerprint of *J. effusus* extract (D), distribution of *J. effusus* in sub-Saharan Africa (GBIF, 2018) (E), chemical structure of dehydroeffusol (F).

Underexplored Medicinal Plants from Sub-Saharan Africa
https://doi.org/10.1016/B978-0-12-816814-1.00027-2

1. General description

1.1 Botanical nomenclature

Juncus effusus L.

1.2 Botanical family

Juncaceae

1.3 Vernacular names

Soft Rush (English)

2. Botanical description

Juncus effusus is a monocot and member of the Juncaceae family. It is a perennial herb that grows from a rhizome, and its soft rushes can reach 0.5—1.5 m in height. It is commonly used in basketry and mat weaving in various locales such as North America, Japan, and Africa. Due to the plants' locality and shape, it provides shelter to a variety of small birds, mammals, fish, and amphibians. The plant limits erosion and is used in wetland rehabilitation and some wastewater treatment applications (plants.usda.gov). Although it has been recorded that animal browsing of *J. effusus* occurs, it may be the contributing plant in marsh or "Vlei" poisoning (Watt and Breyer-Brandwijk, 1962).

3. Distribution

According to the Encyclopedia of Life, *J. effusus* is considered rush that is widely distributed across the world being adapted to moist areas such as lake and river banks, at the edge of some forests, wetlands, marshes, and fen meadows (www.eol.org). It is nonendemic to South Africa being distributed across all provinces except North West and is of "Least Concern" according to the South African National Biodiversity Institute (SANBI—redlist.sanbi.org).

4. Ethnobotanical usage

Medicinal use of *J. effusus* derives mainly from traditional Chinese medicine where it is used to treat fevers, anxiety, physical tension, insomnia, fidgetiness, and, in general, is used as a sedative (Liao et al., 2011; Ma et al., 2015).

5. Phytochemical constituents

Several constituents have been isolated from *J. effusus* some of which have been tested for their bioactivity and in vitro effects. Compounds include dihydrodibenzoxepins, dehydroeffusol, and a number of other phenanthrenes, juncusyl esters, cycloartane terpenes, and floavonoids (Michela Corsaro et al., 1994; Dong-zhe et al., 1996; El-Shamy et al., 2015; Kovács et al., 2008; Della Greca et al., 1993).

6. TLC fingerprinting of plant extract

The plant material was crushed and ground after an air drying process. The dried material was ground into a fine powder and extracted using ethanol in a 1:10 (weight:volume) ratio. The extract was left to shake for 48 h, filtered and dried using rotary evaporation. For the separation of the phytochemicals of *J. effusus*, 2 mg of the ethanolic extract was weighed out and dissolved in 200 μL of ethanol. Thin layer chromatography (TLC) was carried out on a precoated silica gel aluminum plate. Ten microliters of the extract were spotted at the height of 10 mm from the bottom of a 10 × 5 cm TLC plate and develop up to 8 cm from the bottom of the plate using the mobile phase 1% methanol in hexane. The plate was observed under ultraviolet (UV light) (long and short wavelength), followed by spraying with freshly prepared vanillin/sulfuric acid (2%) to detect the bands on the TLC plate.

7. Pharmacological properties

7.1 Antibacterial activity

Monoglycerides have been tested on the freshwater algae *Selenastrum capricornatum*, and some have been found to inhibit its growth. Monoglycerides 3 and 4 showed 40% growth inhibition at 10^{-4} M and compounds 1 and 8 showed a 70% inhibition at 10^{-4} M (Dellagreca et al., 1998).

7.2 Antitumor activity

In vitro anticancer assays were performed on potato discs infected with *Agrobacterium tumerfaciens*. Compounds 1 and 4 showed an 80% inhibition of tumor growth while compound 5 showed an 85% inhibition. This corresponded with the brine shrimp 50 % lethal concentration (LC_{50}) value of 4.6, 3.0, and 3.0 μg/mL, respectively (Della Greca et al., 1993). Dehydroeffusol has been found to have a dose-dependent effect on the vascular growth of gastric tumors up to the highest concentration tested, 48 μM (Liu et al., 2015).

7.3 Sedative activity

Stemming from the antianxiety and sedative properties observed in *J. effusus*, the observed effect was attributed to the compound dehydroeffusol. The study was conducted on mice whose movement, head-dip number, and ability to stay on a rotating rod as well as a number of other factors were measured. It was observed that the dehydroeffusol had similar effects on head-dipping at the same concentration as the positive control diazepam (at 5 mg/kg). Dehydroeffusol, did however, showed lowered effects on locomotion and mice could remain longer on the rotating rod than the positive control at the same concentration (5 mg kg) (Liao et al., 2011)

8. Additional information

8.1 Therapeutic (proposed) usage

Antianxiety and antitumor

8.2 Safety data

A number of phenanthrenes were tested against brine shrimp for toxicity. Samples were prepared by dissolving known concentrations (10, 100, and 1000 μg/mL) onto paper disks. Shrimp were hatched, grown, and separated into groups with 10 individuals per group. Each concentration was tested against one group contained in a volume of 5 mL. The LC_{50} was calculated by assessing the number of dead shrimp after 24 h at each concentration (Meyer et al., 1982). Of the 18 phenanthrenes tested all were found to be toxic at varying concentrations, 14 were toxic below 20 μg/mL while 3 were found to be toxic between 80 and 85 μg/mL (Della Greca et al., 1993).

8.3 Trade information

Not threatened, not endangered, and abundant

8.4 Dosage

Not available

References

Dellagreca, M., et al., 1998. Anti-algal phenylpropane glycerides from *Juncus effusus*. Natural Product Letters 12 (4), 263–270. Available at: http://www.tandfonline.com/doi/abs/10.1080/10575639808048300.

Dong-zhe, J., et al., 1996. Two p-coumaroyl glycerides from *Juncus effusus*. Phytochemistry 41 (2), 545–547.

El-Shamy, A.I., Abdel-Razek, A.F., Nassar, M.I., 2015. Phytochemical review of *Juncus* L. genus (Fam. Juncaceae). Arabian Journal of Chemistry 8 (5), 614–623. Available at: http://www.sciencedirect.com/science/article/pii/S1878535212001542.

Della Greca, M., Fiorentino, A., Molinaro, A., et al., 1993a. A bioactive dihydrodibenzoxepin from *Juncus effusus*. Phytochemistry 34 (4), 1182–1184.

Della Greca, M., Fiorentino, A., Mangoni, L., et al., 1993b. Cytotoxic 9,10-Dihydrophenanthrenes from *Juncus effusus* L. Tetrahedron 49 (16), 3425–3432.

GBIF, 2018. *Juncus effusus* L. In GBIF Secretariat (2017). GBIF Backbone Taxonomy. Checklist dataset. https://doi.org/10.15468/39omei. accessed via GBIF.org on 2019-02-24.

Kovács, A., Vasas, A., Hohmann, J., 2008. Natural phenanthrenes and their biological activity. Phytochemistry 69 (5), 1084–1110. Available at: http://linkinghub.elsevier.com/retrieve/pii/S0031942207007212.

Liao, Y.-J.J., et al., 2011. Anxiolytic and sedative effects of dehydroeffusol from *Juncus effusus* in mice. Planta Medica 77 (5), 416–420. Available at: http://www.ncbi.nlm.nih.gov/pubmed/21104609.

Liu, W., et al., 2015. Dehydroeffusol effectively inhibits human gastric cancer cell-mediated vasculogenic mimicry with low toxicity. Toxicology and Applied Pharmacology 287 (2), 98–110. Available at: https://doi.org/10.1016/j.taap.2015.05.003.

Ma, W., et al., 2015. Four new phenanthrenoid dimers from *Juncus effusus* L. with cytotoxic and anti-inflammatory activities. Fitoterapia 105, 83–88. Available at: http://www.sciencedirect.com/science/article/pii/S0367326X1530023X.

Meggar, 2005. Photo by Meggar. Available online: https://commons.wikimedia.org/wiki/File:Juncus_effuses.jpg. (CC BY-SA 3.0).

Meyer, B., et al., 1982. Brine Shrimp : a convenient general bioassay for active plant constituents. Journal of Medicinal Plants Research 45, 31–34. February.

Michela Corsaro, M., et al., 1994. Cycloartane glucosides from *Juncus effusus*. Phytochemistry 37 (2), 515–519.

Peigimccann, 2008. *Juncus effuses* Loch Kruse 7-8-08. Available online: https://commons.wikimedia.org/wiki/File:Juncus_effuses_Loch_Kruse_7-8-08.jpg. (CC BY-SA 3.0).

Rasbak, 2006. *Juncus effusus* Inflorescnes. Available online: https://commons.wikimedia.org/wiki/File:Pitrus_bloeiwijze_closeup_(Juncus_effusus).jpg. (CC BY-SA 3.0).

Watt, J.M., Breyer-Brandwijk, M.G., 1962. The Medicinal and Poisonous Plants of Southern and Eastern Africa: Being an Account of Their Medicinal and Other Uses, Chemical Composition, Pharmacological Effects and Toxicology in Man and Animal. E. & S. Livingstone. Available at: https://books.google.com/books?id=2ZjwAAAAMAAJ&pgis=1.

Lannea schweinfurthii

Fatimah Lawal, Thilivhali E. Tshikalange

Department of Plant and Soil Sciences, University of Pretoria, Pretoria, Gauteng, South Africa

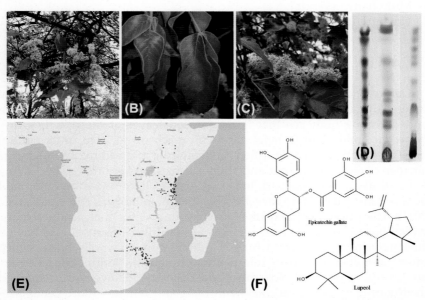

FIGURE 28   Aerial plant parts of *Lannea schweinfurthii* (Grobler, 2015a) (A), leaves of *L. schweinfurthii* (Wursten, 2016) (B), flowers of *L. schweinfurthii* (Grobler, 2015b) (C), TLC chromatogram, Lane 1; *L. schweinfurthii* hexane root bark extract, Lane 2; *L. schweinfurthii* dichloromethane root bark extract, Lane 3; *L. schweinfurthii* ethyl acetate root bark extract (D), distribution within sub-Saharan Africa (GBIF, 2018) (E), chemical structures of lupeol and epicatechin gallate (F).

Underexplored Medicinal Plants from Sub-Saharan Africa
https://doi.org/10.1016/B978-0-12-816814-1.00028-4

1. General description

1.1 Botanical nomenclature

Lannea schweinfurthii (Engl.) Engl.

1.2 Botanical family

Anacardiaceae

1.3 Vernacular names

False marula (English)
Valsmaroela (Afrikaans)
Mmopu (North Sotho)
Mulivhadza (Venda)
Umganunkomo (Zulu)

2. Botanical description

Lannea schweinfurthii is a deciduous tree or shrub belonging to the family Anacardiaceae. The tree is easily identified by the outspread crown and drooping branches that bear crowded leaves at the tips. It grows between 3 and 15 m in height and can reach up to 20 m in its natural habitat. It can be distinguished from marula (*Sclerocarya birrea*) by its smaller sized fruits, bigger and shinier leaves, and shorter stalks having fewer leaflets. The tree bark is fleshy, gray to light brown in color, and occasionally flakes off to reveal a pale orange under bark (Bingham et al., 2011). The origin of the flakes is from young stems that produce hairs, which become gray or brown flakes at maturity. The roots also have a striking appearance with a furlike indumentum of woolly hairs, which often pass off or are mostly referred to as fungus. In South Africa, flowers are produced between November and December. Flowers are contained in drooping spikelike racemes with male and female inflorescence produced on separate trees.

3. Distribution

Geographically, it is found in areas of Eastern Africa in the regions of Kenya, Malawi, Rwanda, Somalia, and Zambia. It also extends through Northern African and Southern African countries including Sudan, Botswana, Zimbabwe, Mozambique, Tanzania, Swaziland, and South Africa. In South Africa, it is found growing in the rural areas of Limpopo, Mpumalanga, and KwaZulu-Natal (Foden and Potter, 2005).

4. Ethnobotanical usage

Several ethnomedicinal uses have been reported by various communities in countries of Eastern and Southern Africa. The decoction of root and stem bark is used for the treatment of malaria and its associated fever symptoms. It is also documented for the treatment of various gastrointestinal discomforts and diseases such as diarrhea, stomachache, dysentery, and constipation. Infusion and decoctions of leaves, stems, and roots are used in the treatment of mild infections such as abscesses and more serious infections such as tuberculosis, venereal diseases including human immunodeficiency virus (HIV), herpes, syphilis, and candidiasis. Infusions from roots are used for neurological disorders, to enhance memory, to cure sterility, to reduce cellulitis, and as a sedative (Adewusi and Steenkamp, 2011; Gathirwa et al., 2011; Kihagi, 2016; Maregesi et al., 2007; Okoth, 2014; Seoposengwe et al., 2013; Stafford et al., 2008).

5. Phytochemical constituents

A mixture of flavonoid, triterpenoids, and novel alkylphenol compounds has been isolated from root and stem bark of *L. schweinfurthii*. Flavonoid compounds include epicatechin, epicatechin gallate, catechin, and rutin. Triterpenoids isolated include β-sitosterol, sitosterol, sitosterol glucoside, lupeol, and lupenone, whereas a mixture of alkyl cardonols, cyclohexenones, and cyclohexenols with the addition of the alkylated phenol group (Okoth, 2014). Studies conducted on the stem bark by Kihagi (2016) resulted in the isolation of five compounds from both polar and nonpolar fractions. These compounds include di-(2′-ethylhexyl) ester phthalic acid and 3-(10′-tridecenyl) phenol, which were isolated for the first time from the dichloromethane (DCM)/hexane fraction. Four known compounds: 1-((E)-heptadec-14′-enyl) cyclohex-4-ene-1,3-diol, 1-((E)-pentadec-12′-enyl)cyclohex-4-ene-1,3-diol, 3-((E)-nonadec-16′-enyl) phenol, and catechin were also reported from the dichloromethane: methanol fraction of the root (Yaouba et al., 2018). No record of compound isolated from the leaves or fruits of this plant has been documented.

6. TLC fingerprinting of plant extract

Dried root samples were extracted with acetone in the ratio of 1 g ground plant material to 10 mL of solvent. The resultant acetone extract was further subjected to liquid—liquid partitioning using a separating funnel to obtain hexane, DCM, and ethyl acetate fractions. Extracts were dried under a fume cupboard to remove excess solvents. Ten milligrams of the dried fractions were reconstituted in 1 mL of solvent respectively. Using a thin layer chromatography (TLC) plate spotter, extracts were loaded as bands on the TLC plates approximately 1 cm from the base of the plate. A solvent front was also indicated at the top of the plate (approximately 1 cm from the top of the plates) using a pencil. The spots were allowed to dry before being developed in TLC tanks, which had been presaturated with solvents. The hexane and dichloromethane fractions were developed in solvent-containing hexane, chloroform, and methanol (1:8:1), whereas the ethyl acetate fraction was developed in a mixture of hexane and ethyl acetate (1:9). Developed plates were allowed to dry, viewed under ultraviolet (UV) light (short and long wavelength), and sprayed with vanillin/sulfuric acid (2%).

7. Pharmacological properties

L. schweinfurthii has not been extensively studied for its in vitro and in vivo biological activities. Several of its traditional uses are yet to be scientifically studied or validated, and those studied have not been fully explored.

7.1 Antibacterial and antifungal activity

Crude extracts and isolated compounds from the stem and root bark of *L. schweinfurthii* were tested for their activity against clinically relevant bacterial and fungi species. In a study by Kihagi (2016), the stem bark of the plant was collected from Bondo, Siaya County in Kenya. The plant materials were dried, grounded, and sequentially extracted with hexane, DCM, ethyl acetate, and methanol. Extracts from the ethyl acetate and methanol fraction showed very high inhibitory activity against *Staphylococcus aureus* American type culture collection (ATCC) 25923, *Bacillus subtilis* ATCC 202368, *Escherichia coli* ATCC 25922, and *Candida albicans* ATCC1 0232. The DCM and hexane fractions were reported to have mild activity on the tested pathogens. In addition, all the crude extracts tested did not inhibit the gram-negative bacteria *Pseudomonas aeruginosa* ATCC 10622. Chromatographic separation was conducted on the ethyl acetate and combined DCM/hexane fractions. From the isolated compounds, only epicatechin showed very good activity against the tested organisms. Epicatechin gallate and some cyclohexanone moieties isolated from this plant have been previously reported to possess good antibacterial, antioxidant, and antiplasmodial activity (Okoth, 2014).

In another study, taraxerol, β-sitosterol, and lupeol isolated from the dichloromethane and ethyl acetate extract showed moderate activity against *E. coli* ATCC 25923. β-Sitosterol was also active against ATCC 25922 (Yaouba et al., 2018).

7.2 Antiviral activity

The activity of a stem bark extract of *L. schweinfurthii* was assessed against the Human Immuno-deficiency Virus (HIV-1, IIIB strain, and HIV-2 ROD strain). The plant material used in this study was collected from the Bunda district in Tanzania. The extraction procedure involved defatting with n-hexane and subsequent extraction with 80% methanol and water. The 80% methanol extract of the plant markedly inhibited HIV-1 and HIV-2 virus with a 50% inhibitory concentration (IC_{50}) lower than 10 µg/mL. The water extract exhibited a moderate activity range against both strains of HIV (Maregesi et al., 2010). In a similar study, an 80% methanol extract of *L. schweinfurthii* showed strong antiviral activity against Semliki forest virus (SF A7) but was inactive against Herpes simplex virus (HSV-1), Vesicular Stomatitis Virus (VSV) T2, and Coxsackie B2 (Cox B2) (Maregesi et al., 2008).

7.3 Antiplasmodial activity

In vitro antiplasmodial and in vivo antimalarial studies were conducted using stem bark extracts of *L. schweinfurthii*. The plant material collected between February and August in Kenya was extracted with water and methanol. Extracts were assessed for their in vitro activity against two strains of *Plasmodium falciparum* (Sierra Leonean CQ-sensitive D6 and Indochinese CQ-resistant W2). Both aqueous and methanol extract showed moderate activity against the D6 strain, whereas a moderate to low activity was observed when the W2 strain was used. In this study, an IC_{50} between 10 and 50 µg/mL was regarded as moderate, whereas 50–100 µg/mL was regarded as low. The extracts were also assessed for their antimalarial activity against mice that were preinfected with *Plasmodium berghei* (strain ANKA). A 100 mg/kg dosage was administered either intraperitoneally or as oral drugs 2–4 h before infection and 24, 48, and 72 h after infection. The mean chemosuppression of parasitemia by both extracts from *L. schweinfurthii* was reported to be higher when administered intraperitoneally and was not significantly different from chloroquine, which was used as the positive control (Gathirwa et al., 2008).

A similar in vitro study was conducted using the *Plasmodium falciparum* K1 strain. The 80% methanol extract of the plant did not show noteworthy activity against the *Plasmodium* strain (minimum inhibitory concentration [MIC] of 125 µg/mL). The antiplasmodial activity of the water extract was not tested in this study (Maregesi et al., 2010). The methanol extract from combined root and bark was also reported to actively inhibit the growth of *Giardia lamblia* trophozoites at a test concentration of 1000 ppm (Johns et al., 1995).

7.4 Antioxidant and neuroprotective activity

This study was conducted in line with the traditional use of *L. schweinfurthii* for the enhancement of memory and as a sedative. In vitro assessment of the potential of the extract from this plant to inhibit rotenone-induced toxicity in a neuronal cell model: SH-SY5Y neuroblastoma cells (ATCC 2266) was determined. Root bark collected from the Venda region in Limpopo South Africa were extracted with methanol and ethyl acetate. Oxidative stress and mitochondrial dysfunction involved in neurological abnormalities associated with Parkinson's disease were assessed in vitro through the determination of intercellular redox (ROS and glutathione content), Caspase-3-activity, and mitochondrial membrane potential (MMP). Methanol and ethyl acetate extract of *L. schweinfurthii* had a rotenone dose-dependent cytoprotective effect on cells. A reduction in rotenone-induced caspase-3 activity and glutathione depletion was also observed. On the other hand, pretreatment of cells with the methanol extract showed a significant ($P < .05$) uncoupling effect, which reduced mitochondrial membrane protection (Seoposengwe et al., 2013).

In an in vitro model of Alzheimer's disease, amyloid-beta peptide was used to induce neurotoxicity in SH-SY5Y (ATCC CRL-2266) cells. The methanol root extract of *L. schweinfurthii* was not found to be toxic to the cells (IC_{50} greater than 100 μg/mL) and reduced the effect of Amyloid-beta induced neural cell death (Adewusi et al., 2013).

In another study, methanol and ethyl acetate extracts from the root were tested for their acetylcholinesterase inhibitory activity. Antioxidant activity was further tested using the 2,2'-azinobis-3-ethylbenzothiazoline-6-sulfonic acid (ABTS) and diphenylpicrylhydrazyl (DPPH) radical scavenging assays. The methanol extract acted as a good radical scavenger but a poor inhibitor of the acetylcholinesterase enzyme, whereas the ethyl acetate fraction only showed noteworthy inhibitory activity against acetylcholinesterase (Adewusi and Steenkamp, 2011).

7.5 Antiinflammatory activity

In an in vivo study, the crude root extracts from *L. schweinfurthii* was evaluated for antiinflammatory activities through the inhibition of carrageenan-induced rat paw oedema. The extract was administered orally at a dosage of 200 mg/kg body weight of the experimental rats. The root extract was able to curb an increase in paw volume and was observed to be most active between 60 and 120 min after carrageenan administration (Yaouba et al., 2018).

8. Additional information

8.1 Therapeutic (proposed) usage

Antiviral, antibacterial, antiinflammatory, neuroprotective activity, antimalarial, and antiprotozoal.

8.2 Safety data

β-Sitosterol was not found to be cytotoxic (50% inhibitory concentration(IC_{50}) of 100 μg/mL) on Vero cells, whereas the root bark extract showed strong toxicity on Vero cells with an IC_{50} value of 7.36 $\pm$ 0.03 μg/mL (Yaouba et al., 2018).

In an in vitro model of Alzheimer's disease, Amyloid-beta peptide was used to induce neurotoxicity in SH-SY5Y (ATCC CRL-2266) cells. The methanol root extract of *L. schweinfurthii* was not found to be toxic to the cells (IC_{50} greater than 100 μg/mL) and reduced the effect of Amyloid-beta induced neural cell death (Adewusi et al., 2013).

An in vitro toxicity study revealed mild toxicity of the methanol extract on Vero cells, but no deaths were observed in the acute toxicity assay using the highest tested concentration (Gathirwa et al., 2008).

8.3 Trade information

Not threatened, not endangered, least concerned, and abundant

8.4 Dosage

Not applicable

References

Adewusi, E.A., Fouche, G., Steenkamp, V., 2013. Effect of four medicinal plants on Amyloid-β Induced neutotoxicty in SH-SY5Y cells. African Journal of Traditional, Complementary and Alternative Medicines 10, 6—11.

Adewusi, E.A., Steenkamp, V., 2011. In vitro screening for acetylcholinesterase inhibition and antioxidant activity of medicinal plants from southern Africa. Asian Pacific Journal of Tropical Medicine 4, 829—835. https://doi.org/10.1016/S1995-7645(11)60203-4.

Bingham, M.G., Willemen, A., Wursten, B.T., Ballings, P., Hyde, M.A., 2011. Flora of Zambia: Species Information: Records of Lannea Schweinfurthii. http://www.zambiaflora.com/speciesdata/citations-display.php?species_id=165920.

Foden, W., Potter, L., 2005. Lannea Schweinfurthii (Engl.) Engl. Var. Stuhlmannii (Engl.) Kokwaro. National Assessment: Red List of South African Plants Version. http://redlist.sanbi.org/species.php?species=864-8.

Gathirwa, J.W., Rukunga, G.M., Mwitari, P.G., Mwikwabe, N.M., Kimani, C.W., Muthaura, C.N., Kiboi, D.M., Nyangacha, R.M., Omar, S.A., 2011. Traditional herbal antimalarial therapy in Kilifi district, Kenya. Journal of Ethnopharmacology 134, 434—442. https://doi.org/10.1016/j.jep.2010.12.043.

Gathirwa, J.W., Rukunga, G.M., Njagi, E.N.M., Omar, S.A., Mwitari, P.G., Guantai, A.N., Tolo, F.M., Ndiege, I.O., 2008. The in vitro antiplasmodial and in vivo anti-malarial efficacy of combinations of some medicinal plants used traditionally for treatment of malaria by the Meru community in Kenya. Journal of Ethnopharmacology 115, 223—231. https://doi.org/10.1016/j.jep.2007.09.021.

GBIF, 2018. Lannea Schweinfurthii Engl. In GBIF Secretariat (2017). GBIF Backbone Taxonomy. Checklist dataset. https://doi.org/10.15468/39omei. accessed via GBIF.org on 2018.07.25.

Grobler, 2015a. Lannea Schweinfurthii (Engl.) Engl. Phalaborwa, South Africa. Available online: https://commons.wikimedia.org/wiki/File:Lannea_schweinfurthii02.jpg. (CC BY-SA 3.0).

Grobler, 2015b. Lannea Schweinfurthii (Engl.) Engl. Phalaborwa, South Africa. Available online: https://commons.wikimedia.org/wiki/File:Lannea_schweinfurthii00.jpg. (CC BY-SA 3.0).

Johns, T., Faubert, G.M., Kokwaro, J.O., Mahunnah, R.L.A., Kimanani, E.K., 1995. Antigiardial activity of gastrointestinal remedies of the Luo of East Africa. Journal of Ethnopharmacology 8741, 17—23.

Kihagi, R.W., 2016. Antibacterial, Antifungal and Phytochemical Screening of the Plant Species Lannea Schweinfurthii. Kenyatta University, Kenya, pp. 18—71.

Maregesi, S., van Miert, S., Pannecouque, C., Haddad, M.H.F., Hermans, N., Wright, C.W., Vlietinck, A.J., Apers, S., Pieters, L., 2010. Screening of tanzanian medicinal plants against Plasmodium falciparum and human immunodeficiency virus. Planta Medica 76, 195—201. https://doi.org/10.1055/s-0029-1186024.

Maregesi, S.M., Ngassapa, O.D., Pieters, L., Vlietinck, A.J., 2007. Ethnopharmacological survey of the Bunda district , Tanzania : plants used to treat infectious diseases. Journal of Ethnopharmacology 113, 457—470. https://doi.org/10.1016/j.jep.2007.07.006.

Maregesi, S.M., Pieters, L., Ngassapa, O.D., Apers, S., Vingerhoets, R., Cos, P., Berghe, D., Vlietinck, A.J., 2008. Screening of some Tanzanian medicinal plants from Bunda district for antibacterial , antifungal and antiviral activities. Journal of Ethnopharmacology 119, 58—66. https://doi.org/10.1016/j.jep.2008.05.033.

Okoth, A.D., 2014. Phytochemistry and Bioactive Natural Products from Lannea Alata, Lannea Rivae, Lannea Schimperi and Lannea Schweinfurthii (Anacardiaceae). University of KwaZulu-Natal, South Africa, pp. 15—122.

Seoposengwe, K., van Tonder, J.J., Steenkamp, V., 2013. In vitro neuroprotective potential of four medicinal plants against rotenone-induced toxicity in SH-SY5Y neuroblastoma cells. BMC Complementary and Alternative Medicine 13, 1—11.

Stafford, G.I., Pedersen, M.E., van Staden, J., Jager, A.K., 2008. Review on plants with CNS-effects used in traditional South African medicine against mental diseases. Journal of Ethnopharmacology 119, 513—537. https://doi.org/10.1016/j.jep.2008.08.010.

Wursten, 2016. Lannea Schweinfurthii Engl. Victoria Falls, Zimbabwe. Available online: https://commons.wikimedia.org/wiki/File:Lannea_schweinfurthii_var._tomentosa04.jpg. (CC BY-SA 3.0).

Yaouba, S., Koch, A., Guantai, E.M., Derese, S., Irungu, B., 2018. Alkenyl cyclohexanone derivatives from Lannea rivae and Lannea schweinfurthii. Phytochemistry Letters 23, 141—148.

Lippia scaberrima

Anna-Mari Kok, Namrita Lall

Department of Plant and Soil Sciences, University of Pretoria, Pretoria, Gauteng, South Africa

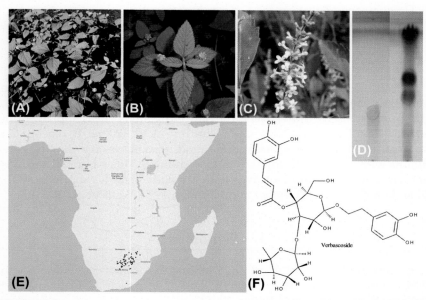

FIGURE 29   Aerial parts of *Lippia scaberrima* (Kenraiz, 2016) (A), close-up view of a related *Lippia* species (Salicyna, 2017) (B), flowers of *L. scaberrima* (Noarovivaio, 2018) (C), TLC chromatogram, Lane 1; verbascoside, Lane 2; *L. scaberrima* ethanolic extract (D), distribution map of *L. scaberrima* in sub-Saharan Africa (GBIF, 2018) (E), chemical structure of verbascoside (F).

1. General description

1.1 Botanical nomenclature

Lippia scaberrima Sond.

1.2 Botanical family

Verbenaceae

1.3 Vernacular names

Beukesbossie (Afrikaans)
Laventelbos (Afrikaans)
Mosukutswane (Tswana)
Umsuzwane (Zulu)

2. Botanical description

Lippia scaberrima is an aromatic, perennial shrub that forms part of the Verbenaceae family. Together with *Lippia javanica, L. rehmannii, L. wilmsii,* and *L. pretoriensis, L. scaberrima* is the only indigenous *Lippia* spp. in South Africa (Regnier et al., 2008; Germishuizen et al., 2006). It reaches an approximate height of 60 cm and is found growing in dry climatic conditions with rainfalls during the summer months. This perennial shrub is known to have deciduous leaves with a woody stem (Combrinck et al., 2006; Retief et al., 2003; Retief and Herman, 1997; Wells et al., 1986).

3. Distribution

L. scaberrima is found distributed among five provinces within South Africa namely, North West, Northern Cape, Mpumalanga, Gauteng, and the Free State (Foden and Potter, 2005).

4. Ethnobotanical usage

L. scaberrima is well known for its medicinal properties among the Tswana, Pedi, Zulu, and Xhosas (Van Wyk et al., 1997; Watt and Breyer-Brandwijk, 1962). It has also been sold as a tea, with health properties namely Mosukudu in Botswana (Shikanga et al., 2010). A tonic created from the leaf infusions is used as a treatment for coughs, fever, colds, and bronchitis (Combrinck et al., 2006; Smith, 1966; Van Wyk et al., 2000; Watt and Breyer-Brandwijk, 1962). According to Pascual et al. (2001), the vast majority of the *Lippia* spp. is used to treat respiratory and gastrointestinal ailments. Some species within the genus *Lippia* have shown to have antimalarial (Gasquet et al., 1993), antiviral (Abad et al., 1995), and cytostatic properties (Lopez et al., 1979).

5. Phytochemical constituents

The essential oil of *L. scaberrima* has been thoroughly investigated for its constituents by various research groups. According to Combrinck et al. (2006), the essential oil (oil extracted from the flowers, leaves, and twigs) is rich in R-(−) carvone, (D)-limonene, and 1, 8-cineole. This was also confirmed in a previous investigation of the essential oil gathered from the flowers and leaves by Terblanche et al. (1998). Some of the other components found in the essential oil of the leaves and flower heads by Combrinck et al. (2006) yielded the following components: α-pinene, β-pinene, camphene, sabinene, myrcene, α-phellandrene, p-cymene, γ-terpinene, linalool, camphor, borneol, α-terpineol, dihydrocarvone, carveol, β-caryophyllene, and α-humulene. No isolated compounds from any plant extract of *L. scaberrima* have been reported except for the components identified within the essential oils.

6. TLC fingerprinting of plant extract

The separation of *L. scaberrima* was observed by weighing out 2 mg of the ethanolic extract, dissolved in 200 μL ethanol. A standard, verbascoside (acteoside) found within various indigenous species of *Lippia* was used by weighing out in the same manner as the plant extract. The thin layer chromatography (TLC) analysis of the ethanolic *L. scaberrima* extract comprised of silica gel 60 F254 TLC plates for the observation of separation of the compounds that may be present within the extract. The plates were marked with a soft pencil, and glass capillaries were used to spot the samples. A reference standard (verbascoside) was spotted to determine its presence within the extract. The spots were left to dry completely before placing the TLC plate within a TLC tank, which contained 10 mL eluent of 9:1 chloroform:methanol as the solvent system. The samples were allowed to separate until the eluent reaches the solvent line, 1 cm from the top of the TLC plate. The plate was observed under ultraviolet (UV light) (long and short wavelength), followed by spraying with freshly prepared vanillin/sulfuric acid (2%) to detect the bands on the TLC plate.

7. Pharmacological properties

Although *L. scaberrima* has not been extensively investigated for its pharmacological properties, many research groups have done initial investigations on the activity of the crude extract. Wide-ranging work has been completed on the activity of the essential oil isolated from *L. scaberrima* especially as a treatment for postharvest pathogens and diseases for economically important fruit.

7.1 Antifungal activity

Regnier et al. (2008) studied the antifungal potential of the essential oil of *L. scaberrima* as well as the major components found within the essential oil, R-(−)-carvone, S-(−)-carvone, limonene, and 1, 8-cineole. These major components including R-(−)-carvone, S-(−)-carvone, showed antifungal potential against *C. gloeosporioides* and *B. parva*. Limonene showed the lowest efficacy against both these pathogens. Regnier et al. (2010) expanded this investigation by including the antifungal properties of the essential oil of *L. scaberrima*. In another study, carvone was tested and found to have activity against three major avocado pathogens, by effectively controlling the growth of these fruit pathogens.

7.2 Antioxidant activity

A phenylethanoid glycoside, verbascoside, is known to occur in measurable amounts within *L. scaberrima* (Olivier et al., 2010). This glycoside is known for its antioxidant properties. Shikanga et al. (2010) measured the free radical scavenging properties of *L. scaberrima* and that of the pure compound, verbascoside. The 50% inhibitory concentration (IC_{50}) values were reported as 1150 µg/mL and 89 µg/mL for *L. scaberrima* and verbascoside, respectively.

7.3 Antibacterial activity

A previous publication by Pennachio (2005) indicated the antibacterial properties that verbascoside may possess. Following the serial microdilution method by Shikanga et al. (2010), both *L. scaberrima* and verbascoside were tested for their antibacterial properties against four human bacterial pathogens namely *Staphylococcus aureus* (American type culture collection [ATCC] 29213), *Enterococcus faecalis* (ATCC 29212), *Pseudomonas aeruginosa* (ATCC 27853) and *Escherichia coli* (ATCC 25922). *L. scaberrima* showed the highest minimum inhibitory concentration (MIC) values against these four pathogens with the highest activity against *E. faecalis* (0.63 mg/mL). The MIC values against the other bacteria were all reported to be 1.3 mg/mL (Shikanga et al., 2010). Verbascoside showed the best activity against these four pathogens with the lowest MIC value reported to be 0.06 mg/mL against *S. aureus* and a slightly higher MIC value of 0.1 mg/mL reported against both *E. faecalis* and *E. coli*. The MIC value against *P. aeruginosa* was reported to be 0.25 mg/mL.

8. Additional information

8.1 Therapeutic (proposed) usage

Antibacterial, antimycobacterial, immunostimulant, and hepatoprotectant

8.2 Safety data

Not available

8.3 Trade information

Not threatened, not endangered, and abundant

8.4 Dosage

Not available

References

Abad, M.J., Sanchez, S., Bermejo, P., Villar, A., Carrasco, L., 1995. Antiviral activity of some medicinal plants. Methods and Findings (Suppl. A), 108.

Combrinck, S., Bosman, A.A., Botha, B.M., Du Plooy, W., McCrindle, R.I., 2006. Effects of post-harvest drying on the essential oil and glandular trichomes of *Lippia scaberrima* Sond. Journal of Essential Oil Research 18, 80−84.

Foden, W., Potter, L., 2005. *Lippia Scaberrima* Sond. National Assessment: Red List of South African Plants Version 2014. Available: http://redlist.sanbi.org/species.php? species=4080-9.

Gasquet, M., Delmas, F., Timo, D.P., Keita, A., guindo, M., Koita, N., Diallo, D., Doumbo, O., 1993. Evaluation in vitro and in vivo of a traditional antimalarial, "Malarial-5". Fitoterapia 64, 423−426.

GBIF, 2018. *Lippia Scaberrima* Sond. In GBIF Secretariat (2017). GBIF Backbone Taxonomy. Checklist dataset. https://doi.org/10.15468/39omei. accessed via GBIF.org on 2019-02-24.

A checklist of South African plants. In: Germishuizen, G., Meyer, N.L., Steenkamp, Y., Keith, M. (Eds.), 2006. Southern African Botanical Diversity Network Report No. 41. SABONET, Pretoria.

Kenraiz, K.Z., 2016. Phyla Scaberrima in Warsaw University Botanical Garden. https://commons.wikimedia.org/wiki/File:Phyla_scaberrima_kz2.jpg. (CC BY-SA 4.0).

Lopez, A.A.M., Rojas, H.N.M., Jimenez, M.C.A., 1979. Plants extracts with cytostatic properties growing in Cuba. Revista Cubana de Medicina Tropical 31, 105—111.

Noarovivaio, 2018. Evergreen Perennial Shrub, Aromatic Foliage, Small White Inflorescences. Available online: https://www.noarovivaio.it/main.php?i=dettaglio-pianta&id_pianta=1223 (No copyright indicated).

Olivier, D.K., Shikanga, E.A., Combrinck, S., Krause, R.W.M., Regnier, T., Dlamini, T.P., 2010. Phenylethanoid glycosides from *Lippia javanica*. South African Journal of Botany 76, 58—63.

Pascual, M.E., Slowing, K., Carretero, E., Mata, D.S., Villar, A., 2001. *Lippia*: traditional uses, chemistry and pharmacology: a review. Journal of Ethnopharmacology 76, 201—214.

Pennachio, M., 2005. Traditional Australian Aboriginal bush medicine. HerbalGram 65, 38—44.

Regnier, T., Du Plooy, W., Combrinck, S., Botha, B., 2008. Fungitoxicity of Lippia Scaberrima essential oil and selected terpenoid components on two mango postharvest spoilage pathogens. Postharvest Biology and Technology 48, 254—258.

Regnier, T., Combrinck, S., Du Plooy, W., Botha, B., 2010. Evaluation of *Lippia scaberrima* essential oil and some pure terpenoid constituents as postharvest mycobiocides for avocado fruit. Postharvest Biology and Technology 57 (3), 176—182.

Retief, E., Herman, P.P.J., 1997. Plants of the Northern Provinces of South Africa: Keys and Diagnostic Characters. National Botanical Institute, Strelitzia Publishers, Pretoria.

Retief, E., 2003. Lippia L. In: Germishuizen, G., Meyer, N.L. (Eds.), Plants of Southern Africa: An Annotated Checklist, Strelitzia, vol. 6. National Botanical Institute, Pretoria, South Africa, p. 943.

Salicyna, 2017. *Lippia* Słodka (Lippia Dulcis), Ogród Botaniczny Uniwersytetu Wrocławskiego. https://commons.wikimedia.org/wiki/File:Lippia_dulcis_2017-09-26_4714.jpg. (CC BY-SA 4.0).

Shikanga, E.A., Combrinck, S., Regnier, T., 2010. South African *Lippia* herbal infusions: total phenolic content and antibacterial activities. South African Journal of Botany 76, 567—571.

Smith, C.A., 1966. Common Names of South African Plants- Memoirs of the Botanical Survey of South Africa, p. 35.

Terblanche, F.C., Kornelius, G., Hasset, A.J., Rohwer, E.R., 1998. Composition of the essential oil of *Lippia scaberrima* Sond. from South Africa. Journal of Essential Oil Research 10, 213—215.

Van Wyk, B.E., Van Oudtshoorn, B., Gericke, N., 1997. Medicinal Plants of South Africa. Briza Publications, Pretoria, South Africa.

Van Wyk, B.E., Van Oudtshoorn, B., Gericke, N., 2000. Medicinal Plants of South Africa, second ed. Briza Publications, Pretoria, South Africa.

Watt, J.M., Breyer-Brandwijk, M.G., 1962. The Medicinal and Poisonous Plants of Southern Africa and Eastern Africa: Being an Account of Their Medicinal Aid and Other Uses, Chemical Composition, Pharmacological Effects and Toxicology in Man and Animals, second ed. E & S Livingstone Ltd, London.

Wells, M.J., Balsinhas, A.A., Joffe, H., Engelbrecht, V.M., Harding, G., Stirton, C.H., 1986. A Catalogue of Problem Plants in Southern Africa, Incorporating the National Weed List of Southern Africa. Memoirs of the Botanical Survey of South Africa No. 53. The Government Printer, Pretoria.

Newtonia buchananii

Katlego Ellena Motlhatlego, Lyndy Joy McGaw

Phytomedicine Programme, Department of Paraclinical Sciences, Faculty of Veterinary Sciences, University of Pretoria, Pretoria, Gauteng, South Africa

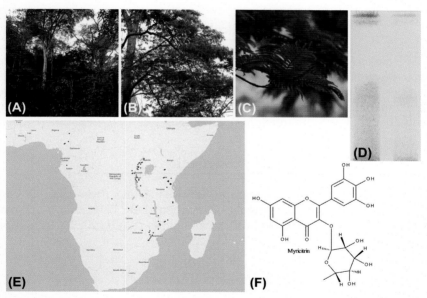

FIGURE 30 Forest dominated by *Newtonia buchananii* (Wursten, 2012) (A), aerial parts of *N. buchananii* (B), closer view of the leaves of *N. buchananii* (C), TLC chromatogram, Lane 1; *N. buchananii* acetone leaf extract, Lane 2; *N. buchananii* MeOH:DCM leaf extracts (D), distribution of *N. buchananii* in sub-Saharan Africa (GBIF, 2018) (E), chemical structure of myricitin (F).

1. General description

1.1 Botanical nomenclature

Newtonia buchananii (Baker) G.C.C. Gilbert & Boutique.

1.2 Botanical family

Fabaceae

1.3 Vernacular names

Forest newtonia (English)
Sangow (Chapman)
Shairu (Chapman)

2. Botanical description

Newtonia buchananii (Baker) G.C.C. Gilbert & Boutique is described as a tall deciduous tree with a height of 10—40 m (Coates-Palgrave, 2002). This species has bipinnate leaves that are linear or falcate. The leaves are 2—9 mm long and tiny, and light green when young. Their pods are brown and about 1.3—2.5 cm and split open on one side.

3. Distribution

Newtonia buchananii is geographically distributed from Nigeria east to Kenya, and south to Angola, Cameroon, DRC, Uganda, Tanzania, Malawi, Zambia, Zimbabwe, and Mozambique (Kakudidi, 2004; Louppe et al., 2008).

4. Ethnobotanical usage

The interest in *N. buchananii* as a potential antidiarrhoeal agent was based on the reported use of *Newtonia* species to treat wounds and other unspecified skin conditions, and for stomach ailments (Fratkin, 1996; Kariba and Houghton, 2001).

5. Phytochemical constituents

Limited phytochemical work has been done on the genus. Isolation of the flavonoid myricetin-3-O-rhamnoside (myricitrin) from *N. buchananii* has been reported (Motlhatlego, 2017). *N. buchananii* also contains phenolics, tannins, flavonols, flavonoids, and proanthocyanins (Motlhatlego, 2017).

6. TLC fingerprinting of plant extract

The chemical constituents of the acetone and methanol:dichloromethane plant extracts were separated on aluminium-backed thin layer chromatography (TLC) plates (Merck). The markings were made with a soft pencil. A volume of 10 μL of the plant extracts resuspended to 10 mg/mL with methanol was spotted onto the TLC plates. In accordance with Kotzé and Eloff (2002) the TLC plates were developed under saturated conditions with eluent systems: ethyl acetate: methanol: water (EMW [40: 5.4:4]), benzene: ethanol: ammonia (BEA [90:10:1]) and chloroform/ethyl acetate/formic acid (CEF [50:40:10]). Separated chemical compounds on the chromatograms were detected by spraying with acidified vanillin (0.1 g vanillin: 28 mL methanol: 1 mL sulfuric acid). Following the spraying procedure, the chromatograms were carefully heated with a heat gun to allow for optimal color development.

7. Pharmacological properties

Newtonia buchananii is distributed across Africa, but pharmacological research for the genus is limited. The recent interest in in vitro research on the species encourages an additional focus on its in vitro potential. This then creates an opportunity for research and development.

7.1 Antibacterial activity and cytotoxicity

The leaves of *N. buchananii* were collected from the Lowveld National Botanical Garden in Nelspruit, South Africa. A voucher specimen was prepared and lodged in the H.G.W.J. Schweickerdt Herbarium (PRU 122348 *N. buchananii*) at the University of Pretoria for reference purposes. The plant material was extracted using acetone. The Gram-positive (*Bacillus cereus* American type culture collection [ATCC] 21366; *Enterococcus faecalis* ATCC 29212; *Staphylococcus aureus* ATCC 29213) and Gram-negative (*E. coli* ATCC 25922; *P. aeruginosa* ATCC 27853; *Salmonella typhimurium* ATCC 39183) bacteria and fungal strains (*Candida albicans* ATCC 10231) and a clinical isolate of *Cryptococcus neoformans* were used in the study. These microorganisms are known to cause diarrheal disease. The cytotoxicity of the plant extracts was determined using an in vitro 1-(4,5-dimethylthiazol-2-yl)-3,5-diphenylformazan (MTT) assay with Vero monkey kidney cells (Mosmann, 1983). Cell growth inhibition for each extract was expressed in terms of 50% lethal concentration (LC_{50}) values. The selectivity index (SI) was also calculated. The cytotoxicity assay was repeated thrice. The results showed that *N. buchananii* extracts were selective for antibacterial activity with the highest SI found to be 19. *N. buchananii* had strong antimicrobial activity against *P. aeruginosa* with minimum inhibitory concentration (MIC) of 20 µg/mL and moderate activity of 40 µg/mL against *B. cereus* (MIC of Gentamicin [Positive control] 7.8×10^{-4} µg/mL) Motlhatlego et al. (2018).

7.2 Antiinflammatory, antioxidant, and acetylcholinesterase activity

The antiinflammatory activity of the extracts was determined by examining the inhibition of nitric oxide (NO) production in lipopolysaccharide (LPS) activated RAW 264.7 macrophages and 15-lipoxygenase enzyme inhibition Motlhatlego et al. (2018). The *N. buchananii* acetone leaf extract and the *N. buchananii* MeOH:DCM leaf extract had the highest lipoxygenase inhibition potential with 50% inhibitory concentration (IC_{50}) values of 13.85 and 14.82 µg/mL, respectively, and the positive control (quercetin) inhibiting at 24.60 ± 0.70 µg/mL. The plant species was found to have low NO inhibitory activity. Antioxidant activity was determined using the diphenylpicrylhydrazyl (DPPH) and 2,2-azino-bis (3-ethyl benzothiazoline-6-sulphonic acid) (ABTS) radical scavenging assays. *N. buchananii* extract was found more active in the ABTS scavenging assay than in the DPPH assay. The *N. buchananii* MeOH:DCM leaf extract and *N. buchananii* MeOH:DCM stem extract were most active in the ABTS scavenging assay with IC_{50} values of 0.09 ± 0.02 and 0.01 ± 0.00 µg/mL, respectively. These antioxidant results were comparable to the standard compounds (trolox and ascorbic acid), which inhibited the free radical formation at 0.37 ± 0.36 and 0.66 ± 0.05 µg/mL, respectively.

7.3 Antibiofilm activity

Bacterial biofilm inhibition of *Newtonia* leaf extracts as well as that of myricitrin was determined. The biofilm inhibition activity of *N. buchananii* extracts was reported for the first time in a PhD thesis (Motlhatlego, 2017).

7.4 Antiviral activity

Newtonia buchananii acetone extracts and isolated myricitrin were evaluated for antiviral mechanisms of action against the H1N1 strain of influenza as a model (Motlhatlego, 2017). The extracts in combination with the influenza virus (PR8/34/H1N1) showed significant antiviral activity ($P < .01$) on viral titer and maintained cell viabilities on the cells ($P < .05$). Myricitrin was effective against influenza virus in a copenetration combined treatment experiment, thereby confirming the efficacy of the antibacterial compound in the viral attachment and entry stages. The work was done in collaboration with Dr. Parvaneh Mehrbod of Influenza and Other Respiratory Viruses Department (Pasteur Institute of Iran) in Tehran, Iran.

8. Additional information

8.1 Therapeutic (proposed) usage

Antibacterial, antibiofilm, and antiviral

8.2 Safety data

Not available

8.3 Trade information

No report provides information on the production, marketing, and trade of this plant species. The plant species is not endangered and not threatened. It is abundant across Africa.

8.4 Dosage

Not available

References

Coates-Palgrave, M., 2002. Keith Coates-Palgrave Trees of Southern Africa, third ed. Struik Publishers, Cape Town, pp. 306–307.

Fratkin, E., 1996. Traditional medicine and concepts of healing among Samburu pastoralists of Kenya. Journal of Ethnobiology 16, 63–97.

GBIF, 2018. Newtonia Buchananii (Baker) G.C.C.Gilbert & Boutique in GBIF Secretariat (2017). GBIF Backbone Taxonomy. Checklist dataset. https://doi.org/10.15468/39omei. accessed via GBIF.org on 2019-02-24.

Kakudidi, E.K., 2004. Cultural and social uses of plants from and around Kibale National Park, Western Uganda. African Journal of Ecology 42, 114–118.

Kariba, R.M., Houghton, P.J., 2001. Antimicrobial activity of Newtonia hildebrandtii. Fitoterapia 72, 415–417.

Kotzé, M., Eloff, J.N., 2002. Extraction of bacterial compounds from Combretum microphyllum (Combretaceae). South African Journal of Botany 68, 62–67.

Louppe, D., Oteng-Amoako, A.A., Martin, B., 2008. Plant Resources of Tropical Africa (TROPA), 7: 392. Wageningen, Netherlands.

Mosmann, T., 1983. Rapid colometric assay for cellular growth and survival: application to proliferation and cytotoxicity assays. Journal of Immunological Methods 65, 55–63.

Motlhatlego, K.E., Njoya, E.M., Abdalla, M.A., Eloff, J.N., McGaw, L.J., 2018. The potential use of leaf extracts of two Newtonia (Fabaceae) species to treat diarrhoea. South African Journal of Botany 116, 25–33.

Motlhatlego, K.E., 2017. The Antimicrobial Activity and Safety of Two Newtonia Species with Potential Antidiarrhoeal Effect. University of Pretoria, South Africa.

Wursten, B., 2012. Rees in Moribane Forest Reserve. The Best-Preserved Parts of the Forest Are Dominated by Newtonia Buchananii. The Marshy Depressions Are Full of Apocynaceae, Including Funtumia Africana, Both Voacanga Africana and V. Thouarsii, Tabernaemontana Ventricosa and Various Lianes like Saba Comorensis, Dictyophleba Lucida, Strophanthus Courmontii and Landolphia. Available online: https://commons.wikimedia.org/wiki/File:Trees_in_Moribane_Forest,_Bart_Wursten.jpg. (CC BY-SA 3.0).

Further reading

Karber, G., 1931. 50% endpoint calculation. Archive for Experimental Pathology and Pharmacology 162, 430–483.

Nymphaea caerulea

Carel B. Oosthuizen, Matthew Fisher, Namrita Lall

Department of Plant and Soil Sciences, University of Pretoria, Pretoria, Gauteng, South Africa

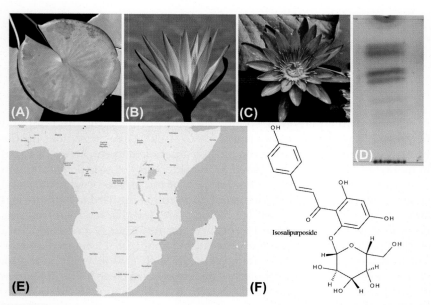

FIGURE 31   Leaf of *Nymphaea caerulea* on the water surface (Peripitus, 2007) (A), flower of *N. caerulea* (Peripitus, 2008) (B), close-up of the flower of *N. caerulea* (Mathieu, 2016) (C), TLC chromatogram, fingerprint of *N. caerulea* extract (D), distribution of *N. caerulea* in sub-Saharan Africa (GBIF, 2018) (E), chemical structure of isoalipurposide (F).

Underexplored Medicinal Plants from Sub-Saharan Africa
https://doi.org/10.1016/B978-0-12-816814-1.00031-4   205

1. General description

1.1 Botanical nomenclature

Nymphaea caerulea Savigny
Synonyms: *N. nouchali Burm. f. var. caerulea (Sav.) Verdc., N. capensis Thunb., N. calliantha Conar., N. mildbraedi Gilg., N. spectabilis Gilg., N. nelsonii Burtt Davy*

1.2 Botanical family

Nymphaeaceae

1.3 Vernacular names

Blue Water Lily (English)
Blou waterlelie (Afrikaans)
iZubu (Zulu)

2. Botanical description

Arising from a perennial, spongy rhizome buried in the mud of pond habitats, *N. caerulea* presents round or oval flat leaves that float on the water surface attached to the rhizome by a petiole and can be up to 40 cm in diameter. The leaves show several characteristics of aquatic plants such as a smooth waxy surface on the top side of the leaf to prevent stomatal clogging, while the leaf margins are slightly rolled upward to help the leaf stay afloat. The flowers of *N. caerulea* are its characteristic feature. Blooming in September until February, the flowers are presented in a starlike pattern when fully open, measuring about 15—20 cm in diameter. The flowers can be found in a range of colors such as blue, white, and pink with blue being the most common. The flowers also close in the afternoon after opening in mid-morning (South African National Biodiversity Institute—SANBI).

3. Distribution

Nymphaea caerulea can be found across South Africa as well as Swaziland, Botswana, Namibia, Zimbabwe, Zambia, Malawi, Angola, Mozambique, the Democratic Republic of Congo, Uganda, Kenya, Tanzania, Sudan, Egypt, and West Africa, usually at altitudes ranging from sea level to 2700 m above sea level (SANBI, 2016).

4. Ethnobotanical usage

Among West African cultures, the rhizome of *N. caerulea* is sometimes eaten during a famine. The rhizome and seed are ingested as a treatment for diabetes. The root and stem are made into an infusion and is used to treat gonorrhea and urinary tract ailments. The rhizome is also made into a tea to treat inflammation of various organs such as the bladder, kidneys, uterus, and intestine, as well as fevers and insomnia, causing drowsiness. The flower can be eaten or made into a decoction and may be considered a narcotic and an aphrodisiac (reduces libido) but has also been used to treat painful urination and coughs (Watt and Breyer-Brandwijk, 1962).

5. Phytochemical constituents

Through nuclear magnetic resonance analysis, a number of compounds have been elucidated from *N. caerulea*. The primary focus in the literature has been compounds derived from the flowers including a variety of glycosides with myricetin, quercetin, and kaempferol aglycones. Further compounds include naringenin, helichrysin B, isosalipurposide, gallic acid, p-coumaric acid, and methoxybenzoic acid (Agnihotri et al., 2008). Delphinidin and its glycosides have also been found specifically in the blue flowers of *N. caerulea* (Fossen and Andersen, 1999).

In some cultures, the flower has been used as an intoxicant with the proposed alkaloid apomorphine being the active metabolite (Bertol et al., 2004). However, the primary source of the metabolite analysis could not be accessed to verify this claim. There is still possible use today with similar intoxicating effects being reported (erowid.org/plants/lotus/), but no studies have been conducted to confirm its presence in *N. caerulea* flowers.

6. TLC fingerprinting of plant extract

The plant material was crushed and ground after an air drying process. The dried material was ground into a fine powder and ethanol was added in a 1:10 (weight:volume) ratio. The extract was shaken for 48 h, filtered and dried using rotary evaporation. The dried extract was collected and stored at 4 C°. To observe the separation of the phytochemicals of *N. caerulea*, 2 mg of the ethanolic extract was weighed out and dissolved in 200 µL of ethanol. Thin layer chromatography (TLC) was carried out on a precoated silica gel aluminum plate. 10 mL of the test solution were spotted at 10 mm from the bottom of a 10 × 5 cm TLC plate and develop up to 8 cm from the bottom of the plate using the mobile phase 100%

ethyl acetate. The plate was observed under ultraviolet light (long and short wavelength), followed by spraying with freshly prepared vanillin/sulfuric acid (2%) to detect the bands on the TLC plate.

7. Pharmacological properties

7.1 Antioxidants

In general, few tests have been performed on the constituents of *N. caerulea*. However, the antioxidant potential of most of the compounds mentioned above has been tested. The antioxidant test was conducted in vitro using myelomonocytic HL-60 cells and the reagent 2',7'-dichlorofluorescin-diacetate (DCFH-DA). This reagent is absorbed into the cells and metabolized to a polar product that remains contained in the cell. The product is then oxidized by intracellular hydrogen peroxide to a fluorescent product (Rosenkranz et al., 1992). Vitamin C was used as a positive control. The kaempferol glycosides, naringenin, p-coumaric acid, and methoxybenzoic acid showed no antioxidant activity, while one myricetin rhamnoside, helichrysin B, the ethanoic, and chloroform extract showed lower antioxidant activity than the control. A number of compounds performed better than the control including a number of the myricetin and quercetin glycosides, gallic acid, and the ethyl acetate fraction of the plant extract (Agnihotri et al., 2008).

7.2 Antitumor

The anthocyanidin delphinidin has been tested for its efficacy for inhibiting cancer cell growth. *In vitro* tests involved the use of lung tumor cells (LXFL529L) and human vulva carcinoma cells (A431). Results showed delphinidin to be effective at inhibiting both cancer cell lines with 50% inhibitory concentration (IC_{50}) values of 33 uM for lung tumor and 18 uM for vulva carcinoma cells at a similar level to the known chemotherapeutic agent epigallocatechin-3-gallate (IC_{50} of 32 uM and 21 uM, respectively) (Meiers et al., 2001).

7.3 Intoxicant

In some cultures, the flower has been used as an intoxicant with the proposed alkaloid apomorphine being the active metabolite (Bertol et al., 2004). However, the primary source of the metabolite analysis could not be accessed to verify this claim. There is still possible use today with similar intoxicating effects being reported (erowid.org/plants/lotus/), but no studies have been conducted to confirm its presence in *N. caerulea* flowers.

8. Additional information

8.1 Therapeutic (proposed) usage

Antioxidant, antitumor, and as a possible intoxicant (anecdotal)

8.2 Safety data

A cytotoxicity test was conducted on myelomonocytes. No cytotoxicity was observed for the myricetin and kaempferol rhamnosides, gallic acid, and p-coumaric acid at 31.25 ug/mL. The ethanolic extract, chloroform, and ethyl acetate fractions showed no cytotoxicity up to 125 ug/mL. Naringenin and helichrysin B showed cytotoxicity above the maximum concentration tested (31.25 µg/mL). The quercetin and myricetin glucosides showed cytotoxicity at higher than 15.6 ug/mL (the maximum dose for these compounds) (Agnihotri et al., 2008).

8.3 Trade information

Least concern. Possibly illegal in some countries, Latvia, Poland, and Russia, although cultivation as an ornamental is common throughout the world.

8.4 Dosage

Not available

References

Agnihotri, V.K., et al., 2008. Antioxidant constituents of *Nymphaea caerulea* flowers. Phytochemistry 69 (10), 2061–2066. Available at: http://www.sciencedirect.com/science/article/pii/S0031942208001921.

Bertol, E., et al., 2004. *Nymphaea* cults in ancient Egypt and the New World: a lesson in empirical pharmacology. Journal of the Royal Society of Medicine 97 (2), 84–85. Available at: http://0-jrs.sagepub.com.innopac.up.ac.za/content/97/2/84.full.

Fossen, T., Andersen, Ø.M., 1999. Delphinidin 3'-galloylgalactosides from blue flowers of *Nymphaea caerulea*. Phytochemistry 50 (7), 1185–1188. Available at: http://www.sciencedirect.com/science/article/pii/S0031942298006499.

GBIF, 2018. *Nymphaea caerulea* Savigny in GBIF Secretariat (2017). GBIF Backbone Taxonomy. Checklist dataset. https://doi.org/10.15468/39omei. accessed via GBIF.org on 2019-02-24.

Mathieu, M.D., 2016. Blue tropical waterlily cultivar *Nymphaea* in botanical garden "Jardin des Martels". Available online: https://commons.wikimedia.org/wiki/File:Jardin_des_Martels_-_N%C3%A9nufars_-_2016-08-07_-_04.jpg. (CC BY-SA 4.0).

Meiers, S., et al., 2001. The anthocyanidins cyanidin and delphinidin are potent inhibitors of the epidermal growth-factor receptor. Journal of Agricultural and Food Chemistry 49 (2), 958–962.

Peripitus, 2007. *Nymphaea caerulea* at the Botanic Garden, Adelaide, South Australia. Available online: https://commons.wikimedia.org/wiki/File:Nymphaea_caerulea_Botanic_Gardens_Adelaide.jpg. (CC BY-SA 3.0).

Peripitus, 2008. Sacred Blue Water-Lily Flower (*Nymphaea caerulea*) with an Amazon Lily Forming the Background. Botanic Garden, Adelaide, South Australia. Available online: https://commons.wikimedia.org/wiki/File:Nymphaea_caerulea_flower.JPG. (CC BY-SA 3.0).

Rosenkranz, A.R., et al., 1992. A microplate assay for the detection of oxidative products using 2 ', 7 ' -dichlorofluorescin-diacetate. Journal of Immunological Methods 156 (1), 39—45.

SANBI, September 14, 2016. *Nymphaea nouchali* Burm. f. var. *caerulea* (Sav.) Verdc. Obtained from URL: http://www.plantzafrica.com/plantnop/nymphnouch.htm.

Watt, J.M., Breyer-Brandwijk, M.G., 1962. The Medicinal and Poisonous Plants of Southern and Eastern Africa: Being an Account of Their Medicinal and Other Uses, Chemical Composition, Pharmacological Effects and Toxicology in Man and Animal. E. & S. Livingstone. Available at: https://books.google.com/books?id=2ZjwAAAAMAAJ&pgis=1.

CHAPTER

32

Ocimum labiatum

Isa A. Lambrechts, Namrita Lall

Department of Plant and Soil Sciences, University of Pretoria, Pretoria, Gauteng, South Africa

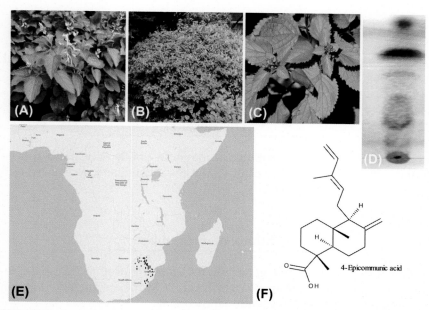

FIGURE 32   Aerial plant parts of *Ocimum labiatum* (JMK, 2015a) (A), bigger plant of *O. labiatum* (JMK, 2015b) (B), closer view of the flowers of *O. labiatum* (Dinkum, 2011) (C), TLC chromatogram, fingerprint of *O. labiatum* extract (D), distribution of *O. labiatum* in sub-Saharan Africa (GBIF, 2017) (E), chemical structure of 4-epicommunic acid (F).

Underexplored Medicinal Plants from Sub-Saharan Africa
https://doi.org/10.1016/B978-0-12-816814-1.00032-6

211

1. General description

1.1 Botanical nomenclature

Ocimum labiatum (N.E.Br.) A.J. Paton

1.2 Botanical family

Lamiaceae

1.3 Vernacular names

Pink sage, shell bush (English)
Pienk salie (Afrikaans)

2. Botanical description

Ocimum labiatum is a fast growing shrub and grows to a height and spread of 1.5 m. It flowers from late summer to autumn (Hankey, 2001).

3. Distribution

Ocimum labiatum is distributed throughout South Africa and can be found scattered through KwaZulu-Natal, Swaziland, and northward into Zimbabwe (Hankey, 2001).

4. Ethnobotanical usage

Plants from the *Ocimum* genus are traditionally used to treat pain, fever, and inflammation (Kapewangolo et al., 2015). There are no reports on *O. labiatum* being used in traditional medicine.

5. Phytochemical constituents

Three compounds have previously been isolated from the ethanolic leaf extract of *O. labiatum*; (+)-trans-ozic acid (4-epicommunic acid), 2α-Hydroxylabda-8(17),12E,14-trien-18-oic acid, and Labda-8(17),12E,14-triene-2R,18-diol (Hussein et al., 2007).

6. TLC fingerprinting of plant extract

For the separation of compounds from *O. labiatum*, 2 mg of an ethanolic extract was weighed out and dissolved in 200 μL ethanol. For the thin layer chromatography (TLC) analysis of *O. labiatum* crude extract, silica gel 60 F254 TLC plates were used to observe the separation of the compounds present within the extract. Plate markings were made with a soft pencil, and glass capillaries were used to spot the samples onto the TLC plate. The spots were left to dry completely before placing the plate in a TLC tank which contained 10 mL eluent 9.5:0.5 dichloromethane: methanol as the solvent system. The samples were allowed to separate until the solvent system reached 1 cm from the top of the TLC plate. The plate was observed under ultraviolet light (long and short wavelength), followed by spraying with freshly prepared vanillin/sulfuric acid (2%) to detect the bands on the TLC plate.

7. Pharmacological properties

7.1 Antioxidant, antiinflammatory activity and cytotoxicity

Leaves of *O. labiatum* were collected in February 2012 from Pretoria, South Africa. An ethanolic leaf extract was prepared from the fresh leaves. The compound Labda-8(17),12E,14-triene-2R,18-diol (LAB) was isolated from the ethanolic crude extract of *O. labiatum*. The antioxidant activity of *O. labiatum* was measured by the diphenylpicrylhydrazyl (DPPH), ferric reducing antioxidant power (FRAP), cupric reducing antioxidant capacity (CUPRAC), and crocin bleaching antioxidant assays, where the crude extract displayed a 50% inhibitory concentration (IC_{50}) at 13 ± 0.8 μg/mL, 53.62 ± 0.57, 47.32 ± 0.76 μg/mL, and 54.86 ± 1.28 μg/mL for the respective antioxidant assays. LAB displayed minimal antioxidant activity.

A cytometric Bead Array (CBA) human Th1/Th2/Th17 cytokine kit was used to analyze seven cytokines: interleukin-2 (IL-2), IL-4, IL-6, IL-10, tumor necrosis factor (TNF), interferon gamma (INF-ɣ), and IL-17A. Peripheral blood mononuclear cells (PBMCs) were exposed to the crude ethanolic extract. The extract significantly reduced the production of IL-2, IL-4, IL-6, and IL-17A proinflammatory cytokines. However, the extract did not significantly reduce the production for IL-10, INF-ɣ, and TNF compared with the control. LAB significantly inhibited the production of all cytokines, except IL-6. The effect of *O. labiatum* extract on phytohemagglutinin (PHA)-induced nitric oxide (NO) production in PBMCs was investigated. A concentration of 25 μM crude extract and isolated compound significantly inhibited the production of NO in PHA-stimulated cells. An abcam c-Jun (Ps73) enzyme-linked immunosorbent assay (ELISA) kit was used to detect PHA-P-induced activator protein 1 (AP-1) from PBMCs. AP-1 is involved in the expression of inflammatory genes. However, cells stimulated with the extract significantly increased the production of AP-1 in PBMC cells. LAB significantly inhibited AP-1 production at a concentration of 50 μM. The viability of PBMCs and TZM-bl cells using the 1-(4,5-dimethylthiazol-2-yl)-3,5-diphenylformazan (MTT) dye was determined for the ethanolic extract. The IC_{50}'s of crude *O. labiatum* extract were $30.1 \pm 0.4\,\mu g/mL$ and $62.6 \pm 0.6\,\mu g/mL$, respectively, for PBMC and TZM-bl cell lines. The labdane diterpenoid compound had an IC_{50} of $21.3\,\mu g/mL$ and $34.3\,\mu g/mL$ for PBMCs and ZM-bl, respectively (Kapewangolo et al., 2015).

7.2 Anti-HIV activity

An ethanolic leaf extract of *O. labiatum* was tested to ascertain its inhibitory activity against the human immunodeficiency virus 1 (HIV-1) enzymes; reverse transcriptase (RT), and protease (PR). A p24 antigen ELISA was used to determine the effect of the crude extract on the replication of HIV-1 in chronically infected U1 cells. The ethanolic crude extract of *O. labiatum* significantly inhibited the HIV-1 PR enzyme with an IC_{50} of $49.8 \pm 0.4\,\mu g/mL$. A significant reduction in HIV-1 replication in U1 cells was also observed after the cells were treated with a noncytotoxic concentration (25 μg/mL) of the crude extract. At the highest concentration tested (100 μg/mL), a weak inhibition of HIV-1 RT enzyme was observed. *O. labiatum* ethanolic extract cytotoxicity was determined on the U1 cell line and displayed a 50% cytotoxic concentration (CC_{50}) of $42.0 \pm 0.13\,\mu g/mL$ (Kapewangolo, 2013).

7.3 Antibacterial and anticancer activity

Aerial parts of *O. labiatum* were collected from Pretoria, South Africa, in September 2004. An ethanolic extract was made from the fresh leaves and the crude extract was subjected to column chromatography. Three compounds were isolated from the ethanolic crude extract of *O. labiatum*; (+)-trans-ozic acid (1), 2R-Hydroxylabda-8(17),12E,14-trien-18-oic acid (2), and Labda-8(17),12E,14-triene-2R,18-diol (3). The isolated compounds 2 and 3 were tested against *Mycobacterium tuberculosis* (strain no. H37Rv American type culture collection (ATCC) 27294) and displayed a minimum inhibitory concentration (MIC) of 157 μM for compound 3. Compound 2 did not display any inhibition of *M. tuberculosis* at the highest concentration tested. Compounds 2 and 3 were tested against a human breast (MCF-7) cancer cell line. Compound 2 had an IC_{50} of 82 μM, while compound 3 had no activity at the highest concentration tested, 650 μM (Hussein et al., 2007).

8. Additional information

8.1 Therapeutic (proposed) usage

Antibacterial, antiinflammatory, and anti-HIV

8.2 Safety data

The IC_{50} values of crude *O. labiatum* extract were 30.1 ± 0.4 μg/mL and 62.6 ± 0.6 μg/mL, respectively, for PBMC and TZM-bl cell lines. The labdane diterpenoid compound had an IC_{50} of 21.3 μg/mL and 34.3 μg/mL for PBMCs and ZM-bl, respectively (Kapewangolo et al., 2015).

8.3 Trade information

Not threatened, not endangered, and abundant

8.4 Dosage

Not available

References

Dinkum, 2011. *Orthosiphon labiatus*. In: Wikimedia Commons. C.C. Available online: https://commons.wikimedia.org/wiki/File:Orthosiphon_labiatus_-_Barcelone.JPG (CC0 1.0).

GBIF, 2017. *Ocimum labiatum* (N.E.Br) A.J.Paton in GBIF Secretariat. GBIF Backbone Taxonomy. Checklist dataset. https://doi.org/10.15468/39omei. Accessed via GBIF.org on 2018-08-07.

Hankey, A., 2001. *Ocimum labiatum*. http://pza.sanbi.org/ocimum-labiatum.

Hussein, A.A., Meyer, J.J., Jimeno, M.L., Rodríguez, B., 2007. Bioactive diterpenes from *Orthosiphon labiatus* and *Salvia africana-lutea*. Journal of Natural Products 70, 293–295.

JMK, 2015a. Flowers of *Ocimum labiatum* in the Manie van der Schijff Botanical Garden at the University of Pretoria. In: Wikimedia Commons. C.C. Available online: https://commons.wikimedia.org/wiki/File:Ocimum_labiatum,_blomme,_Manie_van_der_Schijff_BT.jpg (CC BY-SA 3.0).

JMK, 2015b. Habit of *Ocimum labiatum* in the Manie van der Schijff Botanical Garden at the University of Pretoria. In: Wikimedia Commons. C.C. Available online: https://commons.wikimedia.org/wiki/File:Ocimum_labiatum,_habitus,_Manie_van_der_Schijff_BT.jpg (CC BY-SA 3.0).

Kapewangolo, P., Omolo, J.J., Bruwer, R., Fonteh, P., Meyer, D., 2015. Antioxidant and anti-inflammatory activity of *Ocimum labiatum* extract and isolated labdane diterpenoid. Journal of Inflammation 12, 1.

Kapewangolo, T.P., 2013. Lamiaceae Plant Extracts and Isolated Compounds Demonstrate Activity against HIV/AIDS.

Phyllanthus phillyreifolius

Mohamad Fawzi Mahomoodally[1],
Beebee Noushreen Kissoon[1], Sameerchand Pudaruth[2]

[1] Department of Health Sciences, Faculty of Science, University of Mauritius, Réduit, Mauritius; [2] Department of ICT, Faculty of Information, Communication and Digital Technologies

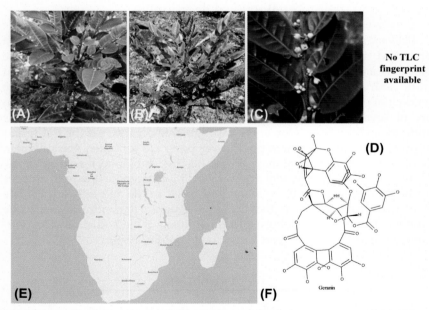

No TLC fingerprint available

FIGURE 33   Aerial parts of *Phyllanthus phillyreifolius* (A,B), close view of the stem with flower buds of *P. phillyreifolius* (C), no TLC fingerprint available (D), distribution of *P. phillyreifolius* in sub-Saharan Africa (GBIF, 2018) (E), chemical structure of geranin (F).

1. General description

1.1 Botanical nomenclature

Phyllanthus phillyreifolius var. *commersonii* Müll. Arg

1.2 Botanical family

Phyllanthaceae

1.3 Vernacular names

Bois de négresse
Bois de cafrine
Bois de ravine
Bois de chien

2. Botanical description

Phyllanthus phillyreifolius is from the Phyllanthaceae family. It is a branched shrub or small tree and can reach 2−6 m tall. Leaves are glabrous and vary in shape. This plant species is reported to be absent from Rodrigues, but other members of the genus are present and have medicinal properties as well. Existing plants from Mauritius and Reunion are of several varieties. *P. phillyreifolius* var. *commersonii* Müll. Arg is endemic to Mauritius. One of the distinguishing features is the triangular stipules with an acuminate tip. Flower parts are arranged spirally or in two whorls of three. The male flower has five subglobose nectary lobes. There are three stamens that are connected into a single one with anthers at the tip. Anthers are three-lobed and fused in the anther head. Female flowers have nectary lobes that are either separate or continuous with one another. The ovary is globose and three-lobed. Style and stigma are variable. Pedicels do not exceed 5 mm long (Coode, 1978).

3. Distribution

Phyllanthus spp. are distributed across tropical and subtropical regions (Grauzdytė et al., 2018b). There are 14 species that grow in the Mascarene Islands, of which 9 are native. *P. phillyreifolius* can be found in Mauritius and Reunion Islands but no record has been made from Rodrigues (Coode, 1978). There are many varieties of this species. There are four variants, namely *P. phillyreifolius* var. *commersonii*, *P. phillyreifolius* var. *gracilipes*, *P. phillyreifolius* var. *stylifer*, and *P. phillyreifolius* var. *telfairianus* that are endemic to Mauritius (National Parks and Conservation Services, n.d.). *P. phillyreifolius* var. *commersonii* can be found in the Black River Gorges National Park, Bar Le Duc mountain, Monvert Nature Walk, besides other locations (Mahomoodally et al., 2018; Pynee et al., 2013).

4. Ethnobotanical usage

Phyllanthus phillyreifolius is commonly used in folk medicine across the Mascarene Islands, against diarrhea and as a diuretic (Poullain et al., 2004). In Reunion Island, the endemic *P. phillyreifolius* Poiret var. *phyllyreifolius* has been found to have chemical components that can regulate tension and diuresis. Although absent in Rodrigues, other members of the genus are used for their medicinal properties.

5. Phytochemical constituents

Geranin has been found to be one of the main compounds present in *P. phillyreifolius*, alongside phyllanthusiin D, elaeocarpusin, and α, β, and γ tocopherol (Grauzdytė et al., 2018a). It is also rich in polyphenols (Grauzdytė et al., 2018b). Ellagitannins, flavonoids, gallic acid, ellagic acid, and granatin B were found in various extracts of this plant during a study in which the pharmacological and polyphenolic profile of this species was carried out (Mahomoodally et al., 2018).

6. TLC fingerprinting of plant extract

Thin layer chromatography (TLC) fingerprint is not available for this plant.

7. Pharmacological properties

This plant is used as a diuretic. It is also used against diarrhea and has been found to be an antioxidant. It exhibits antibacterial, anticancer, and enzyme inhibitory activities. Research is still required for this species to establish the extent of its medicinal properties.

7.1 Antioxidant activity and enzyme-inhibiting property

Different extracts of this species were found to have diphenylpicrylhydrazyl (DPPH) and 2,2′-azinobis-3-ethylbenzothiazoline-6-sulfonic acid (ABTS) scavenging properties to varying extents. Metal chelating effect and ferric and cupric reducing power were also found. Enzyme-inhibiting property was also tested and confirmed against multiple key enzymes. These included two cholinesterases, acetylcholinesterase (AChE) and butyrylcholinesterase (BChE); their inhibition is effective in Alzheimer's diseases. α-amylase and α-glycosidase were also inhibited, effective for diabetes. Lastly, tyrosinase inhibition has multiple benefits for excess melanin formation, neurodegenerative diseases like Parkinson's disease, and management of pigmentation (Mahomoodally et al., 2018).

7.2 Antimicrobial activity

Disc diffusion method was performed to test for antimicrobial activity against four species of bacteria, *Escherichia coli*, *Staphylococcus epidermidis*, *Staphylococcus aureus*, and *Bacillus cereus*. An extract of the plant that was macerated in ethyl acetate was found to have antibacterial activity against *B. cereus* and *E. coli*, while *S. epidermidis* was more receptive to an ethyl acetate-Soxhlet extract (Mahomoodally et al., 2018).

7.3 Anticancer activity

Cytotoxic potential of various extracts of this plant was tested against two cancer cells lines, HeLa (cervical carcinoma) and MDA-MB-231 (human mammary adenocarcinoma). *P. phillyreifolius* has gallic acid as one of its phytochemical constituent, an agent that is known to decrease cell viability. In the study, it has been found that extracts of this plant can reduce cell viability for the HeLa cell line in a time-dependent fashion. For the MDA-MB-231 cell line, a different extract reduced cell viability. The compound quercetin, a flavanol, acts in a time and dose-dependent fashion through various mechanisms (Mahomoodally et al., 2018).

8. Additional information

8.1 Therapeutic (proposed) usage

Antioxidant, anticancer, antibacterial, and as a diuretic

8.2 Safety data

Not available

8.3 Trade information

Not available

8.4 Dosage

Not available

References

Coode, M.J.E., 1978. Notes on Euphorbiaceae in the Mascarene Islands: I. Kew Bulletin 33, 109. https://doi.org/10.2307/4110107.

GBIF, 2018. *Phyllanthus phillyreifolius* poir. In: GBIF Secretariat (2017). GBIF Backbone Taxonomy. Checklist dataset. https://doi.org/10.15468/39omei.

Grauzdytė, D., Pukalskas, A., El Kalamouni, C., Venskutonis, P.R., 2018a. Antioxidant potential and phytochemical composition of extracts obtained from *Phyllanthus phillyreifolius* by different extraction methods. Natural Product Research 1–4. https://doi.org/10.1080/14786419.2018.1493586.

Grauzdytė, D., Pukalskas, A., Viranaicken, W., El Kalamouni, C., Venskutonis, P.R., 2018b. Protective effects of *Phyllanthus phillyreifolius* extracts against hydrogen peroxide induced oxidative stress in HEK293 cells. PLoS One 13, e0207672 e0207672. https://doi.org/10.1371/journal.pone.0207672.

Mahomoodally, M.F., Yerlikaya, S., Llorent-Martínez, E.J., Uğurlu, A., Baloglu, M.C., Altunoglu, Y.C., Mollica, A., Dardenne, K.K., Aumeeruddy, M.Z., Puchooa, D., Zengin, G., 2018. Pharmacological and polyphenolic profiles of *Phyllanthus phillyreifolius* var. *commersonii* Müll. Arg: an unexplored endemic species from Mauritius. Food Research International. https://doi.org/10.1016/j.foodres.2018.10.075.

National Parks and Conservation Services. n.d. Black River Gorges National Park Management Plan 94.

Poullain, C., Girard-Valenciennes, E., Smadja, J., 2004. Plants from reunion island: evaluation of their free radical scavenging and antioxidant activities. Journal of Ethnopharmacology 95, 19–26. https://doi.org/10.1016/j.jep.2004.05.023.

Pynee, K.B., Dubuisson, J.-Y., Hennequin, S., 2013. Flora diversity richness of mount bar Le Duc Volcanic crater (Ripailles Hill), Nouvelle Découverte, Mauritius. Cahiers scientifiques de l'océan Indien occidental 4.

Plantago longissima

Bianca Fibrich, Namrita Lall

Department of Plant and Soil Sciences, University of Pretoria, Pretoria, Gauteng, South Africa

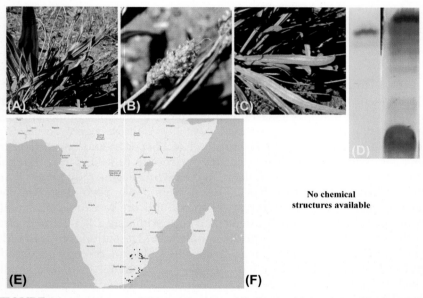

No chemical
structures available

FIGURE 34   Aerial parts of *Plantago longissima* (A), flower of *P. longissima* (B), closer look at the leaves of *P. longissima* (C), TLC chromatogram, Lane 1; *P. longissima* extract pre vanillin spray, Lane 2; *P. longissima* extract post vanillin spray (D), distribution of *P. longissima* in sub-Saharan Africa (GBIF, 2018) (E), no chemical compounds have been reported (F).

Underexplored Medicinal Plants from Sub-Saharan Africa
https://doi.org/10.1016/B978-0-12-816814-1.00034-X

223

1. General description

1.1 Botanical nomenclature

Plantago longissima Decne
Synonyms: *Plantago longissima* Decne. var. *burkei* Pilg., *Plantago longissima* Decne. var. *densiuscula* Pilg

1.2 Botanical family

Plantaginaceae

1.3 Vernacular names

Lamb's tongue (English)
Oorpynwortel (Afrikaans)

2. Botanical description

The Plantaginaceae family comprises of only three genera, of which *Plantago* encompasses over 250 species of perennial or annual herbs with simple leaves that may be arranged in a basal rosette or cauline, spirally with parallel venation (in perennials). *Plantago* is the only genus occurring in southern Africa, and *P. longissima* is 1 of 12 species and one variety in this genus. One inflorescence occurs per rosette (0.4−1.12 m in length) consisting of a dense to lax spike with the peduncle generally longer than the inflorescence (0.15−0.5 m). The flowers have been described as bearing glabrous bracts with acute apices and are bisexual and small. Four deltoid corolla lobes are acute and approximately 2 × 1.2 mm in size with four stamens inserted into the corolla tube. The superior ovary holds two to four loculus each with an ovule and a filiform, often overexerted, style. The fruit occurs as a circumscissile capsule with two to four small, black to dark brown, rounded tetrahedral shaped seeds (approximately 0.6−0.8 mm) per ellipsoid capsule (3 × 1.5 mm) with a hilum at the apex. This is one of the distinguishing features between *P. longissima* and *P. major* (with which it is often confused), as the latter bears more seeds per capsule. Winged, acute, elliptical lobes ±2.5−1 mm in size form the calyx. The narrow leaves are elliptical, ovate, or obovate (±190−175 × 45−150 mm), glabrous with scattered isolated hairs and dry to a brown or black color, a second distinguishing characteristic from *P. major* which dries to an olive-green color. Leaves are often found on woolly bracts and have a flattened petiole 50−400 mm in length. The imbricate calyx has four membranous lobes (Glen, 1998).

3. Distribution

Plantago longissima is endemic to the Eastern Cape, Gauteng, Northern Province, Mpumalanga, and Kwa-Zulu Natal regions of South Africa as well as Swaziland.

4. Ethnobotanical usage

No ethnomedicinal uses have been recorded for *P. longissima*; however, *P. major*, a member of the genus with which it is often confused, has been traditionally reported for the treatment of diseases related to the skin, digestive organs, circulation, pain and inflammation, respiratory ailments, reproduction, and for cancer (Samuelsen, 2000).

5. Phytochemical constituents

No compounds have been reported for this species.

6. TLC fingerprinting of plant extract

For the separation of compounds present within *P. longissima*, 2 mg of the ethanolic extract was weighed out and dissolved in 200 µL ethanol. The separation of compounds present within the crude extract of *P. longissima* was observed using silica gel 60 F254 thin layer chromatography (TLC) plates. The plates were cut to size and, using a soft pencil, a line was drawn 1 cm from both the bottom and top of the plate. On the bottom line, samples were spotted approximately 1 cm apart using a capillary. The spots were allowed to dry completely and the TLC plate was placed in a TLC chamber containing the eluent. Before the addition of the TLC plate, the chamber was left briefly to allow the mobile phase to totally saturate the chamber. 10 mL of eluent (7:3 dichloromethane: methanol) was used. The samples were then allowed to separate until the solvent front reaches the line drawn at the top of the TLC plate. The plate was observed under ultraviolet light (long and short wavelength), followed by spraying with freshly prepared vanillin/sulfuric acid (2%) to detect the bands on the TLC plate.

7. Pharmacological properties

Information surrounding pharmacological or traditional applications of *P. longissima* is minimal. However, it was investigated for its antibacterial activity against methicillin-sensitive *S. aureus* (Heyman et al., 2009).

7.1 Antibacterial activity

Root material was collected from farms in the Northern and northeast regions of Kwa-Zulu Natal in and authenticated at the HGWJ Schweickerdt herbarium at the University of Pretoria. The dried material was extracted using ethanol, filtered and concentrated. The extract showed no significant antibacterial activity against methicillin-sensitive *Staphylococcus aureus*, a superbug responsible for causing a wide range of infections including pneumonia, mastitis, meningitis, urinary tract infection, as well as postoperational infections. The minimum inhibitory concentration was found to be 12.5 mg/mL, while the minimum bactericidal concentration was more than 12 mg/mL (Heyman et al., 2009).

8. Additional Information

8.1 Therapeutic (proposed) usage

Antibacterial

8.2 Safety data

Not available

8.3 Trade information

Not threatened, not endangered, and abundant

8.4 Dosage

Not available

References

GBIF, 2018. *Plantago Longissima* Decne. In GBIF Secretariat (2017). GBIF Backbone Taxonomy. Checklist dataset. https://doi.org/10.15468/39omei.

Glen, H.F., 1998. FSA contributions 12: plantaginaceae. Bothalia 28, 151–157.

Heyman, H.M., Hussein, A.A., Meyer, J.J.M., Lall, N., 2009. Antibacterial activity of South African medicinal plants against methicillin resistant *Staphylococcus aureus*. Pharmaceutical Biology 47, 67–71. https://doi.org/10.1080/13880200802434096.

Plantago longissima Decne Collected from the Rehabilitated Wetland at the University of Pretoria Experimental Farm, November 2016 (Photocredit: Bianca Fibrich).

Samuelsen, A.B., 2000. The traditional uses, chemical constituents and biological activities of *Plantago major* L. A review. Journal of Ethnopharmacology 71, 1—21. https://doi.org/10.1016/S0378-8741(00)00212-9.

Further reading

Cholo, F., Foden, W., 2006. *Plantago Longissima* Decne. National Assessment: Red List of South African Plants Version 2017.1.

Plectranthus ecklonii

Isa A. Lambrechts, Namrita Lall

Department of Plant and Soil Sciences, University of Pretoria, Pretoria, Gauteng, South Africa

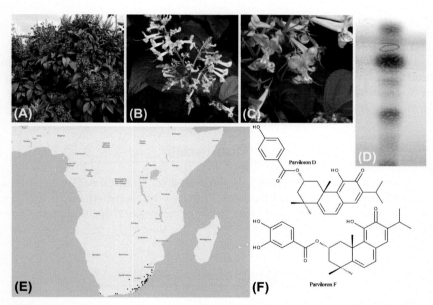

FIGURE 35 Aerial plant parts of *Plectranthus ecklonii* (Wildflowernursery, 2018) (A), flowers of *P. ecklonii* (JMK. 2013a) (B), closer view of the flowers (JMK, 2013b) (C), TLC chromatogram, fingerprint of *P. ecklonii* extract (D), distribution of *P. ecklonii* in sub-Saharan Africa (GBIF, 2018) (E), chemical structures of parviloron D and F (F).

1. General description

1.1 Botanical nomenclature

Plectranthus ecklonii Benth

1.2 Botanical family

Lamiaceae

1.3 Vernacular names

Spur flower (English)
Grootspoorsalie, Persmuishondblaar (Afrikaans)

2. Botanical description

Plectranthus ecklonii is a fast-growing shrub of 1—2 m. The squire stem has tufts of purple hair along the nodes, and the large leaves are arranged in opposite pairs along the stem. In autumn, from March to May, blue, white, or pink flowers can be seen on the plants (Van Jaarsveld, 2011).

3. Distribution

Plectranthus ecklonii is widely distributed in Australia, Mexico, New Zealand, South Africa, and the United States. In South Africa, *P. ecklonii* can be found growing from the Eastern Cape to Mpumalanga (Van Jaarsveld, 2011).

4. Ethnobotanical usage

The aqueous extract of *P. ecklonii* is traditionally used to treat inflammation and as an antifungal agent. In South Africa, it is also traditionally used to treat nausea, vomiting, stomach aches, and meningitis. The leaves are used to treat coughs, chest complaints, and tuberculosis. In Zimbabwe, the aerial parts of the plant are used to treat skin hyperpigmentation and other skin-related diseases (Figueiredo et al., 2010; Nyila et al., 2009). *P. ecklonii* can be used to treat headaches and hay fever. The essential oil of the leaves has been reported to be effective in treating skin infections due to its antibacterial and antifungal properties (Rice et al., 2011).

5. Phytochemical constituents

Two abietane compounds, parvifloron D and parvifloron F, have previously been isolated from the leaves of an ethyl acetate extract and a dichloromethane extract of *P. ecklonii*. Rosmarinic acid has previously been isolated from an aqueous leaf extract of *P. ecklonii* (Falé et al., 2009; Rijo et al., 2013).

6. TLC fingerprinting of plant extract

For observing the separation of compounds from *P. ecklonii*, 2 mg of the ethanolic extract was weighed out and dissolved in 200 μL ethanol. For the thin layer chromatography (TLC) analysis of *P. ecklonii* crude extract, silica gel 60 F254 TLC plates were used to observe the separation of the compounds present within the extract. Plate markings were made with a soft pencil and glass capillaries were used to spot the samples onto the TLC plate. The spot was left to dry completely before placing the plate in a TLC tank which contained 10 mL eluent 9.5:0.5 dichloromethane (DCM): methanol as the solvent system. The samples were allowed to separate until the solvent system reached 1 cm from the top of the TLC plate. The plate was observed under ultraviolet light (long and short wavelength), followed by spraying with freshly prepared vanillin/sulfuric acid (2%) to detect the bands on the TLC plate.

7. Pharmacological properties

7.1 Antibacterial, antityrosinase, and cytotoxicity of crude extract and isolated constituents

The leaves of *P. ecklonii* were collected in Pretoria, South Africa. From the leaves obtained, an ethyl acetate crude extract was prepared. The crude extract was subjected to silica gel column chromatography using hexane/ethyl acetate mixtures of increasing polarity. Five fractions were isolated and tested against *Listeria monocytogenes* (LMG 21263). Two of the five fractions had noteworthy activity with minimum inhibitory concentrations (MICs) of 125 μg/mL and 62.5 μg/mL. Parvifloron D and parvifloron F were isolated from the two active fractions. Parvifloron D and parvifloron F had noteworthy antibacterial activity against *L. monocytogenes* with MIC values of 15.6 μg/mL and 31.2 μg/mL, respectively. Parvifloron F was found to moderately inhibit *Mycobacterium tuberculosis* with an MIC of 95 μg/mL. The crude extract of *P. ecklonii* displayed moderate antibacterial activity against *L. monocytogenes* and exhibited an MIC of 500 µg/mL. *P. ecklonii* crude extract and two active compounds displayed noteworthy antibacterial activities against a range of gram-positive and gram-negative bacteria. The antibacterial activity observed could be linked to the traditional usage of the plant. The crude extract of *P. ecklonii* against the tyrosinase enzyme exhibited a 50% inhibitory concentration (IC_{50}) of 61.7 ± 2.7 µg/mL (Nyila et al., 2009).

7.2 Antiacetylcholinesterase and antioxidant activity

The leaves of *P. ecklonii* were collected during spring (March—June) 2006 in Lisbon, Portugal. Aqueous leaf extracts were prepared as either a decoction or an infusion. *P. ecklonii* infusion and decoction displayed moderate acetylcholinesterase (AChE) inhibition with IC_{50} values of 46.7% and 62.8%, respectively. The antioxidant activity of *P. ecklonii* was measured by the diphenylpicrylhydrazyl (DPPH) and β-carotene/linoleic acid methods. *P. ecklonii* infusion and decoction inhibited the DPPH free radical at IC_{50} of 2.4 ± 0.1 µg/mL and 3.8 ± 0.1 µg/mL, respectively. The opposite was observed for the β-carotene—linoleic acid test compared with the positive control, 2,6-di-tert-butyl-4-hydroxytoluene. The infusion and decoction of *P. ecklonii* displayed IC_{50} values of 142.1 ± 8.0 µg/mL and 109.0 ± 3.1 µg/mL, respectively, for the β-carotene—linoleic acid test (Falé et al., 2009).

7.3 Glucosyltransferase activity and biofilm formation of *Streptococcus sobrinus* and *Streptococcus mutans*

The leaves of *P. ecklonii* were collected in the summer of 2008 in Lisbon, Portugal. A decoction was made with distilled water from the leaves. The aqueous extract of *P. ecklonii* demonstrated antimicrobial activity against *Streptococcus sobrinus* and *Streptococcus mutans* with MIC values of 4.7 mg/mL and 5.0 mg/mL, respectively. *P. ecklonii* displayed inhibition of the biofilm formation at IC_{50} values of 1.0 ± 0.2 mg/mL and 2.7 ± 0.6 mg/mL against *S. sobrinus* and *S. mutans*, respectively. The inhibition of glucosyltransferase of *S. sobrinus* and *S. mutants* involved in biofilm formation was evaluated. The decoction was found to inhibit glucosyltransferase of *S. sobrinus* and *S. mutants* at IC_{50} values of 1.2 ± 0.1 mg/mL and 1.6 ± 0.0 mg/mL (Figueiredo et al., 2010).

8. Additional information

8.1 Therapeutic (proposed) usage

Antibacterial, antibiofilm, and skin hyperpigmentation

8.2 Safety data

The cytotoxicity of the crude extract, parvifloron D and parvifloron F, was determined on a monkey kidney Vero cell lines. Parvifloron D and parvifloron F were found to be toxic on the cell lines. The crude extract displayed moderate toxicity with an IC_{50} value of 30.13 µg/mL (Nyila et al., 2009).

8.3 Trade information

Not threatened, not endangered, and abundant

8.4 Dosage

Not available

References

Falé, P.L., Borges, C., Madeira, P.J.A., Ascensão, L., Araújo, M.E.M., Florêncio, M.H., Serralheiro, M.L.M., 2009. Rosmarinic acid, scutellarein 4′-methyl ether 7-O-glucuronide and (16S)-coleon E are the main compounds responsible for the antiacetylcholinesterase and antioxidant activity in herbal tea of *Plectranthus barbatus* ("falso boldo"). Food Chemistry 114, 798−805.

Figueiredo, N.L., de Aguiar, Sara Raquel, M.M., Falé, P.L., Ascensão, L., Serralheiro, M.L.M., Lino, A.R.L., 2010. The inhibitory effect of *Plectranthus barbatus* and *Plectranthus ecklonii* leaves on the viability, glucosyltransferase activity and biofilm formation of *Streptococcus sobrinus* and *Streptococcus mutans*. Food Chemistry 119, 664−668.

GBIF, 2018. *Plectranthus ecklonii* Benth. In: GBIF Secretariat (2017). GBIF Backbone Taxonomy. Checklist dataset. https://doi.org/10.15468/39omei.

JMK, 2013a. *Plectranthus ecklonii* 'Erma'. Wikimedia commons. C.C. Available online: https://commons.wikimedia.org/wiki/File:Plectranthus_ecklonii,_b,_Manie_van_der_Schijff_BT.jpg. (CC BY-SA 3.0).

JMK, 2013b. *Plectranthus ecklonii* 'Erma'. Wikimedia commons. C.C. Available online: https://commons.wikimedia.org/wiki/File:Plectranthus_ecklonii,_a,_Manie_van_der_Schijff_BT.jpg. (CC BY-SA 3.0).

Nyila, M.A., Leonard, C.M., Hussein, A.A., Lall, N., 2009. Bioactivities of *Plectranthus ecklonii* constituents. Natural product communications 4, 1177−1180.

Rice, L., Brits, G., Potgieter, C., Van Staden, J., 2011. *Plectranthus*: a plant for the future? South African Journal of Botany 77, 947−959.

Rijo, P., Faustino, C., Simões, M.F., 2013. Antimicrobial natural products from *Plectranthus* plants. Microbial pathogens and strategies for combating them: Science, Technology and Education 2, 13.

Van Jaarsveld, E., 2011. *Plectranthus ecklonii* Benth. http://www.plantzafrica.com/plantnop/plectranecklon.htm 2014.

Wildflowernursery, 2018. Available online: https://wildflowernursery.co.za/indigenous-plant-database/plectranthus-ecklonii/.

Plectranthus neochilus

Isa A. Lambrechts, Namrita Lall

Department of Plant and Soil Sciences, University of Pretoria, Pretoria, Gauteng, South Africa

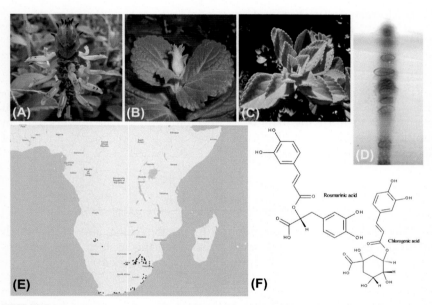

FIGURE 36   Flower of *Plectranthus neochilus* (Kenraiz, 2017) (A), closer view of the leaves of *P. neochilus* (Salicyna, 2017) (B), leaves of *P. neochilus* (JMK, 2012) (C), TLC chromatogram, fingerprint of *P. neochilus* extract (D), distribution of *P. neochilus* in sub-Saharan Africa (GBIF, 2018) (E), chemical structures of rosmarinic acid and chlorogenic acid (F).

1. General description

1.1 Botanical nomenclature

Plectranthus neochilus Schltr

1.2 Botanical family

Lamiaceae

1.3 Vernacular names

Blue Coleus or Lobster Flower (English)
Muskietbossie (Afrikaans)
Ibozane (Zulu)
Boldo-rasteiro (Portuguese)

2. Botanical description

Plectranthus neochilus is a small aromatic herb with succulent gray-green leaves which grows up to 0.5 m high and 1.5 m wide. From September to April, the plant bears deep blue and purple flowers with an unpleasant scent. *P. neochilus* can be used as a ground cover as it is robust and grows fast (Mukoma, 2004).

3. Distribution

Plectranthus neochilus is endemic to South Africa and Namibia. It naturally grows in sandy to rocky areas from the Eastern Cape to Limpopo, KwaZulu-Natal, and Mpumalanga (Mukoma, 2004).

4. Ethnobotanical usage

Plectranthus neochilus is traditionally used in Brazil as a folk medicine. An infusion or aqueous extract from the fresh leaves are used to treat skin infections, disturbed digestion, hepatic insufficiency, dyspepsia, and respiratory ailments (Caixeta et al., 2011; Duarte and Lopes, 2007). In South Africa, *P. neochilus* is used by the Zulu communities in KwaZulu-Natal to treat respiratory diseases with a decoction made from the leaves (York et al., 2011).

5. Phytochemical constituents

Two compounds have previously been isolated from the leaves of *P. neochilus*: chlorogenic acid and rosmarinic acid (Rijo et al., 2014).

The monoterpenoids were found to be 77% of the essential oil. The major constituents of the oils were citronellol that is 29.0%, citronellyl formate which contributes 11.0%, linalool 9.8%, and isomethone that is 9.2% of the monoterpenoids. The main sesquiterpene was found to be citronellyl propionate that contributed 3.4% to the sesquiterpenes (Lawal et al., 2010).

The aerial parts of *P. neochilus* were collected during the vegetative and flowering phases in Lisbon, Portugal. The essential oil was isolated from fresh plant material by hydrodistillation for 3 h, using a Clevenger-type apparatus. The essential oil of *P. neochilus* was analyzed with gas chromatography—mass spectrometry (GCMS), and the major volatile components were found to be α-terpenyl acetate (traces—48%), α-thujone (2%—28%), β-caryophyllene (2%—28%), β-pinene (1%—25%), and α-pinene (1%—19%). However, *P. neochilus* from South Africa was mentioned to predominantly contain monoterpenes (78%), of which citronellol (29%), citronellyl formate (11%), linalool (10%), and isomenthone (9%) were the major compounds present in the oil. The quantitative and qualitative differences in the essential oil composition between South Africa and Portugal were attributed to geographic, climatic, and genetic factors (Mota et al., 2014).

6. TLC fingerprinting of plant extract

For observing the separation of compounds from *P. neochilus*, 2 mg of the ethanolic extract was weighed out and dissolved in 200 μL ethanol. For the thin layer chromatography (TLC) analysis of *P. neochilus* crude extract, silica gel 60 F254 TLC plates were used to observe the separation of the compounds present within the extract. Plate markings were made with a soft pencil, and glass capillaries were used to spot the samples onto the TLC plate. The spot was left to dry completely before placing the plate in a TLC tank which contained 10 mL eluent 9.5:0.5 dichloromethane (DCM): methanol as the solvent system. The sample was allowed to separate until the solvent system reached 1 cm from the top of the TLC plate. The plate was observed under ultraviolet light (long and short wavelength), followed by spraying with freshly prepared vanillin/sulfuric acid (2%) to detect the bands on the TLC plate.

7. Pharmacological properties

Plectranthus neochilus extract and essential oil have not been extensively researched for their pharmacological properties. This provides the potential for further research.

7.1 Antioxidant of essential oils

The essential oil of *P. neochilus* was tested for its antioxidant activity using the diphenylpicrylhydrazyl (DPPH) radical scavenging assay and the thiobarbituric acid reactive substances (TBARS) assay for checking the capacity for preventing lipid oxidation. *P. neochilus* essential oil was found to inhibit 60% lipid oxidation at 1000 mg/L and to have moderate free radical scavenging ability (Mota et al., 2014).

7.2 Anticancer activity

Aerial parts of *P. neochilus* were collected in January 2011 from Campus Universitario Darcy Ribeiro, Universidade de Brasília. Ethanol and hexane crude extracts were made using a passive maceration technique. The crude hexane extract (PNH) was submitted to silica gel 60 G, and five fractions were obtained. The crude ethanol extract (PNE) was submitted to liquid—liquid partition and solvent extraction and four fractions were obtained. Cytotoxicity studies were carried out with the crude extracts and the fractions obtained. Tongue squamous cell carcinoma (SCC-25) and hypopharyngeal carcinoma (FaDu) were used as test cell lines. Human keratinocyte cell line (HaCaT) and a fibroblast cell line (L929) served as the control cell lines. A PNH hexane fraction caused low cell viability in tongue squamous cell carcinoma (SCC-25) of 17% and cell viability of 50% and higher in FaDu, HaCaT, and L929 cell lines. The PNH fraction displayed a 50% cytotoxic concentration (CC_{50}) of 274.2 µg/mL on the SCC-25 cell line. The CC_{50} on the remaining cell lines were 540.9 µg/mL, 550 µg/mL, and 762.1 µg/mL for FaDu, L929, and HaCaT cell lines, respectively. The tumor specificity index (TSI) was determined and found to be HaCat/FaDu; 1.40, L929/FaDu; 1.01, HaCat/SCC-25; 2.77, and L929/SCC-25; 2.00. It was concluded that the TSIs indicated the specificity of the PNH fraction for tongue carcinoma cells when compared with the control cell lines (Borges et al., 2016).

7.3 Antibacterial activity

A moderate antibacterial activity of *P. neochilus* essential oil was observed against gram-positive bacteria. The essential oil from the vegetative phase tested against *Bacillus cereus* showed inhibition of the gram-positive bacteria that was not significantly different ($P < .05$) from the positive antibiotic control (Mota et al., 2014).

In another study, the plant material was collected from Lisbon, Portugal. The dried plant material was powdered, submerged in acetone, and placed in an ultrasonic bath for 2 h at room temperature. The antibacterial activity of *P. neochilus* was performed using the microplate broth microdilution method. The antimicrobial activity of the ultrasound acetone extract was found to inhibit the gram-positive bacteria *Mycobacterium smegmatis* (American type culture collection (ATCC) 607) at a minimum inhibitory concentration (MIC) of 15.62 µg/mL. Moderate antibacterial activity was observed for the ultrasound acetone extract of *P. neochilus* against the gram-positive bacteria, *Bacillus subtilis* (ATCC 6633) and *Staphylococcus epidermidis* (ATCC 12228) at MICs of 125 µg/mL and 62.5 µg/mL, respectively (Pereira et al., 2015).

7.4 Antidiabetic activity

The leaves of *P. neochilus* were collected in Brazil. Crude extracts were obtained by either submerging dried plant material in hexane for 7 days or an infusion was made from the leaves with distilled water. *P. neochilus* hexane and aqueous extracts inhibited α-glucosidase at 30.63 µg/mL and 48.11 µg/mL, respectively (De Souza et al., 2012).

8. Additional information

8.1 Therapeutic (proposed) usage

Antibacterial, antidiabetic, antituberculosis, and anticancer

8.2 Safety data

Cytotoxicity studies were carried out with the hexane and ethanol crude extracts and the fractions obtained from *P. neochilus*. Tongue squamous cell carcinoma (SCC-25) and hypopharyngeal carcinoma (FaDu) were used as test cell lines. Human keratinocyte cell line (HaCaT) and a fibroblast cell line (L929) served as the control cell lines. A hexane extract caused low cell viability in tongue squamous cell carcinoma (SCC-25) of 17% and cell viability of 50% and higher in FaDu, HaCaT, and L929 cell lines. The hexane fraction displayed a 50% cytotoxic concentration (CC_{50}) of 274.2 µg/mL on the SCC-25 cell line. The CC_{50} on the remaining cell lines were 540.9 µg/mL, 550 µg/mL, and 762.1 µg/mL for FaDu, L929, and HaCaT cell lines, respectively (Borges et al., 2016).

8.3 Trade information

Not threatened, not endangered, and abundant

8.4 Dosage

Not available

References

Borges, G.A., Ferreira, J.F., Elias, S.T., Guerra, E.N.S., Silveira, D., Simeoni, L.A., 2016. Cytotoxic effect of *Plectranthus neochilus* extracts in head and neck carcinoma cell lines. African Journal of Pharmacy and Pharmacology 10, 157–163.

Caixeta, S.C., Magalhaes, L.G., de Melo, N.I., Wakabayashi, K.A., de P Aguiar, G., de P Aguiar, D., Mantovani, A.L., Alves, J.M., Oliveira, P.F., Tavares, D.C., 2011. Chemical composition and in vitro schistosomicidal activity of the essential oil of *Plectranthus neochilus* grown in Southeast Brazil. Chemistry and Biodiversity 8, 2149–2157.

De Souza, P.M., de Sales, P.M., Simeoni, L.A., Silva, E.C., Silveira, D., de Oliveira Magalhães, P., 2012. Inhibitory activity of α-amylase and α-glucosidase by plant extracts from the Brazilian cerrado. Planta Medica 78, 393–399.

Duarte, M.d.R., Lopes, J.F., 2007. Stem and leaf anatomy of *Plectranthus neochilus* Schltr. Lamiaceae. Revista Brasileira de Farmacognosia 17, 549–556.

GBIF, 2018. *Plectranthus neochilus* Schltr. In GBIF Secretariat (2017). GBIF Backbone Taxonomy. Checklist dataset. https://doi.org/10.15468/39omei.

JMK, 2012. *Plectranthus neochilus* Schltr. In: Wikimedia Commons. C.C. Available online: https://commons.wikimedia.org/wiki/File:Plectranthus_neochilus,_Pretoria.jpg.

Kenraiz, K.Z., 2017. *Plectranthus neochilus* Schltr. In: Wikimedia Commons. C.C. Available from: https://commons.wikimedia.org/wiki/File:Plectranthus_neochilus_kz2.jpg. (CC BY-SA 4.0).

Lawal, O., Hutchings, A., Oyedeji, O., 2010. Chemical composition of the leaf oil of *Plectranthus neochilus* Schltr. Journal of Essential Oil Research 22, 546–547.

Mota, L., Figueiredo, A.C., Pedro, L.G., Barroso, J.G., Miguel, M.G., Faleiro, M.L., Ascensao, L., 2014. Volatile-oils composition, and bioactivity of the essential oils of *Plectranthus barbatus*, *P. neochilus*, and *P. ornatus* grown in Portugal. Chemistry and Biodiversity 11, 719–732.

Mukoma, T., 2004. PlantZafrica. http://www.plantzafrica.com/plantnop/plectranneochil.htm 2014.

Pereira, M., Matias, D., Pereira, F., Reis, C.P., Simões, M.F., Rijo, P., 2015. Antimicrobial Screening of *Plectranthus madagascariensis* and *P. neochilus* Extracts.

Rijo, P., Matias, D., Fernandes, A.S., Simões, M.F., Nicolai, M., Reis, C.P., 2014. Antimicrobial plant extracts encapsulated into polymeric beads for potential application on the skin. Polymers 6, 479–490.

Salicyna, 2017. *Plectranthus neochilus* Schltr. In: Wikimedia Commons. C.C. Available from: https://commons.wikimedia.org/wiki/File:Plectranthus_neochilus_2017-05-31_2252.jpg.

York, T., De Wet, H., Van Vuuren, S., 2011. Plants used for treating respiratory infections in rural Maputaland, KwaZulu-Natal, South Africa. Journal of Ethnopharmacology 135, 696–710.

Rapanea melanophloeos

Analike Blom van Staden, Namrita Lall

Department of Plant and Soil Sciences, University of Pretoria, Pretoria, Gauteng, South Africa

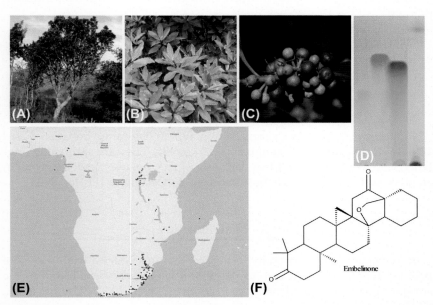

FIGURE 37 *Rapanea melanophloeos* (JMK, 2012) (A), close view of the leaves of *R. melanophloeos* (Shawka, 2010) (B), fruits of *R. melanophloeos* (Venter, 2015) (C), TLC chromatogram, Lane 1; myricetin, Lane 2; quercetin, Lane 3; catechin, Lane 4; *R. melanophloeos* extract (D), distribution of *R. melanophloeos* in sub-Saharan Africa (GBIF, 2018) (E), chemical structure of embelinone (F).

1. General description

1.1 Botanical nomenclature

Rapanea melanophloeos (L.) Mez

1.2 Botanical family

Myrsinaceae

1.3 Vernacular names

Cape beech (English)
Kaapse boekenhout (Afrikaans)
Mudonera, mudongera, mufuro, mukwiramakoko, murwiti, mutomo (Shona)
iGcolo, udzilidzili (Siswati)
IsiCalabi, umaPhipha, iKhubalwane, isiQalaba sehlati (Zulu)
isiQwane sehlati (Xhosa)

2. Botanical description

R. melanophloeos is an evergreen tree, which can range between 4 and 18 m high. The leaves are tough and dark green. They are simple, oblong-lanceolate, and have reddish leafstalks. The yellow flowers grow in clusters and are observable between June to December (Porter, 2005).

3. Distribution

R. melanophloeos is generally located in Southern Africa from the Cape provinces of South Africa up to Zambia. *R. melanophloeos* is found in the coastal areas and the Afromontane region (Porter, 2005; Schmidt et al., 2002).

4. Ethnobotanical usage

Decoctions made from the root, bark, and fruits of *R. melanophloeos* are used as an anthelmintic in humans and livestock. The Sabaots in Kopsiro uses *R. melanophloeos'* bark for stomach aches by drinking an extract after boiling it in water. Additively, *R. melanophloeos* is used for general body aches in Swaziland. Other medicinal uses include for respiratory problems, heart complaints, fever, and muscle pains. Communities in Kenya chew berries and swallow the seeds to remove intestinal worms, whereas berries mixed with milk are drunk for its purgative and anthelmintic action (Amuka et al., 2014; Amusan et al., 2002; Beentje et al., 1994; Kokwaro, 1993; Okello et al., 2010; Schmidt et al., 2002).

5. Phytochemical constituents

Compounds and phytochemical groups previously identified from *R. melanophloeos* are saponins, triterpenes, tannins, flavonoids, benzoquinones, alkyl- and alkenylresorcinols, terpeno-p-hydroxy-benzoic acid, embelin, rapanone, and cardiac glycosides. Embelinine and schimperinone have been isolated from *R. melanophloeos* by Machocho et al. in 2003 (Amenya et al., 2014; Githiori et al., 2002; Gwala, 2011; Machocho et al., 2003; Mashimbye, 1993; Ohtani et al., 1993).

6. TLC fingerprinting of plant extract

For observing the separation of the compounds from *R. melanophloeos*, 2 mg of the ethanolic extract was weighed out and dissolved in 200 µL ethanol. For the standards, myricetin, quercetin, and catechin (Sigma-Aldrich Co. St Louis, MO, USA) were weighed out in the same manner as the extract and dissolved in 600 µL of ethanol. For the thin layer chromatography (TLC) analysis of *R. melanophloeos* crude extract, silica gel 60 F254 TLC plates were used to observe the separation of the compounds present within the extract. Plate markings were made with a soft pencil, and glass capillaries were used to spot the samples onto the TLC plate. Reference standards, myricetin, quercetin, and catechin, were spotted to determine whether it was present in the extract. The spots were left to dry completely before placing the plate in a TLC tank which contained 10 mL eluent 9:1 dichloromethane: methanol as the solvent system. The plate was observed under ultraviolet light (long and short wavelength), followed by spraying with freshly prepared vanillin/sulfuric acid (2%) to detect the bands on the TLC plate.

7. Pharmacological properties

R. melanophloeos has been moderately researched for its in vitro and in vivo medicinal properties. Although it is a widely distributed and well-known plant in South Africa, there is still an opportunity for research and development regarding this plant.

7.1 Antibacterial and antifungal activity

In one study, the leaves and stems of *R. melanophloeos* were collected (February to March 2015) from the Manie van der Schijff botanical garden of the University of Pretoria. An ethanolic extract was prepared. The ethanol crude extract showed growth inhibitory activity against *Propionibacterium acnes*, American type culture collection (ATCC) 6919 and ATCC 11827 strains, with a minimum inhibitory concentration of 125 µg/mL (Blom van Staden and lall, 2018). A bactericidal effect was observed for *R. melanophloeos* at >250 µg/mL and 125 µg/mL for ATCC 11827 and ATCC 6919 strains, respectively. *R. melanophloeos* has shown antifungal activity against *Cladosporium cucumerinum* (Ohtani et al., 1993).

7.2 Anthelmintic activity

R. melanophloeos was evaluated for its activity against *Heligmosomoides polygyrus*. The effect on both the total worm count (TWC) and percentage fecal egg (FEC) reduction was determined. The mice treated with *R. melanophloeos* led to a statistically significant reduction in FEC, but did not significantly reduce the numbers of *H. polygyrus* (Githiori et al., 2002).

7.3 Phytochemical content and antioxidants

The leaf and stem ethanol extracts of *R. melanophloeos*, obtained from the University of Pretoria, were screened for its phytochemical constituents. The extract was tested for total tannins, saponins, alkaloids, cardiac glycosides, terpenes, flavonoids, and total phenolics. The ethanol extracts of *R. melanophloeos* showed the presence of tannins, saponins, alkaloids, cardiac glycosides, terpenes, and total phenolics. The hexane, chloroform, ethyl acetate, methanol, and water extracts of *R. melanophloeos* exhibited antioxidant activity against diphenylpicrylhydrazyl (DPPH) with 50% inhibitory concentration (IC_{50}) values of 3.05 mg/mL, 4.32 mg/mL, 4.83 mg/mL, 3.31 mg/mL, and 3.89 mg/mL, respectively. The same extracts of *R. melanophloeos* also exhibited antioxidant activity against 2,2'-azinobis-3-ethylbenzothiazoline-6-sulfonic acid (ABTS) with IC_{50} values of 3.31 mg/mL, 3.22 mg/mL, 2.79 mg/mL, 1.44 mg/mL, and >5 mg/mL, respectively. The hexane, chloroform, ethyl acetate, methanol, and water extracts of *R. melanophloeos* exhibited chelating activity against Fe^{2+} with IC_{50} values of 4.23 mg/mL, 3.55 mg/mL, 0.93 mg/mL, 3.22 mg/mL, and >5 mg/mL, respectively (Mosa et al., 2011).

8. Additional information

8.1 Therapeutic (proposed) usage

Antibacterial and anthelmintic

8.2 Safety data

Not available

8.3 Trade information

Declining

8.4 Dosage

Not available

References

Amenya, H.Z., Gathumbi, P.K., Mbaria, J.M., Thaiyah, A.G., Thoithi, G.N., 2014. Sub-acute toxicity of the chloroformic extract of *Rapanea melanophloeos* (L.) Mez in rats. Journal of Ethnopharmacology 154 (3), 593–599.

Amuka, O., Mbugua, P.K., Okemo, P.O., 2014. Ethnobotanical survey of selected medicinal plants used by the Ogiek communities in Kenya against microbial infections. Ethnobotany Research and Applications 12, 627–641.

Amusan, O.O., Dlamini, P.S., Msonthi, J.D., Makhubu, L.P., 2002. Some herbal remedies from Manzini region of Swaziland. Journal of Ethnopharmacology 79 (1), 109–112.

Beentje, H., Adamson, J., Bhanderi, D., 1994. Kenya trees, shrubs, and lianas. In: National Museums of Kenya.

Blom van Staden, A., Lall, N., 2018. Medicinal plants as alternative treatments for progressive macular hypomelanosis. In: Medicinal Plants for Holistic Health and Well-Being, pp. 145–182.

GBIF, 2018. *Rapanea melanophloeos* (L.) Mez. In: GBIF Secretariat (2017). GBIF Backbone Taxonomy. Checklist dataset. https://doi.org/10.15468/39omei. Accessed 30 July 2018.

Githiori, J.B., Höglund, J., Waller, P.J., Baker, R.L., 2002. Anthelmintic activity of preparations derived from *Myrsine africana* and *Rapanea melanophloeos* against the nematode parasite, *Haemonchus contortus*, of sheep. Journal of Ethnopharmacology 80 (2), 187–191.

Gwala, P.E., 2011. The Antiplatelet Aggregation Activity of *Rapanea melanophloeos*-A Zulu Medicinal Plant.

JMK, 2012. Habit of the Cape Beach, Near Louwsburg, KwaZulu-Natal. Available online: https://commons.wikimedia.org/wiki/File:Rapanea_melanophloeos,_habitus,_Louwsburg.jpg (CC BY-SA 3.0). Accessed 30 July 2018.

Kokwaro, J.O., 1993. Medicinal Plants of East Africa. Kenya Literature Bureau, Nairobi, 401pp. ISBN, 9966, 44: 190.

Machocho, A.K., Kiprono, P.C., Grinberg, S., Bittner, S., 2003. Pentacyclic triterpenoids from *Embelia schimperi*. Phytochemistry 62 (4), 573–577.

Mashimbye, M.J., 1993. Chemical constituents of plants native to Venda. University of Natal.

Mosa, R., Lazarus, G., Gwala, P., Oyedeji, A., Opoku, A., 2011. In vitro antiplatelet aggregation, antioxidant and cytotoxic activity of extracts of some Zulu medicinal plants. Journal of Natural Products 4, 136–146.

Ohtani, K., Mavi, S., Hostettmann, K., 1993. Molluscicidal and antifungal triterpenoid saponins from *Rapanea melanophloeos* leaves. Phytochemistry 33 (1), 83–86.

Okello, S., Nyunja, R., Netondo, G.W., Onyango, J.C., 2010. Ethnobotanical study of medicinal plants used by Sabaots of Mt. Elgon Kenya. African Journal of Traditional, Complementary and Alternative Medicines 7, 1.

Porter, H., 2005. *Rapanea melanophloeos*. Plantzafrica. http://www.plantzafrica.com/plantqrs/rapanmelan.htm. Accessed 30 July 2018.

Schmidt, E., Lotter, M., McCleland, W., Burrows, J.E., 2002. Trees and shrubs of Mpumalanga and Kruger national park. Jacana.

Shawka, A., 2010. *Rapanea melanophloeos* Tree. Detail of Foliage. Photo Taken in Cape Town. Available online: https://commons.wikimedia.org/wiki/File:Rapanea_melanophloeos_-_foliage_7.JPG (Public domain). Accessed 30 July 2018.

Venter, 2015. *Rapanea melanophloeos* (L.) Mez — Nature's Valley, Cape Province, South Africa — Fruits in Various Stages of Maturity. Available online: https://commons.wikimedia.org/wiki/File:Rapanea_melanophloeos00.jpg (CC BY-SA 3.0). Accessed 30 July 2018.

Ravenala madagascariensis

Shanoo Suroowan, Fawzi Mahomoodally

Department of Health Sciences, Faculty of Science, University of Mauritius,
Réduit, Mauritius

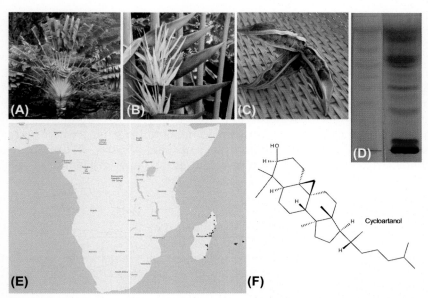

FIGURE 38 Aerial plant parts of *Ravenala madagascariensis* (A), flowers of *R. madagascariensis* (B), seeds of *R. madagascariensis* (Jeffdelonge, 2005) (C), TLC chromatogram, Lane 1; *R. madagascariensis* leaf extract pre vanillin, Lane 2; *R. madagascariensis* leaf extract post vanillin (D), distribution of *R. madagascariensis* in sub-Saharan Africa (GBIF, 2018) (E), chemical structure of cycloartanol (F).

Underexplored Medicinal Plants from Sub-Saharan Africa
https://doi.org/10.1016/B978-0-12-816814-1.00038-7

1. General description

1.1 Botanical nomenclature

Ravenala madagascariensis Sonn

1.2 Botanical family

Strelitziaceae

1.3 Vernacular names

Traveler's tree (English)
Arbre du voyageur
Ravenale (Mauritius)

2. Botanical description

The tree grows as tall as 30—60 feet (9—18 m). The leaves are green, oblong, and have a broad margin pinnate with an evergreen venation of over 36 inches long. The flowers originating from the plant are white/cream/gray, while the fruits occur as hard brown fruits around 5 to 1 inch in length. The fruits do not attract wildlife. Both the fruits and the leaves are nonshowy ("Botanical Journeys Plant Guides" 2008—2010). Further characteristics of the plant can be found in the paper of Handique et al. (2013).

3. Distribution

In Madagascar, *R. madagascariensis* is endemic. It is also widely found in parts of North America, as well as in many tropical and subtropical regions where it is cultivated mostly for its ornamental value (Reyad-ul-Ferdous et al., 2014). *R. madagascariensis* is an invasive plant in Mauritius, continually threatening the native forests.

4. Ethnobotanical usage

Natives in Madagascar employ the plant for its numerous therapeutic applications mostly against diabetes, diarrhea, edema, hypertension, and kidney stones while the seeds are antiseptic Razafindraibe et al. (2013);

Jain and Srivastava (2005). On the other hand, the plant is used for its therapeutic benefits to assuage cough, stomachache, and urine retention (Rabearivony et al., 2015). In Mauritius, a decoction of the heart and leaves is used orally against diabetes. The seeds are also employed against mucous discharge where six seeds of the plant are decocted in one cup of water and administered twice a day for 3 days (Adjanohoun, 1983; Mootoosamy and Mahomoodally, 2014; Suroowan and Mahomoodally, 2016).

5. Phytochemical constituents

The plant is rich in numerous phytochemicals mostly anthraquinones, cardiac glycosides, cyanogenic glycosides, flavonoids, phlobatannins, saponins, steroids, tannins, terpenoids, and triterpenoids (Reyad-ul-Ferdous et al., 2014). The cycloartanol triterpene and (2E, 7R, 11R) phytyl-3, 7, 11, 15-tetramethylhexadec-2-enyl pentadecanoate as well as (24S, 31S)-cycloartan-31, 32-diol have been isolated from the plant (Ramiarantsoa et al., 2014).

6. TLC fingerprinting of plant extract

R. madagascariensis leaves were collected and shed dried. The plant material was ground into a fine powder and extracted using ethanol at a ratio of 1:10 (weight:volume). After 24 h, the extract was filtered and dried using rotary evaporation. Two milligrams of the dried extract was weighed out and dissolved in 1 mL of acetone. For the thin layer chromatography (TLC) analysis of *R. madagascariensis* crude extract, silica gel 60 F254 TLC plates were used to observe the separation of the compounds present within the extract. Plate markings were made with a soft pencil, and glass capillaries were used to spot the samples onto the TLC plate. The spot was left to dry completely before placing the plate in a TLC tank which contained 10 mL eluent 9:1 dichloromethane: methanol as the solvent system. The plate was observed under ultraviolet light (long and short wavelength), followed by spraying with freshly prepared vanillin/sulfuric acid (2%) to detect the bands on the TLC plate.

7. Pharmacological properties

An earlier study showed that the ethanolic and aqueous extracts of the leaves displayed antidiabetic activity in vitro and in vivo rats where diabetes was induced through the administration of alloxan. The leaves have been reported to be hypolipidemic and renoprotective (Priyadarsini et al., 2010). Phytochemicals identified in the plant are known to exert antiasthmatic, -cancer, -diabetic, -diarrheal, -analgesia, cardioprotective, hepatoprotective, and lipid-lowering activities (Reyad-ul-Ferdous et al., 2014).

7.1 Antidiabetic activity

Priyadarsini et al. (2010) investigated the effect on glucose diffusion across the gastrointestinal tract of the ethanol, ethylacetate, and n-Hexane leaf extracts of *R. madagascariensis* in vitro. The concentration of each extract employed was 50 g per liter. The results were compared with the results when no extracts were employed in a similar system. The aqueous and ethanolic extracts demonstrated a significant inhibitory effect on glucose diffusion. The same assay was extended to an in vivo alloxan-induced diabetic rat model, and the concentration of the extracts employed was 200 and 400 mg/kg, by weight. The results demonstrated that both extracts displayed a significant ($P < .001$) antidiabetic activity. The conventional drug, glibenclamide, was employed as the standard reference at a concentration of 10 mg/kg of body weight. The antidiabetic effect displayed by the ethanolic extract was comparable with that exhibited by the standard hence validating the traditional claim of the plant.

7.2 Antimicrobial activity

The ethanolic and n-hexane extract of *R. madagascariensis* was assayed on *Citrobacter freundii*, *Klebsiella pneumoniae* (American type culture collection (ATCC) 13883), *Proteus mirabilis* (ATCC 25933), *Proteus vulgaris*, *Serratia marcescens* (ATCC 39006), and *Shigella flexneri* (ATCC 12022) for their antimicrobial potential. It suppressed the growth of *C. freundii*, *K. pneumoniae*, *P. mirabilis*, *P. vulgaris*, *S. marcescens*, and *S. flexneri* remarkably. The ethanolic extract was most active on *P. mirabilis*, while being least active against *P. vulgaris* with inhibition zones (10.80 ± 0.04 mm) and (4.6 ± 0.01 mm), respectively. On the other hand, the n-hexane extract displayed antimicrobial activity on *K. pneumoniae* and *S. marcescens* solely with 24% inhibition. The highest minimum inhibitory concentration (MIC) was noted for the ethanolic extract (150 mg/mL) against *K. pneumoniae* and *P. vulgaris*, while the lowest MIC recorded for the n-hexane extract (100 mg/mL) was against *S. marcescens* and *K. pneumoniae* for n-hexane extract (Onifade et al., 2015).

Another antimicrobial investigation assayed the aqueous soluble partitionates, carbon tetrachloride, chloroform, crude methanolic, and hexane extracts of the aerial parts of *R. madagascariensis* for disc diffusion assay against *Bacillus cereus*, *B. megaterium*, *B. subtilis*, *Staphylococcus aureus*, and *Sarcina lutea*. The samples exhibited a weak antimicrobial activity with inhibition zones between 2.0 and 9.0 mm (Sharmin et al., 2014).

7.3 Antithrombolytic activity

The antithrombolytic activity of the aqueous soluble partitionates, carbon tetrachloride, chloroform, crude methanolic, and hexane extracts of *R. madagascariensis* was investigated for their antithrombolytic and membrane-stabilizing activities. The methanolic crude leaf extract and aqueous soluble fraction exhibited percentage cloy lysis activity of 45.32 ± 0.82 and 32.67 ± 0.74%, respectively (Chowdhury et al., 2013).

8. Additional information

8.1 Therapeutic (proposed) usage

Antidiabetic, antimicrobial, and antithrombolytic

8.2 Safety data

Not available

8.3 Trade information

Not threatened and not endangered

8.4 Dosage

Not available

References

Adjanohoun, E., 1983. Contribution aux études ethnobotaniques et floristiques à Maurice (Iles Maurice et Rodrigues). Agence de cooperation culturelle et technique.

Botanical Journeys Plant Guides, 2008-2010 (Retrieved Feb 28: 2011). www.botanical-journeys-plant-guides.com.

Chowdhury, S.R., Sharmin, T., Hoque, M., Sumsujjaman, M., Das, M., Nahar, F., 2013. Evaluation of thrombolytic and membrane stabilizing activities of four medicinal plants of Bangladesh. International Journal of Pharmaceutical Sciences and Research 4 (11), 4223.

GBIF, 2018. *Ravenala madagascariensis* Sonn. In GBIF Secretariat (2017). GBIF Backbone Taxonomy. Checklist dataset. https://doi.org/10.15468/39omei.

Handique, L., Parkash, V., Hazarika, A.D., 2013. Phylogeny of *Musa paradisiaca, Ravenala madagascariensis* and *Heliconia rostrata* based on morphological, biochemical, amino acid sequences of rbcl protein and matK DNA sequences. International Journal of Theoretical and Applied Sciences 5, 69−78.

Jain, S.K., Srivastava, S., 2005. Traditional Uses of Some Indian Plants Among Islanders of the Indian Ocean.

Jeffdelonge, 2005. *Ravenala madagascariensis* (Open Fruit with Seeds). Available online: https://upload.wikimedia.org/wikipedia/commons/2/20/Ravenala_madagascariensis2.jpg. (CC BY-SA 1.0).

Mootoosamy, A., Mahomoodally, M.F., 2014. Ethnomedicinal application of native remedies used against diabetes and related complications in Mauritius. Journal of Ethnopharmacology 151 (1), 413−444.

Onifade, A.K., Bello, M.O., Fadipe, D.O., 2015. Bioassay directed fractionation of antibacterial compounds from traveller's tree (*Ravenala madagascariensis* sonnerat) and its phytochemical constituents. International Journal of Bioassays 4 (9), 4299−4304.

Priyadarsini, S.S., Vadivu, R., Jayshree, N., 2010. In vitro and in vivo antidiabetic activity of the leaves of *Ravenala madagascariensis* Sonn., on alloxan induced diabetic rats. Journal of Pharmaceutical Science Technology 2 (9), 312−317.

Rabearivony, A.D., Kuhlman, A.R., Razafiariso, Z.L., Raharimalala, F., Rakotoarivony, F., Randrianarivony, T., Rakotoarivelo, N., Randrianasolo, A., Bussmann, R.W., 2015. Ethnobotanical Study of the Medicinal Plants Known by Men in Ambalabe, vol. 14. Ethnobotany Research and Applications, Madagascar, pp. 123−138.

Ramiarantsoa, H., Yao-Kouassi, P.A., Kanko, C., Assi, K.M., Djakoure, A.L., Tonzibo, F.Z., 2014. Chemical constituents of the antidiabetic plant *Ravenala madagascariensis*. International Journal of Pharmaceutical Sciences and Research 5 (12), 5503.

Razafindraibe, M., Kuhlman, A.R., Rabarison, H., Rakotoarimanana, V., Rajeriarison, C., Rakotoarivelo, N., Randrianarivony, T., Rakotoarivony, F., Ludovic, R., Randrianasolo, A., Bussmann, R.W., 2013. Medicinal plants used by women from Agnalazaha littoral forest (Southeastern Madagascar). Journal of Ethnobiology and Ethnomedicine 9 (1), 73.

Reyad-ul-Ferdous, M., Uddin, N., Shahjahan, D.S., Hossen, M., Arman, M.S.I., Islam, A., 2014. Preliminary in Vitro Potential Phytochemicals Investigation of Barks of *Ravenala madagascariensis* Sonnerat.

Sharmin, T., Chowdhury, S.R., Mian, M.Y., Hoque, M., Sumsujjaman, M., Nahar, F., 2014. Evaluation of antimicrobial activities of some Bangladeshi medicinal plants. World Journal of Pharmaceutical Sciences 2 (2), 170−175.

Suroowan, S., Mahomoodally, M.F., 2016. A comparative ethnopharmacological analysis of traditional medicine used against respiratory tract diseases in Mauritius. Journal of Ethnopharmacology 177, 61−80.

Further reading

Omale, J., Okafor, P.N., 2008. Comparative antioxidant capacity, membrane stabilization, polyphenol composition and cytotoxicity of the leaf and stem of Cissus multistriata. African Journal of Biotechnology 7 (17).

Prasad, S., Kashyap, R.S., Deopujari, J.Y., Purohit, H.J., Taori, G.M., Daginawala, H.F., 2007. Effect of Fagonia arabica (Dhamasa) on in vitro thrombolysis. BMC Complementary and Alternative Medicine 7 (1), 36.

Searsia lancea

Murunwa Madzinga, Quenton Kritzinger

Department of Plant and Soil Sciences, University of Pretoria, Pretoria, Gauteng, South Africa

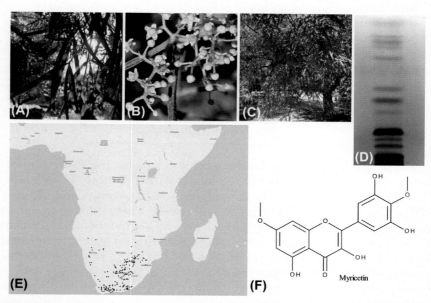

FIGURE 39 Leaves of *Searsia lancea* (Jackson, 2008) (A), flowers of *S. lancea* (Venter, 2016) (B), aerial parts of *S. lancea* (Kenraiz, 2016) (C), TLC chromatogram, fingerprint of *S. lancea* extract (D); distribution map of in sub-Saharan Africa (GBIF, 2018) (E) chemical structure of myricetin (F).

Underexplored Medicinal Plants from Sub-Saharan Africa
https://doi.org/10.1016/B978-0-12-816814-1.00039-9

1. General description

1.1 Botanical nomenclature

Searsia lancea (L.f.) F.A.Barkley

1.2 Botanical family

Anacardiaceae

1.3 Vernacular names

Karree (English)
Rooikaree (Afrikaans)
Mokalabata, Monhlohlo, Motshakhutshakhu (Northern Sotho)
Inhlangutshane (Siswati)
Mosinabele, Mosilabele (Southern Sotho)
Mosabele, Mosilabele (Tswana)
Mushakaladza (Venḓa)
Umhlakotshane (Xhosa)

2. Botanical description

Searsia lancea, previously known as *Rhus lancea*, is a tree indigenous to South Africa. It is a member of the family Anacardiaceae (Mango family), the fourth largest family in southern Africa (Aganga and Mosase, 2001). The Karree is an evergreen and drought tolerant tree found in most parts of southern Africa. It usually grows to a height of 7 and 7 m in width, but it can, however, grow larger depending on the environmental factors. It is single-stemmed, branching and has a soft, round, and dense canopy. The bark is coarse-textured, and the young trees are red to brown while the older trees are dark grayish. The tree has hairless compound leaves that are further divided into three leaflets (trifoliate) and are lancea-shaped. The leaves are leathery and are dark olive green adaxially and pale green abaxially (Gundiza et al., 2008; Stern, 2008; Van Wyk et al., 2008). The small, inconspicuous flowers are produced from June to September with male and female flowers found on different trees. Dull yellow-to-brown, small, slightly flattened and round fruits of about 5 mm are seen from September to January (Gundiza et al., 2008; Stern, 2008; Van Wyk et al., 2008). The seeds are small with a tough small mesocarp consisting of fibrous material (Aganga and Mosase, 2001).

3. Distribution

Searsia lancea occurs from north Zambia to South Africa where it grows in all provinces of South Africa, except for Kwazulu-Natal (Stern, 2008). It is often found on calcareous substrates, and it occurs naturally in Acacia woodland and along rivers, streams, and drainage lines (Stern, 2008; Van Wyk et al., 2008).

4. Ethnobotanical usage

The leaves and fruits of the Karree tree are said to be used in Lesotho for the treatment of diabetes and herpes. The leaves and fruits are mixed with milk from a young cow to cure diabetes (Kose et al., 2015). The leaves are also traditionally used to treat headache, fever, colds, pustules, and papules in South Africa (Kose et al., 2015; Mulaudzi et al., 2012). Vhavenda people (North of Limpopo province) use a decoction of boiled fresh leaves as a steam (and a drinking decoction) for a person suffering from colds, headaches, and related fevers. The decoction is also used to bathe a baby with smallpox-related disease and to wash animals with skin infections (Mabogo, 1990; Personal communication).

5. Phytochemical constituents

The plant is reported to contain flavonoids and tannins (Van der Merwe et al., 2001). Nair et al. (1983) reported on the isolation of a flavonoid, myricetin 7,4-dimethyl ether, and its 3-O-galactoside from a 95% ethanolic leaf extract. The essential oil from the leaves of this plant contains α-pinene, benzene, δ-3-carene, isopropyl toluene, and trans-caryophyllene (Gundiza et al., 2008). Profisetinidin tetraflavanoids have also been isolated from the heartwood of this plant (Young et al., 1985).

6. TLC fingerprinting of plant extract

Two milligrams of the ethanolic extract was weighed out and dissolved in 1 mL of ethanol. Separation of the compounds of the crude ethanolic extract was observed using silica gel 60 F254 thin layer chromatography (TLC) plates. Markings on the TLC plates were made using a blunt pencil and capillaries were used to spot the TLC plates with the sample.

Once the spot was dry, the TLC plate was placed in a TLC developing tank containing hexane:dichloromethane (2:3) as the solvent system. The TLC plate was allowed to develop until the solvent system was 1 cm from the top of the plate. The plate was observed under ultraviolet (UV light) (long and short wavelength), followed by spraying with freshly prepared vanillin/sulfuric acid (2%) to detect the bands on the TLC plate.

7. Pharmacological properties

7.1 Antimicrobial activity

Leaves of *S. lancea* were collected in Harare, Zimbabwe. One kilogram of the leaves was steam distilled for about 3 h. The obtained essential oil was dried using anhydrous sodium sulfate and stored at 4°C after filtration. The essential oil was tested for its antibacterial activity using the disc diffusion assay against 12 different bacterial species, namely: *Acinetobacter calcoaceticus* (NCIB 8250), *Bacillus subtilis* (NCIB 3610), *Citrobacter freundii* (NCIB 11,490), *Clostridium perfringens*, *Clostridium sporogenes* (NCIB 10696), *Escherichia coli* (NCIB 8879), *Klebsiella pneumoniae* (NCIB 4184), *Proteus vulgaris* (NCIB 4175), *Pseudomonas aeruginosa* (NCIB 950), *Salmonella typhii*, *Staphylococcus aureus* (NCIB 6751), and *Yersinia enteroco litica* (NCIB 10460). The *S. lancea* essential oil was found to have significant activity against all bacterial species with the highest noted activity against *E. coli* (19.2 mm zone of inhibition) (Gundiza et al., 2008). The antibacterial activity was also noted when the organic (petroleum ether, dichloromethane, and 80% ethanol), and water extracts were tested against *E. coli, S. aureus, B. subtilis*, and *K. pneumoniae* using the microdilution assay (Mulaudzi et al., 2012). The dichloromethane extract was found to have a good antibacterial activity, exhibiting the minimum inhibitory concentration (MIC) of 0.01 µg/mL against *B. subtilis* (Mulaudzi et al., 2012).

The essential oil was also tested for antifungal activity against *Candida albicans, Aspergillus niger, Aspergillus flavus*, and *Penicillium notatum*. The highest activity was observed against *A. flavus* (74.2 cm inhibition zone when 100.0 µg/mL was tested). This antifungal activity may be attributed to a high concentration of α-pinene (86.95%) found in the essential oils (Gundiza et al., 2008). The antifungal activity of leaf extracts against *C. albicans* was also evaluated by Mulaudzi et al. (2012). The aqueous and organic (petroleum ether, dichloromethane, 80% ethanol) extracts were tested using the microdilution assay, and the 80% ethanol extract was found to exhibit a minimum inhibitory concentration of 1.25 µg/mL activity as compared to the other extracts that showed higher MIC values.

7.2 Anticancer activity

The dichloromethane (DCM) extracts of the stem and fruits have been reported to exhibit moderate in vitro anticancer activity against renal TK10, breast MCF7, and melanoma UACC62 cell lines (Fouche et al., 2008).

7.3 Antioxidant and antiinflammatory activity

In a study by Gundiza et al., (2008), the dilutions of essential oils extracted from *S. lancea* leaves were spotted on silica gel sheets and developed, and thereafter sprayed with 0.2% of the stable radical, diphenylpicrylhydrazyl (DPPH). The essential oil exhibited a mean zone of color of 19.2 mm; this activity was almost the same as that of ascorbic acid, which was used as a positive control. The noted antioxidant activity may be due to a monoterpene, α-pinene, which acts as a radical scavenging agent (Gundiza et al., 2008).

Mulaudzi et al. (2012) evaluated the aqueous and organic extracts (petroleum ether, dichloromethane, and 80% ethanol) of the leaves of *S. lancea* for their antiinflammatory activity. The activity was tested on the cyclooxygenase (COX) enzymes, namely, COX-1 and COX-2. The dichloromethane extract was found to have an antiinflammatory activity against the COX-1 enzyme.

7.4 Anticholinesterase activity

Cholinesterases are a group of enzymes that catalyzed the hydrolysis of neurotransmitter acetylcholine into choline and acetic acid (Colovic et al., 2013). The inhibitors of acetylcholinesterase have been used in the treatment of degenerative disease such as Alzheimer's disease (Oh et al., 2004). The acetylcholinesterase activity bioassay was carried using the methanolic and water extract of the *S. lancea* leaves. The extracts were tested on an enzyme isolated from electric eels. The methanolic extract showed $59.8 \pm 3.7\%$ inhibitory concentration, and the water extract showed the lowest inhibitory concentration of 35% (Mulaudzi et al., 2012).

8. Additional information

8.1 Therapeutic (proposed) usage

Antibacterial, antifungal, and anticancer

8.2 Safety data

Toxic to bovine dermis and Vero cell lines (Tshidzumba, 2018)

8.3 Trade information

Not threatened nor endangered, and it is abundant.

8.4 Dosage

Not available

References

Aganga, A.A., Mosase, K.W., 2001. Tannin content, nutritive value and dry matter digestibility of *Lonchocarpus capassa, Zizyphus mucronata, Sclerocarya birrea, Kirkia acuminata* and *Rhus lancea* seeds. Animal Feed Science and Technology 91 (1–2), 107–113.

Colovic, M.B., Krstic, D.Z., Lazarevic-Pasti, T.D., Bondzic, A.M., Vasic, V.M., 2013. Acetylcholinesterase inhibitors: pharmacology and toxicology. Current Neuropharmacology 11 (3), 315–335.

Fouché, G., Cragg, G.M., Pillay, P., Kolesnikova, N., Maharaj, V.J., Senabe, J., 2008. In vitro anticancer screening of South African plants. Journal of Ethnopharmacology 119 (3), 455–461.

GBIF, 2018. *Searsia lancea* (L.f.) F.A. Barkley in GBIF Secretariat (2017). GBIF Backbone Taxonomy. Checklist dataset. https://doi.org/10.15468/39omei.

Gundidza, M., Gweru, N., Mmbengwa, V., Ramalivhana, N.J., Magwa, Z., Samie, A., 2008. Phytoconstituents and biological activities of essential oil from *Rhus lancea* L. F. African Journal of Biotechnology 7 (16), 2787–2789.

Jackson, J.S, 2008. Foliage Cultivated, Berkeley, California. Online. Available online: https://commons.wikimedia.org/wiki/Searsia_lancea#/media/File:Searsia_lancea_Berkeley3.jpg (CC BY 2.0).

Kenraiz, K.Z., 2016. *Searsia lancea* in Clovis Botanical Garden. Online. Available online: https://commons.wikimedia.org/wiki/Category:Searsia_lancea#/media/File:Searsia_lancea_kz1.jpg (CC BY-SA 4.0).

Kose, L.S., Moteetee, A., Van Vuuren, S., 2015. Ethnobotanical survey of medicinal plants used in the Maseru district of Lesotho. Journal of Ethnopharmacology 170, 184–200.

Mabogo, D.E.N., 1990. The Ethnobotany of the Vhavenda. PhD thesis. University of Pretoria, South Africa.

Mulaudzi, R.B., Ndhlala, A.R., Kulkarni, M.G., Van Staden, J., 2012. Pharmacological properties and protein binding capacity of phenolic extracts of some venda medicinal plants used against cough and fever. Journal of Ethnopharmacology 143 (1), 185–193.

Nair, A.R., Kotiyal, J.P., Bhardwaj, D.K., 1983. Myricetin 7, 4'-dimethyl ether and its 3-galactoside from *Rhus lancea*. Phytochemistry 22 (1), 318–319.

Oh, M.H., Houghton, P.J., Whang, W.K., Cho, J.H., 2004. Screening of Korean herbal medicines used to improve cognitive function for anticholinesterase activity. Phytomedicine 11 (6), 544–548.

Stern, M., 2008. *Searsia lancea* (L.f.) F.A.Barkley. Online. Available at: http://pza.sanbi.org/searsia-lancea.

Tshidzumba, P.W., 2018. An Inventory and Pharmacological Evaluation of Medicinal Plants Used as Antidiabetes and Anti-arthritis in Vhembe District Municipality, Limpopo Province. PhD thesis. University of Venda, South Africa.

Van der Merwe, D., Swan, G.E., Botha, C.J., 2001. Use of ethnoveterinary medicinal plants in cattle by Setswana-speaking people in the Madikwe area of the North West Province of South Africa. Journal of the South African Veterinary Association 72 (4), 189–196.

Van Wyk, B., Van Wyk, P., Van Wyk, B.E., 2008. Photo Guide to Trees of Southern Africa. Briza Publications, Pretoria, p. 281.

Venter, P., 2016. The Small Yellow Flowers of a Female Tree. Online. Available online: https://en.wikipedia.org/wiki/Searsia_lancea#/media/File:Searsia_lancea01.jpg (CC BY-SA 4.0).

Young, D.A., Kolodziej, H., Ferreira, D., Roux, D.G., 1985. Synthesis of condensed tannins. Part 16. Stereochemical differentiation of the first 'angular' (2 S, 3 R)-profisetinidin tetra-flavanoids from *Rhus lancea* (karree) and the varying dynamic behaviour of their derivatives. Journal of the Chemical Society, Perkin Transactions 1, 2537—2544.

40

Siphonochilus aethiopicus

Anna-Mari Kok, Namrita Lall

Department of Plant and Soil Sciences, University of Pretoria, Pretoria, Gauteng, South Africa

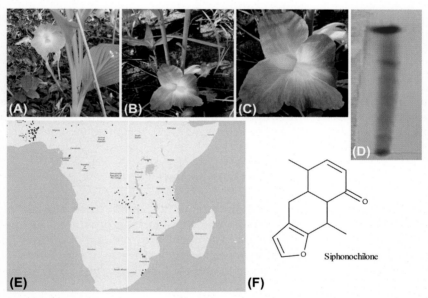

FIGURE 40   Aerial parts of *Siphonochilus aethiopicus* (Rulkens, 2013a) (A), flower of *S. aethiopicus* (Rulkens, 2013b) (B), flower of *S. aethiopicus* (Rulkens, 2013c) (C), TLC chromatogram, fingerprint of *S. aethiopicus* extract (D), distribution of *S. aethiopicus* in sub-Saharan Africa (GBIF, 2018) (E), chemical structure of siphonochilone (F).

261

1. General description

1.1 Botanical nomenclature

Siphonochilus aethiopicus (Schweif.) B. L. Burt.

1.2 Botanical family

Zingiberaceae

1.3 Vernacular names

Natal ginger (English)
Wild ginger (English)
Wildegemmer (Afrikaans)
Indungulo isiphephetho (Zulu)

2. Botanical description

Siphonochilus aethiopicus (Schweif.) B. L. Burt. is a deciduous, aromatic, and rhizomatous plant that grows at a height of approximately 1m. The leaves are glabrous, with bright pink to white flowers and yellow markings in bloom from October to February (Kiew, 1980; Pooley, 1998).

3. Distribution

Siphonochilus aethiopicus is not endemic to South Africa but can be found distributed in the Limpopo and Mpumalanga province. The species is also found in the Letaba catchment area of Limpopo Lowveld through to Swaziland. Once a prominent species in the province of KwaZulu-Natal, it has now since thought to be extinct due to over usage.

4. Ethnobotanical usage

Siphonochilus aethiopicus is well known for its medicinal properties among the Zulu and Swati. The Zulu use this plant as protection against lightning and snakes. The rhizomes are favored and are freshly chewed for treatment against asthma, hysteria, colds, and coughs especially against any flu symptoms. For the Swati culture, this plant is used by the women to treat menstrual pain and to treat malaria (Van Wyk et al., 1997).

5. Phytochemical constituents

Little is known about the secondary chemistry of this species. A report of the volatile oil composition of an unidentified *Kaempferia* (now *Siphonochilus*) species appeared in 1915 and ongoing work has identified α-terpineol and a sesquiterpene as constituents of the oil in the rhizome of *S. aethiopicus*. Another sesquiterpenoid, siphonochilone, has been patented for the application of various activities including antiinflammatory activities (Gericke, 2011). The isolation of derivatives of furanoterpenoids, namely 4aaH-3,5a,8ab-trimethyl-4,4a,9-tetrahydronaphtho[2,3-b]-furan-8-one and 2-hydroxy-4aaH-3,5a,8ab-trimethyl-4,4a,9-tetrahydronaptho[2,3-b]-furan-8-one, was reported (10, 149, 150). Viljoen et al. (2002) described the essential oil content of *S. aethiopicus*. A study done by Igoli and Obanu (2011) showed that the volatile oil of both fresh and roasted rhizomes of *S. aethiopicus* mostly consisted of terpenes.

6. TLC fingerprinting of plant extract

The separation of *S. aethiopicus* was observed by weighing out 2 mg of an ethanolic extract, dissolved in 200 μL ethanol. The thin layer chromatography (TLC) analysis of the ethanolic *S. aethiopicus* extract comprised of silica gel 60 F254 TLC plates for the observation of separation of the compounds that may be present within the extract. The plates were marked with a soft pencil, and glass capillaries were used to spot the sample. The spot was left to dry completely before placing the TLC plates within a TLC tank which contained 10 mL eluent of 95:5 chloroform: methanol as the solvent system. The sample was allowed to separate until the eluent reached the solvent line, 1 cm from the top of the TLC plate. The plate was observed under ultraviolet light (long and short wavelength), followed by spraying with freshly prepared vanillin/sulfuric acid (2%) to detect the bands on the TLC plate.

7. Pharmacological properties

A few studies were conducted on *S. aethiopicus* which involved comparing the bioactivity of the plant leaves with the rhizomes. Many biological properties were investigated but no significant activity has been found for most properties. Only the biological properties tested with noteworthy results were noted below.

7.1 Antiplasmodial activity

Lategan et al. (2009) studied the antiplasmodial potential of the ethyl acetate extract of *S. aethiopicus*. The study found that the ethyl acetate extract was active against both chloroquine-sensitive and chloroquine-resistant strains of *Plasmodium falciparum*. Further in vivo studies showed the active nature of the ethyl acetate extract of *S. aethiopicus*.

7.2 Antiinflammatory activity

The diethyl extract showed potent inhibition of the nuclear factor kappa-light-chain-enhancer of activated B cells (NF-KB) transcription process as seen in an NF-KB transcription response cellular assay (Fouche et al., 2013). Furthermore, Fouche et al. (2013) showed the inhibition of interleukin (IL-8) by the ethanol extract of *S. aethiopicus*, an important cytokine involved in the inflammatory process. As shown by Zschocke and Van Staden (2000), the leaves of *S. aethiopicus* are known for their antiinflammatory activity and were also confirmed by the cyclooxygenase (COX)-1 and COX-2 inhibition study conducted by Light et al. (2002).

7.3 Antifungal activity

A study by Coopoosamy et al. (2010) investigated the antifungal activity of both the ethanolic and aqueous extracts of leaves, rhizomes, and combinations thereof. It was noted that the ethanol had shown better activity than the aqueous extracts, suggesting isolation of certain compound from these extracts may reveal the compound in question with even more activity than the crude extracts.

7.4 Antibacterial activity

A study conducted by Light et al. (2002) indicated the antibacterial activity of various parts of *S. aethiopicus* tested. The ethyl acetate extract of the roots of *S. aethiopicus* had shown very effective antibacterial activity with a minimum inhibitory concentration (MIC) value of 780 µg/mL against *Bacillus subtilis*, whereas the ethanol root extract had shown the same MIC value against *Staphylococcus aureus*.

8. Additional information

8.1 Therapeutic (proposed) usage

Antibacterial, antifungal, and immunostimulant

8.2 Safety data

No visible toxicity was observed on vervet monkey kidney (Vero) cells (Light et al., 2002).

8.3 Trade information

Siphonochilus aethiopicus is currently listed in the Red Data Book of South African plants as critically endangered.

8.4 Dosage

Not available

References

Coopoosamy, R.M., Naidoo, K.K., Buwa, L., Mayekiso, B., 2010. Screening of *Siphonochilus aetiopicus* (Schweinf.) B. L. Burtt for antibacterial and antifungal properties. Journal of Medicinal Plants Research 4 (12), 1228−1231.

Fouche, G., Van Rooyen, S., Faleschini, T., 2013. *Siphonochilus aethiopicus,* a traditional remedy for the treatment of allergic asthma. The International Journal Genuine Traditional Medicine (TANG) 3 (1), 1−6.

GBIF, 2018. *Siphonochilus aethiopicus* (Schweinf.) B.L.Burtt in GBIF Secretariat (2017). In: GBIF Backbone Taxonomy. Checklist dataset. https://doi.org/10.15468/39omei.

Gericke, N., 2011. Muthi to medicine. South African Journal of Botany 77 (4), 850−856.

Igoli, N.P., Obanu, Z., 2011. The volatile components of wild ginger (*Siphonochilus aethiopicus* (Schweinf) B. I Burtt). African Journal of Food Science 5 (9), 541−549.

Kiew, K.Y., 1980. Taxonomic studies in the genus *Kaempferia* (Zingiberaceae). Notes of the Royal Botanic Garden (Edinburgh) 38 (1), 1−12.

Lategan, C.A., Campbell, W.E., Seaman, T., Smith, P.J., 2009. The bioactivity of novel furano-terpenoids isolated from *Siphonochilus aethiopicus.* Journal of Ethnopharmacology 121 (1), 92−97.

Light, M.E., McGaw, L.J., Rabe, T., Sparg, S.G., Taylor, M.B., Erasmus, D.G., Jager, A.K., Van Staden, J., 2002. Investigation of the biological activities of *Siphonochilus aethiopicus* and the effect of seasonal senescence. South African Journal of Botany 68, 55−61.

Pooley, E., 1998. A Field Guide to Wild Flowers KwaZulu- Natal and the Eastern Region. Natal Flora Publications Trust, Durban.

Rulkens, 2013a. A Wild Member of the Ginger Family (Zingiberaceae). Available online: https://commons.wikimedia.org/wiki/File:Siphonochilus_aethiopicus_(9710468874).jpg. (CC BY-SA 2.0).

Rulkens, 2013b. *Siphonochilus aethiopicus* 1. Available online: https://commons.wikimedia.org/wiki/File:Siphonochilus_aethiopicus_1_(11668847913).jpg. (CC BY-SA 2.0).

Rulkens, 2013c. In the Wild in Metuge District in Northern Mozambique, about 50 m.a.S. In Heavy Clay Soil. Early Rainy Season. Available online: https://commons.wikimedia.org/wiki/File:Siphonochilus_aethiopicus_2_(11668821403).jpg. (CC BY-SA 2.0).

Van Wyk, B.E., Oudtshoorn, B., Gericke, N., 1997. Medicinal plants of South Africa. Briza, Pretoria.

Viljoen, A.M., Demirci, B., Baser, K.H.C., Van Wyk, B.E., 2002. The essential oil composition of the roots and rhizomes of *Siphonochilus aethiopicus*. South African Journal of Botany 68 (1), 115—116.

Zschocke, S., Van Staden, J., 2000. *Cryptocarya* species- substitute plants for *Ocotea bullata*? a pharmacological investigation in terms of cyclooxygenase-1 and -2 inhibition. Journal of Ethnopharmacology 71, 473—478.

Further reading

Holzapfel, C.W., Marais, W., Wessels, P.L., Van Wyk, B.,E., 2002. Furanoterpenoids from *Siphonochlus aethiopicus*. Phytochemistry 59 (4), 405—407.

41

Stillingia lineata subsp. lineata

Nawraj Rummun[1,2], Cláudia Baider[3],
Theeshan Bahorun[1],
Vidushi S. Neergheen-Bhujun[1,2]

[1] ANDI Centre of Excellence for Biomedical and Biomaterials Research, University of Mauritius, Réduit, Republic of Mauritius; [2] Department of Health Sciences, Faculty of Science, University of Mauritius, Réduit, Republic of Mauritius; [3] The Mauritius Herbarium, Agricultural Services, Ministry of Agro-Industry and Food Security, Réduit, Republic of Mauritius

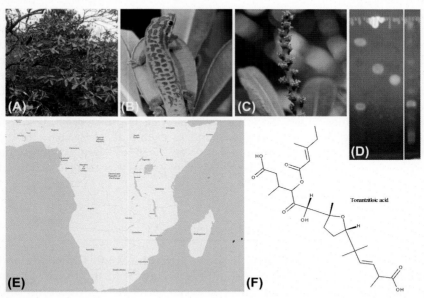

FIGURE 41 A specimen of *Stillingia lineata* (A), leaves showing midrib and margin (with an endemic *Phelsuma cepediana*) (B), inflorescence of *S. lineata* (C), TLC chromatogram, Lane 1 bottom; rutin, top; quercitrin; Lane 2 bottom; hyperoside, top; quercetin; Lane 3; chlorogenic acid; Lane 4; *S. lineata* hydromethanolic extract (D); distribution map of *S. lineata* in sub-Saharan Africa (GBIF, 2018) (E), chemical structure of tonantzitloic acid (F).

1. General description

1.1 Botanical nomenclature

Stillingia lineata (Lam.) Müll. Arg. subsp. *lineata*

1.2 Botanical family

Euphorbiaceae

1.3 Vernacular names

Mauritius: Fangame
Réunion: Bois de lait; Tanguin de pays

2. Botanical description

Shrub to tree up to 12 m high, latex abundant in the bark, branches, and leaves. Branchlet with many leaf scars. Leaves alternated, simple, at branchlet apex, variable, 3—15·(—24) × 2—4 cm; blade elliptical, elliptical-obovate, or obovate; base cunated, rounded, or truncate; tip rounded, obtuse, or acute; young leaves more coriaceous and also on smaller plants, becoming more papyraceous with age and on large plants; large and distinct midrib, secondary venation not very visible; margin entire to slightly serrated or crenated, with no gland. Inflorescence terminal, one spike per group of leaves, 2—13 cm long; flowers shortly pedicellated, female flowers at the base, usually solitary, few; male flowers at the apex, many, sometimes all flowers of the inflorescence are male; bract, 1—2 mm thick, variable shape; one visible gland in each side of the base of the inflorescence. Fruit 3 rounded lobes, 5—6 × 7—8 mm dehiscing explosively. Seeds oblong, 4—5 × 3—3.5 mm, gray with caruncle (Adapted from Coode, 1982).

3. Distribution

S. lineata (Lam.) Müll. Arg. is found from the South China Sea and Pacific Ocean (subsp. *pacifica* (Müll. Arg.) Stennis) to the Indian Ocean (subsp. *lineata*). The latter subspecies is endemic to Mauritius and Réunion. A relatively common species, on Mauritius, is found across the island as in North mountain range (Le Pouce, Pieter Both), in the Southwest native remnants of Pétrin, Magenta, Mt Rempart, among others, and the Southeast vegetation of Mt Bambous (Coode, 1982).

4. Ethnobotanical usage

In Mauritius, a bath of the leaf decoction is used to treat skin diseases (Gurib-Fakim and Guého, 1996), whereas in Réunion, the species is used in the treatment of furuncles and more recently against the Chikungunya virus (Dorla et al., 2018).

5. Phytochemical constituents

The isolated phytochemicals reported from this subspecies are mainly of terpenoid origin. Tonantzitlolone derivatives having C20-flexibilane and tigliane skeleton, as well as tonantzitloic acid, were reported from the ethyl acetate, leaf extract (Olivon et al., 2015). In addition to the C15-flexibilane skeleton tonantzitlolone derivatives, the ethyl acetate extract obtained from the bark also contained the pimarane derivative, ent-12a-hydroxy-3,7-dioxoisopimara-8,15-diene (Techer et al., 2015). Thin layer chromatography (TLC) revealed the presence of rutin and chlorogenic acid among the different flavonoid compounds present in *S. lineata* subsp. *lineata* hydromethanolic leaf extract.

6. TLC fingerprinting of plant extract

The air-dried leaf was extracted with aqueous methanol (80%, v/v) and partitioned with dichloromethane. The aqueous phase was lyophilized, and 5 mg of the powdered extract was dissolved in 1 mL of aqueous methanol (80%, v/v). For the reference standards quercitrin, quercetin, rutin, hyperoside, and chlorogenic acid were purchased from Extrasynthèse (France), and 1 mg of each standard was dissolved in 1 mL methanol. For the chromatographic separation, 10 µL of extract and 5 µL of reference standard were spotted on a silica gel 60 F254 thin layer chromatography (TLC) plate (20 × 20 cm). The spots were left to dry, and the plate was placed in a TLC tank, presaturated with 100 mL mobile phase. The mobile phase comprises ethyl acetate, formic acid, and water in ratio 8:1:1 (v/v). The samples were allowed to separate until the solvent front reached about 15 cm from the baseline. The plate was dried and sprayed with 1% methanolic diphenyl boric acid aminoethyl ester (DPBAE) and examined under ultraviolet light at 365 nm to detect the bands on the TLC plates.

7. Pharmacological properties

The reported scientific evaluation of its therapeutic potential is limited to in vitro antimicrobial, antidiabetic, and cancer cytotoxicity activities.

7.1 Antibacterial activity

The ethyl acetate extract of *S. lineata* leaf showed 2.5-fold higher growth inhibitory activity as compared with the clinical antibiotic, chloramphenicol, against *Staphylococcus aureus* as determined by the paper disc diffusion method (Dorla et al., 2018).

7.2 Antiviral activity

The ethyl acetate extract of *S. lineata* leaf and bark showed potent antiviral activity against chikungunya virus strain 899 (Olivon et al., 2015; Techer et al., 2015). The leaf extracts further inhibited replication of the human immunodeficiency virus (HIV)-1 and HIV-2 virus (Olivon et al., 2015).

7.3 Cancer cell cytotoxicity

Dichloromethane extract of leaf of *S. lineata* ssp. *lineata* collected from Mauritius showed cytotoxicity against the human colon carcinoma (Co115) cell line (Chapuis et al., 1988).

7.4 Antidiabetic activity

The methanolic extract of *S. lineata* showed potent inhibitory activity against α-glucosidase enzyme with a 50% inhibitory concentration (IC_{50}) value of 1.0 ± 0.0, 1.8 ± 0.3, and $19.3 \pm 3.6\,\mu g/mL$, respectively, compared with, the clinically used α-glucosidase inhibitor, acarbose (IC_{50} of $5115.7 \pm 3.9\,\mu g/mL$) (Picot et al., 2014). Furthermore, the extract also exhibited a potent glucose diffusion retardation index, highlighting its ability to delay glucose absorption following oral administration (Picot et al., 2014).

8. Additional information

8.1 Therapeutic (proposed) usage

Chikungunya virus and antidiabetic

8.2 Safety data

The ethyl acetate bark extract was found to be moderately cytotoxic against the host Vero (African green monkey kidney) cells (Techer et al., 2015).

8.3 Trade information

The species would be classified under Least Concerned following the International Union for Conservation of Nature (IUCN) Red List category (IUCN, 2001).

8.4 Dosage

Not available

References

Chapuis, J.C., Sordat, B., Hostetmann, K., 1988. Screening for cytotoxic activity of plants used in traditional medicine. Journal of Ethnopharmacology 23, 273—284. https://doi.org/10.1016/0378-8741(88)90006-2.

Coode, M.J.E., 1982. 160. Euphorbiacées. In: Bosser, J., Cadet, T., Guého, J., Marais, W. (Eds.), Flore des Mascareignes — La Reunion, Maurice, Rodrigues. MSIRI/ORSTOM/KEW. Imprimerie du Gouverment, Mauritius.

Dorla, E., Grondin, I., Hue, T., Clerc, P., Dumas, S., Gauvin-Bialecki, A., Laurent, P., 2018. Traditional uses, antimicrobial and acaricidal activities of 20 plants selected among Reunion Island's Flora. South African Journal of Botany. https://doi.org/10.1016/j.sajb.2018.04.014.

GBIF, 2018. *Stillingia lineata* Müll.Arg. In GBIF Secretariat (2017). GBIF Backbone Taxonomy. Checklist dataset. https://doi.org/10.15468/39omei.

Gurib-Fakim, A., Gueho, J., 1996. Plantes medicinales de Maurice, Tome 2. Editions de l'Ocean Indien, Mauritius.

IUCN, 2001. IUCN Red List Categories and Criteria, Version 3.1. IUCN Species Survival Commission, Gland, Switzerland and Cambridge, United Kingdom.

Olivon, F., Palenzuela, H., Girard-Valenciennes, E., Neyts, J., Pannecouque, C., Roussi, F., Grondin, I., Leyssen, P., Litaudon, M., 2015. Antiviral activity of flexibilane and tigliane diterpenoids from *Stillingia lineata*. Journal of Natural Products 78, 1119—1128. https://doi.org/10.1021/acs.jnatprod.5b00116.

Picot, C.M.N., Subratty, A.H., Mahomoodally, M.F., 2014. Inhibitory potential of five traditionally used native antidiabetic medicinal plants on α-amylase, α-glucosidase, glucose entrapment, and amylolysis kinetics in vitro. Advances in Pharmacological Sciences 2014, 1—7. https://doi.org/10.1155/2014/739834.

Techer, S., Girard-Valenciennes, E., Retailleau, P., Neyts, J., Guéritte, F., Leyssen, P., Litaudon, M., Smadja, J., Grondin, I., 2015. Tonantzitlolones from *Stillingia lineata* ssp. *lineata* as potential inhibitors of chikungunya virus. Phytochemistry Letters 12, 313—319. https://doi.org/10.1016/j.phytol.2015.04.023.

Terminalia bentzoe subsp. bentzoe

Nawraj Rummun[1,2], *Cláudia Baider*[3],
Theeshan Bahorun[1],
Vidushi S. Neergheen-Bhujun[1,2]

[1] ANDI Centre of Excellence for Biomedical and Biomaterials Research,
University of Mauritius, Réduit, Republic of Mauritius; [2] Department of
Health Sciences, Faculty of Science, University of Mauritius, Réduit,
Republic of Mauritius; [3] The Mauritius Herbarium, Agricultural Services,
Ministry of Agro-Industry and Food Security, Réduit, Republic of Mauritius

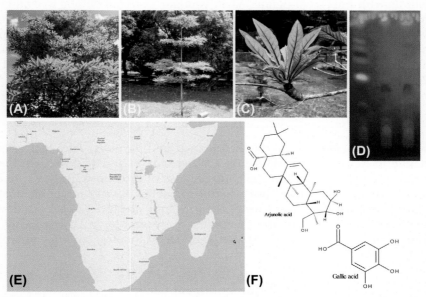

FIGURE 42   Aerial part of *Terminalia bentzoe* (Shawka, 2012a) (A), a specimen of *T. bentzoe* (Shawka, 2012b) (B), close-up view of the leaves of *T. bentzoe* (Molteno, 2017) (C), TLC chromatogram, Lane 1; *T. bentzoe* leaf extract, Lane 2; *T. bentzoe* flower extract, Lane 3; *T. bentzoe* bark extract (D), distribution map of *T. bentzoe* in sub-Saharan Africa (GBIF, 2018) (E), chemical structures of gallic acid and arjunolic acid (F).

1. General description

1.1 Botanical nomenclature

Terminalia bentzoe (L.) L.f. subsp. *bentzoe*

1.2 Botanical family

Combretaceae

1.3 Vernacular names

Mauritius: Bois benjoin, Bois benzoin
Réunion: Benjoin; Benjoin pays

2. Botanical description

Tree reaches the canopy, 10—20 (-30) m tall, sometimes with buttress. Branches are arranged horizontally, thickening toward the apex. Leaves are simple, in a cluster at the end of branches, heterophyllous, linear to nearly elliptic with pubescent petiole when younger, becomes elliptic to oval or oboval with glabrous petiole; margin is largely crenulated, palid green; venation, especially the midrib, red in younger leaves, becoming green in older leaves. Flowers are pentamerous, white or pale yellow, inflorescence axillary, as long as the leaves. Fruit samara with two wings, indehiscent, 2—3.5 cm diameter, green, seed 1 (Adapted from Wickens, 1990).

3. Distribution

T. bentzoe is endemic to the Mascarenes, and the subspecies *bentzoe* is native to Réunion and Mauritius. Once common and widespread, the species declined in all three islands because of direct use (priced wood and medicinal properties) but also due to habitat destruction of its most suitable habitat. It is a species of the lowlands and drier forests, today found on Mauritius in native remnants, for example, in Powder Mills, Corps de Garde, Yemen, Magenta, Trois Mamelles, and Chamarel (Page, 1998; Wickens, 1976).

4. Ethnobotanical usage

In Mauritius, *T. bentzoe* bark is used as part of a polyherbal formulation against dysentery and gonorrhea (Daruty, 1886; Rouillard and Guého, 1999). A decoction prepared by mixing *T. bentzoe* bark with leaves of *Aphloia theiformis* (Vahl) Benn. (Aphloiaceae) is administered two to three times daily to treat dysentery (Gurib-Fakim and Guého, 1996). Its bark decoction alone was also said to be used by the slaves against diarrhea and dysmenorrhea (Bouton, 1864).

In Réunion, many more uses have been recorded, for example, the leaf and stem are used against fever, cold, cough, influenza, asthma, dysmenorrhea, and pleuritic pain (Jonville et al., 2011; Poullain et al., 2004), whereas the whole plant is also used against bronchitis and reproductive disorders (spermatozoids) (Dorla et al., 2018).

5. Phytochemical constituents

The phytochemical and polysaccharide composition of *T. bentzoe* leaves are reported from cultivated trees in Cairo (Egypt). The polyphenolic profile comprises of gallic acid (36.3%), ellagic acid (12.2%), pyrogallol (2.8%), (+) catechin (5.2%), chlorogenic acid (4.7%), synergic acid (5.5%), pyrocatechol (9.7%), cinnamic acid (3.0%), p-Coumaric acid (1.3%), caffeic acid (1.5%), quercetin (5.5%), and rutin (2.0%) (El-Rafie et al., 2016). Only three triterpenes including oleanolic acid, masilinic acid, and arjunolic acid have been reported from *T. bentzoe* (Elsayed et al., 2015). Similarly, the polysaccharide profile of *T. bentzoe* includes xylose, glucose, mannose, ribose, rhamnose, arabinose, galactose, fructose, and mannitol (Mohamed El-Rafie and Abdel-Aziz Hamed, 2014). Methyl hexadecanoate (40.0%) and methyl octadecanoate (6.6%) are the major fatty acid methyl esters present in *T. bentzoe* leaves (El-Rafie et al., 2016). The phytochemical profile of *T. bentzoe* flower and bark has not been reported.

6. TLC fingerprinting of plant extract

The air-dried plant material was extracted with aqueous methanol (80%, v/v) and partitioned with dichloromethane. The aqueous phase was lyophilized, and 5 mg of the powdered extract was dissolved in 1 mL of aqueous methanol (80%, v/v). For the reference standards, quercitrin, quercetin, rutin, hyperoside, and chlorogenic acid were purchased from extrasynthèse (France), and 1 mg of each standard was dissolved in 1 mL methanol. For the chromatographic separation, 10 µL of extract and 5 µL of reference standard were spotted on a silica gel 60 F254 thin layer chromatography (TLC) plate (20 × 20 cm). The spots were left to dry, and the plate was placed in a TLC tank, presaturated with 100 mL mobile phase. The mobile phase comprised of ethyl acetate, formic acid, and water in a ratio of 8:1:1 (v/v). The samples were allowed to separate until the solvent front reached about 15 cm from the baseline. The plate was dried and sprayed with 1% methanolic diphenyl boric acid aminoethyl ester (DPBAE) and examined in ultraviolet light at 365 nm to detect the bands on the TLC plates.

7. Pharmacological properties

Although widely incorporated in the traditional medicinal system of both Réunion and Mauritius, research toward evaluating the *T. bentzoe* clinical efficacy in human subjects is limited. Only a few reports of its in vitro and in vivo bioactivities are available.

7.1 Anticancer

The methanolic leaf extract of *T. bentzoe* showed antimigratory activity against the metastatic human breast cancer MDA-MB-231 cells in the wound-healing assay (Elsayed et al., 2015). The bioactive antimigratory components were identified as oleanolic acid and mesalinic acid. Both triterpene acids showed potent dose-dependent growth inhibition of MDA-MB-231 as evaluated by the 3-(4,5-dimethylthiazol-2-yl)-2,5-diphenyltetrazolium bromide (MTT) assay. Moreover, both oleanolic acid and maslinic acid were relatively less toxic to the nontumorigenic immortalized human mammary epithelial, MCF-10A, cells (Elsayed et al., 2015). Adding to this, Jonville et al. (2011) reported the moderate cytotoxic activity, against human lung carcinoma A-549 cells, of dichloromethane extract of *T. bentzoe* bark (50% inhibitory concentration (IC_{50}) of 80 μg/mL) compared with etoposide (IC_{50} of 0.7 μg/mL).

7.2 Antiplasmodial activity

Methanolic leaf extracts of *T. bentzoe* exhibited promising in vitro antiplasmodial activity against both the 3D7 chloroquine—sensitive strain and the W2 chloroquine—resistant strain of *Plasmodium falciparum* (Jonville et al., 2008). Similarly, the methanolic bark extract of *T. bentzoe* also displayed promising activity against the 3D7 chloroquine—sensitive strain (Jonville et al., 2011). The effect was further corroborated in female Swiss mice infected with *Plasmodium berghei*. At a dose equivalent to 50 mg/kg, intraperitoneally administered (200 μL/mouse), *T. bentzoe* leaf extract showed a noticeable effect on day 7 postinfection by inhibiting 83% of the parasitic load (Jonville et al., 2008). Furthermore, at the same dose, the extract prolonged the longevity of the mice by 60% at day 15 postinfection compared with physiological serum (0% viability). However, at the higher doses, these extracts were found to be toxic (Jonville et al., 2008).

7.3 Antibacterial activity

The plant leaf ethyl acetate extract exhibited in vitro antibacterial activity against the gram-negative bacteria *Streptococcus pyogenes*, *Listeria monocytogenes*, and *Staphylococcus aureus* (Dorla et al., 2018).

7.4 Antioxidant

The methanolic extract of *T. bentzoe* leaf and stem exhibit moderate diphenylpicrylhydrazyl (DPPH) radical scavenging activity and β-carotene bleaching activity in comparison with known antioxidant standards including butylated hydroxyanisole, ascorbic acid, and Trolox (Poullain et al., 2004). Using similar methods, El-Rafie et al. (2016) reported the in vitro antioxidant potential of a hydroalcoholic extract of *T. bentzoe* leaves. Furthermore, *T. bentzoe* leaf extract mitigated oxidative stress in hyper-cholesterolemic male albino rats by ameliorating oxidative stress markers namely malondialdehyde, superoxide dismutase, and glutathione by 114.1%, 52.7%, and 19.5%, respectively (El-Rafie et al., 2016).

7.5 Antihyperlipidemic activity and hepatoprotective activity

The antihyperlipidemic effect of *T. bentzoe* leaf hydroalcoholic extract, in male albino rats, was comparable with the clinically used drug, lipanthyl. Treatment with extract and drug improved rat's body weight by 28% and 31%, respectively, showing a reduction in cholesterol and fat deposition in the liver (El-Rafie et al., 2016). Extract treatment at a dose equivalent to 500 mg/kg body weight improved the lipid profile in terms of total cholesterol, high-density lipoproteins, low-density lipoproteins, and triglycerides. *T. bentzoe* extract treatment further enhanced the liver function enzymes namely alanine transaminase and aspartate trans-aminase while decreasing degenerative changes in hyperlipidemic rats (El-Rafie et al., 2016).

8. Additional information

8.1 Therapeutic (proposed) usage

Antiplasmodial, antibacterial, anticancer, and hepatoprotective

8.2 Safety data

T. bentzoe bark methanolic extract showed low cytotoxicity against human skin fibroblast WS1 cells with an IC_{50} value greater than 200 µg/mL

(Jonville et al., 2011). Similarly, low toxicity was reported for *T. bentzoe* leaf methanolic extract against human normal fetal lung fibroblasts, WI-38 (IC_{50} of 115 µg/mL) (Jonville et al., 2008). Moreover, oral administration of *T. bentzoe* leaf hydroalcoholic extract to male albino rats at a dose equivalent to 500 mg/kg body weight did not result in animal mortality after 15 days and were considered safe (El-Rafie et al., 2016).

8.3 Trade information

This subspecies is considered threatened to extinction in the vulnerable category of the Red List of the International Union for Conservation of Nature (Page, 1998).

8.4 Dosage

Not available

References

Bouton, L., 1864. *Plantes médicinales de Maurice*, second ed. Typographie E. Dupuy et P. Dubois, Port-Louis, Mauritius.

Daruty, C., 1886. Plantes médicinales de l'île Maurice et des pays intertropicaux. General Steam Printing Company, Mauritius.

Dorla, E., Grondin, I., Hue, T., Clerc, P., Dumas, S., Gauvin-Bialecki, A., Laurent, P., 2018. Traditional uses, antimicrobial and acaricidal activities of 20 plants selected among reunion Island's flora. South African Journal of Botany. https://doi.org/10.1016/j.sajb.2018.04.014.

El-Rafie, H.M., Mohammed, R.S., Hamed, M.A., Ibrahim, G.E., Abou Zeid, A.H., 2016. Phytochemical and biological studies of total ethanol and petroleum ether extracts of *Terminalia bentzoe* (L.) leaves. International Journal of Pharmacognosy and Phytochemical Research 8, 592–603.

Elsayed, H.E., Akl, M.R., Ebrahim, H.Y., Sallam, A.A., Haggag, E.G., Kamal, A.M., El Sayed, K.A., 2015. Discovery, optimization, and pharmacophore modelling of oleanolic acid and analogues as breast cancer cell migration and invasion inhibitors through targeting Brk/Paxillin/Rac1 axis. Chemical Biology and Drug Design 85, 231–243. https://doi.org/10.1111/cbdd.12380.

GBIF, 2018. *Terminalia bentzoe* (L.) L.F. In GBIF Secretariat (2017). GBIF Backbone Taxonomy. Checklist dataset. https://doi.org/10.15468/39omei.

Gurib-Fakim, A., Gueho, J., 1996. Plantes medicinales de Maurice, Tome 2. Editions de l'Ocean Indien, Mauritius.

Jonville, M.C., Kodja, H., Humeau, L., Fournel, J., De Mol, P., Cao, M., Angenot, L., Frédérich, M., 2008. Screening of medicinal plants from reunion Island for antimalarial and cytotoxic activity. Journal of Ethnopharmacology 120, 382–386. https://doi.org/10.1016/j.jep.2008.09.005.

Jonville, M.C., Kodja, H., Strasberg, D., Pichette, A., Ollivier, E., Frédérich, M., Angenot, L., Legault, J., 2011. Antiplasmodial, anti-inflammatory and cytotoxic activities of various plant extracts from the Mascarene Archipelago. Journal of Ethnopharmacology 136, 525–531. https://doi.org/10.1016/j.jep.2010.06.013.

Mohamed El-Rafie, H., Abdel-Aziz Hamed, M., 2014. Antioxidant and anti-inflammatory activities of silver nanoparticles biosynthesized from aqueous leaves extracts of four *Terminalia* species. Advances in Natural Sciences: Nanoscience and Nanotechnology 5. https://doi.org/10.1088/2043-6262/5/3/035008.

Molteno, S., 2017. Available online: https://commons.wikimedia.org/wiki/File:Terminalia_bentzoe_subsp_bentzoe_-_Vallee_dOosterlog_2.jpg. (CC BY-SA 4.0.

Page, W., 1998. *Terminalia benzoin* ssp. benzoin. The IUCN Red List of Threatened Species 8235 e.T30745A9575875.

Poullain, C., Girard-Valenciennes, E., Smadja, J., 2004. Plants from Réunion island: evaluation of their free radical scavenging and antioxidant activities. Journal of Ethnopharmacology 95, 19—26. https://doi.org/10.1016/j.jep.2004.05.023.

Rouillard, G., Guého, J., 1999. Les plantes et leur histoire à l'Ile Maurice. MSM, Mauritius.

Shawka, A., 2012a. Terminalia Bentzoe — Bois Benjoin — Mauritian Tree. Available online: https://commons.wikimedia.org/wiki/File:Terminalia_bentzoe_-_Bois_Benjoin_-_Mauritian_tree_11.jpg. (CC BY-SA 3.0).

Shawka, A., 2012b. Terminalia Bentzoe — Bois Benjoin — Mauritian Tree. Available online: https://commons.wikimedia.org/wiki/File:Terminalia_bentzoe_-_Bois_Benjoin_-_Mauritian_tree_2.jpg. (CC BY-SA 3.0).

Wickens, G.E., 1976. Notes on *Terminalia* (Combretaceae) and *Memecylon* (Melastomataceae) for the "Flore des Mascareignes". Kew Bulletin 31, 1—4. https://doi.org/10.2307/4108990.

Wickens, G.E., 1990. 91. Combrétacées. In: Bosser, J., Cadet, T., Guého, J., Marais, W. (Eds.), Flore des Mascareignes — La Réunion, Maurice, Rodrigues. MSIRI/ORSTOM/KEW. Imprimerie de Montligeon, France.

Terminalia prunioides

Fatimah Lawal, Thilivhali E. Tshikalange

Department of Plant and Soil Sciences, University of Pretoria, Pretoria, Gauteng, South Africa

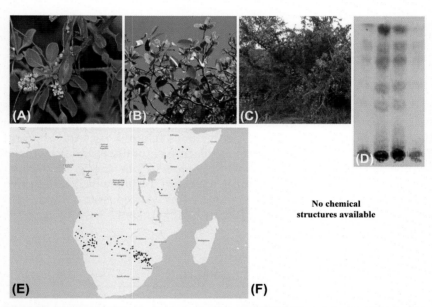

No chemical
structures available

FIGURE 43 Seeds of *Terminalia prunioides* (Dupont, 2013a) (A), aerial parts of *T. prunioides* (Aardvark, 2008) (B), a specimen of *T. prunioides* (Dupont, 2013b) (C), TLC chromatogram, Lane 1; *T. prunioides* acetone extract, Lane 2; *T. prunioides* hexane extract, Lane 3; *T. prunioides* dichloromethane extracts, Lane 4; *T. prunioides* methanol extracts (D), distribution of *T. prunioides* within sub-Saharan Africa (GBIF, 2018) (E), no chemical compounds have been reported (F).

Underexplored Medicinal Plants from Sub-Saharan Africa
https://doi.org/10.1016/B978-0-12-816814-1.00043-0

1. General description

1.1 Botanical nomenclature

Terminalia prunioides M.A. Lawson

1.2 Botanical family

Combretaceae

1.3 Vernacular names

Purple-pod terminalia/purple-pod cluster leaf (English)
Bloedboom/Hardekoolboom (Afrikaans)
Mutsiara (North Sotho)
Mutwari (Venda)

2. Botanical description

T. prunioides exists as a small shrub or medium-sized tree (2.5–15 m) which sometimes bears more than one stem (multistemmed) and droopy branches that spread outward. Spines are sometimes seen to be present on the branches or long shoots. It is sometimes referred to as the Lowveld *Terminalia* or Lowveld cluster leaf as they are naturally found growing in bushvelds. In South Africa, flowering occurs from spring to summer producing oval, flat-winged, purple to deep red fruits which turn brown when dried. The species name *prunioides* was derived from a Latin word used to describe its brightly colored plumlike fruits (Orwa et al., 2009; Tropical Plant Database).

3. Distribution

T. prunioides is native to South Africa, found in the areas of Limpopo and Mpumalanga (Foden and Potter, 2005). It is also native to several other Southern and Eastern African countries such as Lesotho, Mozambique, Swaziland, Tanzania, Zambia, Zimbabwe, Ethiopia, Botswana, Kenya, and Angola. It is found growing on frost-free sandy soils, coastal bushland, stony slopes, alluvial planes, riverine thickets, or saline areas (Strohbach, 2000).

4. Ethnobotanical usage

In Southern African traditional medicine, *T. prunioides* has been reported to be used in the treatment of several human ailments. The stem bark and hypogenous organs are used in the treatment of common colds, cough, sore throat, diarrhea, constipation, and stomach ache (Urso et al., 2016). Decoctions from the plant are used for postnatal abdominal pain and backaches (Adebayo et al., 2015).

5. Phytochemical constituents

To the best of our knowledge, no studies have been conducted on the phytochemistry and chemical constituent of this plant. However, several bioactive compounds have been isolated from other species in the *Terminalia* genus. Thin layer chromatography (TLC) fingerprinting also revealed that *T. prunioides* may share some similar constituents with other *Terminalia* species (Masoko et al., 2005). A preliminary phytochemical screening by Adebayo et al. (2015) indicated the presence of a higher amount of phenolic content (79 mg/g gallic acid equivalent) in the acetone leaf extract.

6. TLC fingerprinting of plant extract

Leaf material was extracted separately with hexane, dichloromethane (DCM), acetone, and methanol. The filtrate was placed under a fume hood at room temperature to remove excess solvent. A preweighed quantity of the resultant extracts was dissolved in a suitable solvent and used for TLC fingerprinting. One hundred micrograms of each reconstituted extract (10 mg/mL) were spotted as bands on thin layer chromatography (TLC) plates. The bands were spotted at least 1 cm from the base of the plates to avoid washback of the loaded samples. The TLC plate was placed in saturated TLC tanks using a solvent system which included; chloroform/ethyl acetate/formic acid (CEF; 5:4:1). The TLC plates were left in the developing tank until the solvent reached a solvent front at least 1 cm from the top of the plate. Once developed, the plates were allowed to dry and then observed under ultraviolet (UV) light at 254 and 360 nm. To detect compounds not visible under UV light, the TLC plates were sprayed with a solution of vanillin/sulfuric acid (2%) and heated using a heat gun (Masoko et al., 2005).

7. Pharmacological properties

T. prunioides has not been extensively studied for its biological activity and phytochemistry. A few studies on the biological activities recorded for leaves of this plant are thus highlighted. No studies were found on stem or root bark of the plant.

7.1 Antifungal and antioxidant activity

Leaves of *T. prunioides* were collected from the Lowveld Botanical Garden, Nelspruit, South Africa. Shade-dried leaves were milled and extracted using hexane, DCM, acetone, and methanol. The antifungal activity of the extracts was tested using five clinically important fungal species (*Aspergillus fumigatus*, *Candida albicans*, *Cryptococcus neoformans* var. *gattii*, *Sporothrix schenckii*, and *Microsporum canis*) which have been implicated in several animal diseases. All extracts from *T. prunioides* showed very good antifungal activity against the tested species with minimum inhibitory concentration (MIC) ranging between 0.02 and 0.64 mg/mL. However, at 48 h incubation time, the inhibition of *A. fumigatus* was reversed (MIC of 2.5 mg/mL) which was attributed to the possible degradation of antifungal compounds with time (Masoko et al., 2005).

A follow-up study by Masoko and Eloff (2005) reported on a bio-autographic investigation of antifungal compounds present in hexane, DCM, acetone, and methanol leaf extracts of *T. prunioides*. TLC plates were spotted with 100 µg of the extracts and developed using three solvent systems. The plates were sprayed with five fungal microorganisms as listed above. A varying degree of antifungal activity was observed for the different compounds which were eluted with the solvent systems. A compound with an RF value of 0.46 eluted in the benzene/ethanol/ammonium hydroxide (BAE) system was reported to be very active on all the tested microorganisms. Another compound from the acetone extract with an RF value of 0.97 eluted in the CEF solvent system showed potent inhibition against *C. albicans*.

Another study was conducted by the same group (Masoko and Eloff, 2007) to determine the antioxidant potential of the hexane, DCM, acetone, and methanol extracts of the leaves using the diphenylpicrylhydrazyl (DPPH) radical scavenging assay. A strong radical scavenging activity was observed with the acetone extracts, while the methanol extract showed moderate activity. Both the hexane and DCM extract did not show significant DPPH scavenging activity.

7.2 Antibacterial activity

Antibacterial activities of the acetone leaf extract were tested against *Staphylococcus aureus* (American type culture collection (ATCC) 29123), *Escherichia coli* (ATCC 27853), *Enterococcus faecalis* (ATCC 29212), and *Pseudomonas aeruginosa* (ATCC 25922). Moderate antibacterial activity was observed with the best inhibitory activity against *S. aureus* and *E. faecalis* (MIC: 0.3 mg/mL). However, storage of the plant extract (6 week duration) resulted in a sharp decline (MIC: 2.3 mg/mL) in antibacterial activity (Eloff, 1999).

7.3 Antiinflammatory

The 15-lipoxygenase (15-LOX) inhibitory activity of the acetone extract from leaves of *T. prunioides* was assessed. Leaves used in the study were collected from the Manie van der Schijff Botanical Garden situated at the University of Pretoria, South Africa. 15-LOX activity was tested in the presence of a suitable substrate (linoleic acid), and the ability of the extract to inhibit product formation was monitored at 234 nm. Acetone extract of *T. prunioides* showed moderate inhibitory effect on the enzyme activity. The 50% inhibitory concentration (IC_{50}) was graphically represented to be within the range of 37–40 µg/mL (Adebayo et al., 2015).

8. Additional information

8.1 Therapeutic (proposed) usage

Antiinflammatory, antibacterial, antifungal, and antioxidant

8.2 Safety data

Not available

8.3 Trade information

Not threatened, not endangered, least concerned, and very abundant

8.4 Dosage

Not applicable

References

Aardvark, 2008. *Terminalia porphyrocarpa* Foliage and Flowers.Jpg, Mount Archer National Park, Rockhampton. Available online: https://commons.wikimedia.org/wiki/File: Terminalia_porphyrocarpa_foliage_and_flowers.jpg. (CC BY-SA 3.0).

Adebayo, S.A., Dzoyem, J.P., Shai, L.J., Eloff, J.N., 2015. The anti-inflammatory and antioxidant activity of 25 plant species used traditionally to treat pain in Southern African. BMC Complementary and Alternative Medicine 15, 159. https://doi.org/10.1186/s12906-015-0669-5.

Dupont, 2013a. Bobbejaan Krans, H7 Road West of Satara, Kruger NP, South Africa. Available online: https://commons.wikimedia.org/wiki/File:Purple-pod_Cluster-leaf_(Terminalia_prunioides)_(12026220083).jpg. (CC BY-SA 2.0).

Dupont, 2013b. Bobbejaan Krans, H7 Road West of Satara, Kruger NP, South Africa. Available online: https://commons.wikimedia.org/wiki/File:Purple-pod_Cluster-leaf_(Terminalia_prunioides)_(12026190183).jpg. (CC BY-SA 2.0).

Eloff, J.N., 1999. The antibacterial activity of 27 southern African members of the Combretaceae. South African Journal of Science 95, 148–152.

Foden, W., Potter, L., 2005. Terminalia Prunioides M.A.Lawson. National Assessment: Red List of South African Plants Version 2017.1. http://redlist.sanbi.org/species.php?species=2037-3.

GBIF, 2018. Terminalia Prunioides M.A.Lawson in GBIF Secretariat (2017). GBIF Backbone Taxonomy. Checklist dataset. https://doi.org/10.15468/39omei.

Masoko, P., Eloff, J.N., 2005. The diversity of antifungal compounds of six South African *Terminalia* species (Combretaceae) determined by bioautography. African Journal of Biotechnology 4, 1425–1431.

Masoko, P., Eloff, J.N., 2007. Screening of twenty-four South African medicinal *Combretum* and six *Terminalia* species (Combretaceae) for antiloxidant activities. African Journal of Traditional, Complementary and Alternative Medicines 4, 231–239.

Masoko, P., Picard, J., Eloff, J.N., 2005. Antifungal activities of six South African *Terminalia* species (Combretaceae). Journal of Ethnopharmacology 99, 301–308. https://doi.org/10.1016/j.jep.2005.01.061.

Orwa, C., Mutua, A., Kindt, R., Jamnadass, R., Anthony, S., 2009. Agroforestree Database: A Tree Reference and Selection Guide Version 4.0. http://www.worldagroforestry.org/sites/treedbs/treedatabases.asp.

Strohbach, B.J., 2000. Vegetation degradation trends in the northern Oshikoto Region : III. The Terminalia *prunioides* woodlands and Andoni grasslands Vegetation degradation trends in the northern Oshikoto Region : III. The *Terminalia prunioides* woodlands and Andoni grasslands. Dinteria 26, 77–92.

Tropical Plants Database, 2018. http://www.tropical.theferns.info/viewtropical.php?id=Terminalia+prunioides.

Urso, V., Adele, M., Tonini, M., Bruschi, P., 2016. Wild medicinal and food plants used by communities living in Mopane woodlands of southern Angola: results of an ethnobotanical field investigation. Journal of Ethnopharmacology 177, 126–139.

Vigna unguiculata

Sipho H. Chauke, Quenton Kritzinger

Department of Plant and Soil Sciences, University of Pretoria, Pretoria, Gauteng, South Africa

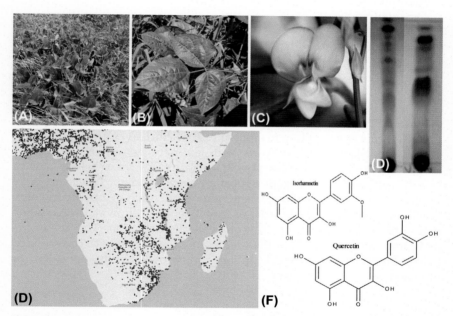

FIGURE 44   Aerial parts of *Vigna unguiculata* (CSIRO, 2006) (A), leaves of *V. unguiculata* (CSIRO, 2006) (B), flower of *V. unguiculata* (Rose, 2011) (C), TLC chromatogram, Lane 1; *V. unguiculata* leaf extract, Lane 2; *V. unguiculata* seed extract (D), distribution of *V. unguiculata* in sub-Saharan Africa (GBIF, 2017) (E), chemical structures of isorhamnetin and quercetin (F).

Underexplored Medicinal Plants from Sub-Saharan Africa
https://doi.org/10.1016/B978-0-12-816814-1.00044-2

1. General description

1.1 Botanical nomenclature

Vigna unguiculata (L.) Walp

1.2 Botanical family

Fabaceae/Leguminosae

1.3 Vernacular names

Cowpea (English)
Akkerboon (Afrikaans)
Imbumba (Zulu)
Dinawe (Ndebele)
Monawa (Pedi)
Munawa (Venda)

2. Botanical description

V. unguiculata is a dicotyledonous annual herb, which varies in growth forms from trailing to erect or bushy. The leaves are usually dark green, linear lanceolate to ovate, with leaf petioles ranging between 5 and 25 cm long. The leaves are alternate except for the first pair of leaves, which are arranged opposite to each other. The flowers of *V. unguiculata* can be yellow, white, pale blue, pink, or purple in color. The fruit occurs in pods, which are usually either yellow or brown when ripe. The seeds often vary in color, shape, and size. The seeds are 2—12 mm long. The testa of the seeds can either be smooth or wrinkled in combination with a black, green, red, brown, white, speckled, or blotched color (DAFF, 2011).

3. Distribution

V. unguiculata is widely cultivated in Niger, Cameroon, Ghana, Mali, Zimbabwe, Burkina Faso, United States of America, Brazil, West Indies, India, Myanmar, Nigeria, and Senegal. In South Africa, it is widely cultivated in the Limpopo, Mpumalanga, North-West and KwaZulu Natal provinces, but mostly at the hands of smallholder farmers (Brader, 2002; DAFF, 2011).

4. Ethnobotanical usage

In Zimbabwe, a decoction of cowpea seeds together with the roots of *Euclea divinorum* or *T. sericea* is taken orally for the treatment of urinary schistosomiasis (Bilharzia) (Nyameza, 1987). In South Africa, the leaves are chewed and applied onto burns and taken in a powder form as a snuff for the treatment of headaches (Gestner, 1939 as cited by Hutchings et al., 1996). Other ethnobotanical uses include emetics (made from the leaves), which are taken for relief of fevers. The seeds are used to treat liver complaints associated with jaundice and as an anthelmintic and as a diuretic (Noorwala et al., 1995). The root paste is also used as an antidote for snake bites, whereas the root infusion is used for the relief of constipation in infants (van Wyk and Gericke, 2000).

5. Phytochemical constituents

A few compounds have been isolated from cowpea leaves and seeds. The compounds which have been isolated from the methanolic seed extracts include 3-O-[α-L-rhamnopyranosyl-(1 → 4)-β-D-galactopyranosyl-(1 → 4)-β-D-glucunopyranosyl]-soyaspogenal B, cycloartenol, stigmasterol, 3-O-acetyloleonic acid, and sitosterol 3-β-D-glucoside. The compounds which have been isolated from the leaf extracts include quercetin, kaempferol, isorhamnetin, caffeic acid, vanillic acid, p-coumaric acid, ferulic acid, cinnamic acid, sinapinic acid, protocatechuic acid, and apigenin (Cai et al., 2003; Lattanzio et al., 2000). Compounds such as coumestrol, daidzein, and genistein have also been isolated from the root extracts of cowpeas (Isobe et al., 2001).

In a study by Zia-Ul-Haq et al. (2013), methanolic seed extracts were evaluated for the total phenolic content and condensed tannin content. The extracts showed higher total phenolic content (11.9–19.32 mg/g) and higher condensed tannin content (14.9–25.4 mg/g) when compared with the content of *Cicer arietinum* (chickpea) seed extracts (Zia-Ul-Haq et al., 2013).

6. TLC fingerprinting of plant extract

The separation of the different phytochemicals present in the leaf and seed extracts of *V. unguiculata* was observed by weighing out 2 mg of each of the leaf- and seed-dried ethanolic extracts. The extracts were dissolved in 200 μL of ethanol. The analysis of the leaf and seed extracts of *V. unguiculata* was done using silica gel 60 F254 thin layer chromatography (TLC) plates. The plates were marked with a soft pencil 1 cm from the top and 1 cm from the bottom of the plate. The extracts were spotted along the bottom line of the TLC plate using glass capillaries. The spots were allowed to dry completely before placing the TLC plates in a chromatography tank containing 10 mL eluent of 7:3 hexane:ethyl acetate as the solvent system. The developed plates were allowed to dry and then viewed under ultraviolet light (short and long wavelength). The plates were sprayed with vanillin\sulfuric acid (2%) solution.

7. Pharmacological properties

The in vivo and in vitro medicinal properties of *V. unguiculata* have not been extensively studied. However, because it is widely cultivated, there are research opportunities regarding this plant.

7.1 Antibacterial activity and antifungal activity

The leaf extracts of two cowpea cultivars (Bechwana white [BW] and Kpodjiguegue [Kpod]) were investigated by Kritzinger et al. (2005) for their antimicrobial activity. Seeds of the two cultivars were obtained from the Agricultural Research Council-Grain Crops Institute, Potchefstroom (South Africa) and a market in Cotonou (Benin), respectively. The seeds were then planted in a greenhouse, and the leaves from the plants were collected after 2 months.

The crude acetone and ethanol extracts were investigated for their antibacterial activity against gram-positive bacteria, including *Bacillus cereus*, *B. pumilus*, *B. subtilis*, *Staphylococcus aureus*, and *Enterococcus faecalis*, and gram-negative bacteria, namely *Enterobacter cloacae*, *Escherichia coli*, *Klebsiella pneumoniae*, *Pseudomonas aeruginosa*, and *Serratia marcescens*. The ethanolic extracts of BW showed moderate (<5.0 mg/mL) activity against *E. faecalis* and *E. cloacae*, whereas the acetone extract showed moderate (<5.0 mg/mL) activity against *B. cereus*, *B. subtilis*, *S. aureus*, *E. faecalis*, and *E. cloacae*. The acetone and ethanol leaf extracts of the Kpod cultivar showed no activity against all the treated bacteria (Kritzinger et al., 2005).

Furthermore, the crude acetone and ethanol extracts were evaluated for their antifungal activity against plant pathogens including *Aspergillus flavus*, *Alternaria alternata*, *Fusarium equiseti*, *Fusarium proliferatum*, and *Penicillium chrysogenum*. The extracts of both cultivars showed moderate (≤5.0 mg/mL) fungal growth inhibition against all the test fungal cultures except for *F. equiseti*. However, the ethanolic extract of BW is the only extract that showed moderate antifungal activity against *F. equiseti*.

The acetone and ethanolic extracts of BW were able to reduce the growth of *A. alternata* at an extract concentration of 2.5 mg/mL. Similarly, the ethanolic extract of BW was able to reduce the growth of *F. proliferatum* at the same concentration. The pod acetone extract was also able to reduce the growth of *A. alternata* at the same concentration (2.5 mg/mL) when compared with the control (Kritzinger et al., 2005).

7.2　Antidiabetic activity

The antidiabetic activity of cowpea seeds was evaluated by Ashraduzzaman et al. (2011). The cowpea seeds were collected from Rajshahi City, Bangladesh, in 2007 and the seed oil was extracted from the collected seeds using the Soxhlet method. The oil extracted from the seeds was then formulated into an oral hypoglycemic drug, which was orally administered to alloxan-induced diabetic rats. This study indicated that the cowpea seed oil extracts decrease the blood glucose level in alloxan-induced diabetic rats when compared with the control rats (Ashraduzzaman et al., 2011).

7.3　Antioxidant activity

The methanolic seed extract of *V. unguiculata* was evaluated for its antioxidant activity using the ferric-reducing antioxidant power assay (FRAP), oxygen radical absorbing capacity assay (ORAC), and diphenylpicrylhydrazyl (DHHP) radical scavenging bioassays (Zia-Ul-Haq et al., 2013). The FRAP values were reported to range between 13.2 and 19.4 mM Fe^{2+}/g, while the ORAC values ranged between 83.8 and 96.2 μM Trolox/g. The DPPH antioxidant scavenging capacity values ranged between 25.1 and 32.5 μM Trolox/g (Zia-Ul-Haq et al., 2013).

8.　Additional information

8.1　Therapeutic (proposed) usage

Antibacterial and antidiabetic

8.2　Safety data

Not available

8.3　Trade information

Not evaluated (not threatened, not endangered, and abundant)

8.4 Dosage

Not available

References

Ashraduzzaman, M.D., Ashraful Alam, M.D., Khatun, S., Banu, S., Absar, N., 2011. *Vigna unguiculata* Linn. Walp. seed oil exhibiting antidiabetic effects in alloxan induced rats. Malaysian Journal of Pharmaceutical Sciences 9, 13–23.

Brade, L., 2002. Foreword. In: Fatokun, C.A., Tarawali, S.A., Singh, B.B., Kormawa, P.M., Tamo, M. (Eds.), Challenges and Opportunities for Enhancing Sustainable Cowpea Production, Proceedings of the 3rd World Cowpea Conference, 4-8 September 2000, Ibadan. International Institute of Tropical Agriculture (IITA), Ibadan, pp. 351–366.

Cai, R., Hettiarachchy, H.S., Jalaluddin, M., 2003. High performance liquid chromatography determination of phenolic constituents in 17 varieties of cowpeas. Journal of Agricultural and Food Chemistry 51, 1623–1627.

CSIRO, 2006. Cowpea Flower. https://commons.wikimedia.org/wiki/File:CSIRO_Science1 Image_2927_Cowpea_flower.jpg.

DAFF (Department of Agriculture, Forestry and Fisheries), 2011. Production Guidelines for Cowpeas, pp. 1–5. www.arc.agric.za/arcgci/Fact%20Sheets%20Library/Cowpea%20%20Production%20guidelines%20for%20cowpea.pdf.

GBIF, 2017. *Vigna unguiculata* Walp. In: GBIF Secretariat. GBIF Backbone Taxonomy. Checklist dataset. https://doi.org/10.15468/39omei. Accessed via GBIF.org.

Gestner, J., 1939. In: Hutchings, A., Haxton Scott, A., Lewis, G., Cunningham, A.B. (Eds.), Zulu Medicinal Plants: An Inventory, vol. 146. University of Natal Press, Scottsville, South Africa, ISBN 086-980-893-1.

Hutchings, A., Haxton Scott, A., Lewis, G., Cunningham, A.B., 1996. Zulu Medicinal Plants: An Inventory. University of Natal Press, Scottsville, p. 146.

Isobe, K., Tateishi, A., Nomura, K., Inoue, H., Tsuboki, Y., 2001. Flavonoids in the extract and exudates of the roots in leguminous crops. Plant Production Science 4, 278–279.

Kritzinger, Q., Lall, N., Aveling, T.A.S., 2005. Antimicrobial activity of cowpea (*Vigna unguiculata*) leaf extracts. South African Journal of Botany 71, 45–48.

Lattanzio, V., Arpaia, S., Cardinalli, A., Di Venere, D., Linsalata, V., 2000. Role of endogenous flavonoids in resistance mechanisms of Vigna to aphids. Journal of Agricultural and Food Chemistry 48, 5316–5320.

Noorwala, M., Mohammad, F.V., Ahmad, V.U., 1995. A new monodesmosidic terpenoid saponin from the seeds of *Vigna unguiculata* subsp. *unguiculata*. Journal of Natural Products 58, 1070–1074.

Nyazema, N.Z., 1987. Medicinal plants of wide use in Zimbabwe. In: Leewenberg, A.J.M. (Ed.), Medicinal and Poisonous Plants of the Tropics: Proceedings of the Symposium of the 14th International Botanical Congress, Berlin, Pudoc, Wageningen, ISBN 902-200-921-1, pp. 36–43.

Rose, H., 2011a. *Vigna unguiculata* Leaf1. https://commons.wikimedia.org/wiki/File:Vigna_unguiculata_leaf1_(10737426723).jpg.

Rose, H., 2011b. *Vigna unguiculata* Habitat7. https://commons.wikimedia.org/wiki/File:Vigna_unguiculata_habit7_(10736971714).jpg.

van Wyk, B.-E., Gericke, N., 2000. People's Plants: A Guide to Useful Plants in Southern Africa. Briza Publications, Pretoria, ISBN 187-509-319-2, p. 192.

Zia-Ul-Haq, M., Ahmad, S., Amarowicz, R., De Feo, V., 2013. Antioxidant activity of the extracts of some cowpea (*Vigna unguiculata* (L.) Walp.) cultivars commonly consumed in Pakistan. Molecules 18, 2005–2017.

Further reading

ARC (Agricultural Research Council), 2014. Cowpeas (*Vigna unguiculata*). www.arc.agric.za/arc-gci/Pages/Cowpeas.aspx.

Lattanzio, V., Cardinalli, A., Linsalata, V., Perrino, P., Ng, N.Q., 1997. Flavonoid HPLC fingerprints of wild Vigna species. In: Singh, B.B., Mohan Raj, D.R., Dashiell, K.E., Jackai, L.E.N. (Eds.), Advances in Cowpea Research. Co-publication of the International Institute of Tropical Agriculture (IITA) and Japan International Research Center for Agricultural Sciences (JIRCA), IIA, Ibadan, Nigeria, ISBN 978-131-110-X, pp. 66—74.

SANBI, 2017. *Vigna unguiculata* (L.) Walp. subsp. *unguiculata*. National Assessment: Red List of South African Plants. www.redlist.sanbi.org. http://redlist.sanbi.org/species.php?species=417-4012.

CHAPTER

45

Wikstroemia indica

Shanoo Suroowan, Fawzi Mahomoodally

Department of Health Sciences, Faculty of Science, University of Mauritius, Réduit, Mauritius

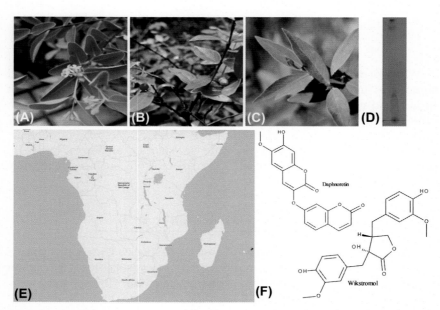

FIGURE 45   Aerial plant parts of *Wikstroemia indica* (A, B), close-up view of the leaves (Marathon, 2016) (C), TLC chromatogram of *W. indica* (D), distribution of *W. indica* in sub-Saharan Africa (GBIF, 2018) (E), chemical structures of daphnoretin and wikstromol (F).

Underexplored Medicinal Plants from Sub-Saharan Africa
https://doi.org/10.1016/B978-0-12-816814-1.00045-4

1. General description

1.1 Botanical nomenclature

Wikstroemia indica (L.) C.A. Mey

1.2 Botanical family

Thymelaeaceae

1.3 Vernacular names

Liaogewang (China)
Indian stringbush
Tiebush (Australia)
Herbe tourterelle (Mauritius)

2. Botanical description

W. indica develops as a shrub growing between 1 and 2 m in height and sometimes taller. The branches originating from the plant are reddish brown and glabrous. The plant bears leaves which are opposite to each other, obovate, elliptic-oblong or lanceolate, papery to thinly leathery with both surfaces being glabrous, base broadly or narrowly cuneate, apex obtuse or acute; lateral veins dense, slender, at narrow angle to midrib. The leaves become reddish brown on both surfaces when dry (MOBOT, 2002).

3. Distribution

The genus *Wikstroemia* consists of around 70 species widely distributed in Oceania, Southeastern Asia, and the Pacific islands. *W. indica* is resident in several countries including Australia, China, India, Indonesia, Malaysia, Papua New Guinea, Philippines, Taiwan, Thailand, and Vietnam. In China, the plant is common in the Fujian, Guangdong, Hunan, Jiangxi, and Zhejiang provinces (Li et al., 2009). In addition, the plant has been naturalized in Mauritius and Rodrigues Island (NGRP, 2002; Lorence and Sussman, 1988).

4. Ethnobotanical usage

In China, the residents widely employ the plant for diverse ailment conditions mostly for the treatment of arthritis, cancer, syphilis, and whooping cough (Lu et al., 2012). In Southern China, it was a common practice to add *W. indica* to broth to maintain overall health. The leaves are cooked in lentils and consumed as a soup in Mauritius and given to anemic individuals (Sussman, 1980; Gurib-Fakim, 2002). They are also employed as an abortifacient in clinical practice (Rahman 2015).

5. Phytochemical constituents

Plants from the genus *Wikstroemia* are reported to be rich in coumarins, flavonoids, lignans, and sesquiterpenes. Initial investigations on the plant led to the isolation of daphnoretin and the central nervous system depressant (+)-nortrachelogenin. In furtherance, the following antileukemic agents were also isolated from the plant: tricin and kaempferol-3-0-pDglucopyranoside (Lee et al., 1981). Other secondary metabolites extracted from the roots include genkwanol A, wikstrol A, wikstrol B, and daphnodorin B (Hu et al., 2000). The stem rind of the plant was found to contain daphnoretin-7-O-beta-D-glucoside, quercitin, physcion, kaempferol 3-rutinoside, D-primev-ersyl genkwanine, and anabellamide (Geng et al., 2006). Recently, six novel compounds namely acetylwikstresinol, bis-5',5'-(+)-matairesinol, bis-5,5'-(+)-matairesinol, wikstronin A, wikstronin B, and wikstresinol have been isolated from the dichloromethane extract of the roots of *W. indica* (Chang et al., 2017).

6. TLC fingerprinting of plant extract

Thin layer chromatography (TLC) fingerprint is provided in Figure 45 (D).

7. Pharmacological properties

According to available literature, the plant is reported to exert a wide array of pharmacological properties including antibacterial, -diarrheal, -inflammatory, -malarial, and -viral as well as being cytotoxic (Chang et al., 2017; Lu et al., 2011).

7.1 Antidiarrheal activity

Rahman (2015) investigated the antidiarrheal potential of the leaf extract of *W. indica* in vivo. Diarrhea was induced in Wistar albino rats employing castor oil and enteropooling assays. Using the gastrointestinal motility assays, the antidiarrheal activity of the leaf extracts was determined. The methanolic extract showed significant antidiarrheal activity at a dose of 200 and 400 mg/kg by inhibiting diarrhea by 18.64% and 28.96% respectively.

7.2 Anti-inflammatory activity

The antiinflammatory activity of the *W. indica* was evaluated employing the mice RAW264.7 cell model and was based on the production of nitric oxide stimulated by lipopolysaccharide following which nitrogen monoxidum was released. The ethyl acetate extract of the root of *W. indica* demonstrated good antiinflammatory activity (50% inhibitory concentration (IC$_{50}$) of 40.19 µg/mL) in comparison with the n-butanol and water-soluble fractions (IC$_{50}$ for both extracts was greater than 100 µg/mL) which demonstrated no activity. This concludes that the ethyl acetate extract of the root significantly inhibits the biosynthesis of nitric oxide in mouse monocyte macrophage (RAW264.7) cells stimulated by lipopolysaccharide (Lu et al., 2012).

7.3 Antimicrobial activity

A study characterized the antimicrobial activity of the rhizome of *W. indica* both qualitatively and quantitatively. Crude flavonoids in three different concentrations (0.106, 0.425, and 0.85 g/mL) from *W. indica* were assayed for their antimicrobial activities on three different bacterial species; *Staphylococcus aureus*, *Escherichia coli*, and *Mucor racemosus*, respectively. The extracts were completely inactive against *M. racemosus* and were ineffective at their lowest concentration employed (0.106 g/mL) against *S. aureus* and *E. coli*. Nonetheless, while the extract concentration was increased from 0.425 to 0.85 g/mL, growth of *S. aureus* and *E. coli* was inhibited in a dose-dependent manner. In addition, minimum inhibitory concentration (MIC) noted against *S. aureus* and *E. coli* were 53 and 106.25 mg/mL, respectively (Lu et al., 2012).

7.4 Anticancer activity

The rhizome of *W. indica* is rich in the bis-coumarin daphnoretin. This metabolite was assayed for its cytotoxic activity against four types of cancer cell lines: adenocarcinomic human alveolar basal epithelial cells (A549), nasopharyngeal carcinoma cell line (CNE), cervical carcinoma (HeLa), and human epithelial type 2 (HEp-2), respectively. Interestingly, significant inhibitory activity was noted against CNE and HeLa cell lines in a dose-dependent fashion between the concentrations of 15.6 and

125 µg/mL. In addition, the proliferation of A549 was restrained at a concentration of 31.25 µg/mL.

On the other hand, daphnoretin was active against HEp-2 only at its highest concentration of 125 µg/mL employed in the study (Lu et al., 2012). Previously, studies had enabled establish the pathways through which daphnoretin exerts its cytotoxic activity. Indeed, an in vitro study conducted by Abou-Karam and Thomas Shier (1999) demonstrated that it is an inhibitor of the tyrosine-specific protein kinase of human epidermal growth factors. In another in vitro investigation by Handa et al. (1983), it was depicted to inhibit the P-388 lymphocytic leukemia. In furtherance, Chen et al. (1996) demonstrated that it strongly restrains human hepatoma Hep 3B cells from expressing the hepatitis B surface antigen.

8. Additional information

8.1 Therapeutic (proposed) usage

Antidiarrheal, anti-inflammatory, antimicrobial, anti-anemia, and anticancer

8.2 Safety data

A novel chalchone-flavone biflavonoid 3′-hydroxydaphnodorin A was isolated from the rhizome of the plant and showed moderate cytotoxic activity against the cellosaurus cell line (CNE-2) and liver hepatocellular carcinoma (HepG2) cell lines with 50% inhibitory concentration (IC_{50}) values of 53.6 ± 10.1 and 65.5 ± 11.4 µM, respectively (Shao et al., 2016).

When the toxicity of the herb was investigated, the aqueous and ethanolic extracts were assessed in mice. None of the samples demonstrated toxicity with maximal tolerance doses higher than 18.7, 11.7, and 25.0 g/kg p.o., respectively (Huang et al., 2009).

8.3 Trade information

Not threatened and not endangered

8.4 Dosage

Not available

References

Abou-Karam, M., Thomas Shier, W., 1999. Inhibition of oncogene product enzyme activity as an approach to cancer chemoprevention. Tyrosine-specific protein kinase inhibition by purpurogallin from *Quercus* sp. Nutgall. Phytotherapy Research: An International Journal Devoted to Pharmacological and Toxicological Evaluation of Natural Product Derivatives 13 (4), 337–340.

Chang, H., Wang, Y., Gao, X., Song, Z., Awale, S., Han, N., Liu, Z., Yin, J., 2017. Lignans from the root of *Wikstroemia indica* and their cytotoxic activity against PANC-1 human pancreatic cancer cells. Fitoterapia 121, 31–37.

Chen, H.C., Chou, C.K., Kuo, Y.H., Yeh, S.F., 1996. Identification of a protein kinase C (PKC) activator, daphnoretin that suppresses hepatitis B virus gene expression in human hepatoma cells. Biochemical Pharmacology 52 (7), 1025–1032.

GBIF, 2018. Wikstroemia Indica C.A.Mey. In GBIF Secretariat (2017). GBIF Backbone Taxonomy. Checklist dataset. https://doi.org/10.15468/39omei.

Geng, L.D., Zhang, C., Xiao, Y.Q., 2006. Studies on the chemical constituents in stem rind of *Wikstroemia indica*. Zhongguo Zhong yao za zhi= Zhongguo zhongyao zazhi. China journal of Chinese materia medica 31 (10), 817–819.

Gurib-Fakim, A., 2002. Mauritius through its Medicinal Plants. Editions La Printemps, Vacoas, Mauritius.

Handa, S.S., Kinghorn, A.D., Cordell, G.A., Farnsworth, N.R., 1983. Plant anticancer agents. XXVI. Constituents of *Peddiea fischeri*. Journal of Natural Products 46 (2), 248–250.

Hu, K., Kobayashi, H., Dong, A., Iwasaki, S., Yao, X., 2000. Antifungal, antimitotic and anti-HIV-1 agents from the roots of Wikstroemia indica. Planta medica 66 (06), 564–567.

Huang, W., Li, Y., Wang, H., Su, M., Jiang, Z., Ooi, V.E., Chung, H.Y., 2009. Toxicological study of a Chinese herbal medicine, *Wikstroemia indica*. Natural product communications 4 (9), 1227–1230.

Lee, K.H., Tagahara, K., Suzuki, H., Wu, R.Y., Haruna, M., Hall, I.H., Huang, H.C., Ito, K., Iida, T., Lai, J.S., 1981. Antitumor agents. 49. Tricin, kaempferol-3-0-β-D-gluco pyranoside and (+)-nortrachelogenin, antileukemic principles from *Wikstroemia indica*. Journal of Natural Products 44 (5), 530–535.

Li, Y.M., Zhu, L., Jiang, J.G., Yang, L., Wang, D.Y., 2009. Bioactive components and pharmacological action of *Wikstroemia indica* (L.) CA Mey and its clinical application. Current Pharmaceutical Biotechnology 10 (8), 743–752.

Lorence, D.H., Sussman, R.W., 1988. Diversity, density, and invasion in a Mauritian wet forest. Monographs of the Systematics of the Missouri Botanical Garden 25, 187–204.

Lu, C.L., Li, Y.M., Fu, G.Q., Yang, L., Jiang, J.G., Zhu, L., Lin, F.L., Chen, J., Lin, Q.S., 2011. Extraction optimisation of daphnoretin from root bark of *Wikstroemia indica* (L.) CA and its antitumour activity tests. Food Chemistry 124 (4), 1500–1506.

Lu, C.L., Zhu, L., Piao, J.H., Jiang, J.G., 2012. Chemical compositions extracted from *Wikstroemia indica* and their multiple activities. Pharmaceutical Biology 50 (2), 225–231.

Marathon, M., 2016. Wikstroemia Indica Foliage. Available online: https://commons.wikimedia.org/wiki/File:Wikstroemia_indica_foliage.jpg. (CC BY-SA 4.0).

Mobot, 2002. Missouri Botanic Garden (Mobot) W3TROPICOS. http://www.mobot.org/MOBOT/Research/alldb.shtml.

NGRP, 2002. World Economic Plants in GRIN (Germplasm Resources Information Network). United States Department of Agriculture, Agricultural Resources Service, National Germplasm Resources Program (NGRP), Beltsville.

Rahman, M.K., 2015. Antidiarrheal and thrombolytic effects of methanol extract of *Wikstroemia indica* (L.) CA Mey leaves. International Journal of Green Pharmacy 9 (1), 08–13.

Shao, M., Huang, X.J., Liu, J.S., Han, W.L., Cai, H.B., Tang, Q.F., Fan, Q., 2016. A new cytotoxic biflavonoid from the rhizome of *Wikstroemia indica*. Natural Product Research 30 (12), 1417–1422.

Sussman, L.K., 1980. Herbal medicine on Mauritius. Journal of Ethnopharmacology 2 (3), 259–278.

Further reading

National Center for Biotechnology Information, 2018. PubChem Compound Database, p. CID=394845. https://pubchem.ncbi.nlm.nih.gov/compound/394845.

Zantedeschia aethiopica

Karina Szuman, Namrita Lall

Department of Plant and Soil Sciences, University of Pretoria, Pretoria, Gauteng, South Africa

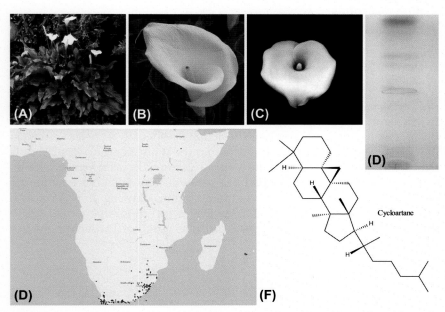

FIGURE 46   Aerial parts of *Zantedeschia aethiopica* (Dall'Orto, 2008a) (A), characteristic white spathe of *Z. aethiopica* (Heyde, 2007; Dall'Orto, 2008b) (B and C), TLC chromatogram, fingerprint of *Z. aethiopica* extract (D), distribution of *Z. aethiopica* in sub-Saharan Africa (GBIF, 2018) (E), chemical structure of cycloartane (F).

Underexplored Medicinal Plants from Sub-Saharan Africa
https://doi.org/10.1016/B978-0-12-816814-1.00046-6

303

1. General description

1.1 Botanical nomenclature

Zantedeschia aethiopica (L.) Spreng

1.2 Botanical family

Araceae

1.3 Vernacular names

White arum lily (English)
Wit varkoor (Afrikaans)
Intebe (Xhosa)
Ihlukwe (Zulu)
Mothebe (Sesotho)

2. Botanical description

Z. aethiopica is a perennial aquatic herb with fleshy rhizomes and stems. It thrives in very rich, well-drained soils. It is easily identifiable by its distinct white "flower" (spathe). The actual flower of *Z. aethiopica* exists on the yellow spadix (central column within the white spathe), which holds many tiny flowers arranged in a spiral pattern. *Z. aethiopica* has large evergreen leaves that are shaped like arrowheads which increase in size when grown in the shade. A unique adaption allowing *Z. aethiopica* to grow in wet environments is that its leaves can discharge excess water through their stomata in a process known as guttation, preventing water logging (Aubrey and Reynolds, 2001).

3. Distribution

The genus *Zantedeschia* is restricted to the African continent, making *Z. aethiopica* indigenous to South Africa. It is commonly found growing along the edges of streams, marshes, ponds, and swamps (areas where water is abundant). *Z. aethiopica* grows across South Africa, from the Western Cape through to the Eastern Cape and from KwaZulu-Natal to Mpumalanga and into the Northern Province (Aubrey and Reynolds, 2001; Khumbula Nursery, 2014).

4. Ethnobotanical usage

The washed leaves of Z. *aethiopica* are heated and used as a dressing for wounds, boils, minor burns, insect bites, and sores. Patients suffering from gout or rheumatism also use the warmed leaves as a poultice to reduce the pain. Traditional communities located in the Cape powder the dried rhizome of Z. *aethiopica* and use it as a poultice for inflamed wounds. The plant can be boiled and eaten by mixing it with honey or syrup as a treatment for asthma and bronchitis; it can also be gargled for the relief of sore throats. The plant must be boiled or cooked in some way as the raw plant material causes swelling of the throat due to the presence of microscopic calcium oxalate crystals (Watt and Breyer-Brandwijk, 1962; Roberts, 1990; Rood, 2008; Wink and van Wyk, 2008).

5. Phytochemical constituents

At present, several chemical constituents present within Z. *aethiopica* have been identified using spectroscopy, including 2 cycloartane triterpenes, 10 sterols, 3 lignans, and 10 phenylpropanoids (Della Greca et al., 1998). Bioactive phytochemicals such as tannins, alkaloids, saponins, steroids, phenols, and glycosides were found to be present within the rhizome of Z. *aethiopica* (Pratush et al., 2013).

6. TLC fingerprinting of plant extract

For observing the separation of compounds from Z. *aethiopica*, 2 mg of an ethanolic extract was weighed out and dissolved in 200 µL ethanol.

For the thin layer chromatography (TLC) analysis of Z. *aethiopica* crude extract, silica gel 60 F254 TLC plates were used to observe the separation of the compounds present within the extract. Plate markings were made with a soft pencil, and glass capillaries were used to spot the samples onto the TLC plate. The spot was left to dry completely before placing the plate in a TLC tank which contained 10 mL eluent 9.5:0.5 methanol:dichloromethane as the solvent system. The sample was allowed to separate until the solvent system reached 1 cm from the top of the TLC plate. The plate was observed under ultraviolet light (long and short wavelength), followed by spraying with freshly prepared vanillin/sulfuric acid (2%) to detect the bands on the TLC plate.

7. Pharmacological properties

Z. aethiopica has been relatively understudied. A few publications have looked into the pharmacological properties of this plant; however, there is still much left unknown about the medicinal properties of this plant which could lead to further research.

7.1 Antibacterial and antifungal activity

The methanolic extracts of the leaves and stems of *Z. aethiopica* were tested against various bacteria (*Mycobacterium*, gram-positive and gram-negative) and two fungal strains. The plant material used in this study was collected around the University of Pretoria campus during August of 2007.

The tested bacterial organisms included *Mycobacterium smegmatis* (American type culture collection [ATCC] 700084), methicillin-resistant *Staphylococcus aureus* (LMP805) (gram-positive bacterium), and four gram-negative bacteria namely β-lactamase positive (βL+) *Escherichia coli* (LMP701), ampicillin-resistant *Klebsiella pneumoniae* (LMP803), carbenicillin-resistant *Pseudomonas aeruginosa* (CRPA, LMP804), and chloramphenicol-resistant *Citrobacter* (CRCF, LMP802). The tested fungi included *Candida albicans* (LMP709U) and *Microsporum audouinii* (LMP725D).

The results showed that the methanolic crude extract of *Z. aethiopica* had no antibacterial activity against *M. smegmatis*, methicillin-resistant *S. aureus*, ampicillin-resistant *K. pneumoniae*, and chloramphenicol-resistant *Citrobacter* at the highest tested concentration of 2500 µg/mL. The extracts did, however, inhibit β-lactamase positive (βL+) *E. coli* and carbenicillin-resistant *P. aeruginosa* with a minimum inhibitory concentration (MIC) of 625 and 312.50 µg/mL, respectively (Nielsen et al., 2012). The plant extracts also showed antifungal activity against both *C. albicans* and *M. audouinii* with an MIC of 312.50 µg/mL, against both fungi.

7.2 Anticoagulant and antithrombotic activity

In a previous report, the leaves of *Z. aethiopica* were collected from the Eastern Cape, South Africa. Thereafter, aqueous (distilled water) and methanol extracts were prepared and tested for their antithrombotic activity using the thrombin assay, whereas the anticoagulant activity was tested using clotting time assays (thrombin-induced and $CaCl_2$-induced). Results indicated that in the presence of tannins, the aqueous leaf extracts showed antithrombotic activity with a 50% inhibitory concentration (IC_{50}) of 4.74 mg/mL; however, when the tannins from the extract were removed, the data could not be determined. Similarly with anticoagulant activity, in the presence of tannins, the aqueous and methanol leaf extracts of *Z. aethiopica* exhibited an IC_{50} of 2.45 and 5.27 mg/mL (thrombin-induced), respectively. However, when the tannins were removed, the aqueous extract showed anticoagulant activity through the inhibition of thrombin-induced clotting with an IC_{50} value of 3.05 mg/mL; no activity was observed in either case for $CaCl_2$-induced clotting (Kee et al., 2008).

8. Additional information

8.1 Therapeutic (proposed) usage

Antibacterial, antifungal, and anticoagulant

8.2 Safety data

Due to the presence of microscopic calcium oxalate crystals, before eating, *Z. aethiopica* must be boiled or cooked in some way as the raw plant material causes swelling of the throat (Aubrey and Reynolds, 2001).

8.3 Trade information

Not threatened, not endangered, and abundant

8.4 Dosage

Not available

References

Aubrey, A., Reynolds, Y., 2001. *Zantedeschia aethiopica* (L.) Spreng. Available online: http://www.plantzafrica.com/plantwxyz/zantedeschaeth.htm.

Dall'Orto, G., 2008a. Bush of Calla Lilies. Available online: https://commons.wikimedia.org/wiki/File:Pianta_di_calla._Foto_Giovanni_Dall%27Orto,_1-June-2006.jpg (The copyright holder of this file allows anyone to use it for any purpose, provided that the copyright holder is properly attributed. Redistribution, derivative work, commercial use, and all other use is permitted).

Dall'Orto, G., 2008b. Inflorescence of *Calla lily*. Picture by Giovanni Dall'Orto, June 1 2008. Available online: https://commons.wikimedia.org/wiki/File:Fiore_di_calla._Foto_Giovanni_Dall%27Orto,_1-June-2006_4.jpg (The copyright holder of this file allows anyone to use it for any purpose, provided that the copyright holder is properly attributed. Redistribution, derivative work, commercial use, and all other use is permitted).

GBIF, 2018. *Zantedeschia aethiopica* Spreng. In: GBIF Secretariat (2018). GBIF Backbone Taxonomy. Checklist dataset. https://doi.org/10.15468/39omei. Accessed via GBIF.org.

Della Greca, M., Ferrara, M., Fiorentino, A., Monaco, P., Previtera, L., 1998. Antialgal compounds from *Zantedeschia aethiopica*. Phytochemistry 49 (5), 1299—1304.

Heyde, M., 2007. Château de Cheverny, Loir-et-Cher, France - gardens, Zantedeschia. Available online: https://commons.wikimedia.org/wiki/File:Cheverny25.jpg.(CCBY-SA4.0).

Kee, N.L.A., Mnonopi, N., Davids, H., Naudé, R.J., Frost, C.L., 2008. Antithrombotic/anticoagulant and anticancer activities of selected medicinal plants from South Africa. African Journal of Biotechnology 7 (3), 217—223.

Khumbula Nursery, 2014. Zantedeschia aethiopica. http://kumbulanursery.co.za/plants/zantedeschia-aethiopica.

Nielsen, T.R.H., Kuete, V., Jäger, A.K., Meyer, J.J.M., Lall, N., 2012. Antimicrobial activity of selected South African medicinal plants. BMC Complementary and Alternative Medicine 12 (1), 74.

Pratush, A., Dogra, S., Gupta, A., 2013. Antimicrobial and phytochemical screening of rhizome extracts of some native medicinal plant of Himachal Pradesh (India). Applied Biological Research 15 (2), 149—153.

Roberts, M., 1990. Indigenous Healing Plants. Southern Book Publishers, South Africa.

Rood, B., 2008. Uit Die Veldepteek. Protea Boekhuis, Pretoria.

Watt, J.M., Breyer-Brandwijk, M.G., 1962. The Medicinal and Poisoness Plants of Southern and Eastern Africa, second ed. Livingstone, London.

Wink, M., van Wyk, B.E., 2008. Mind Altering and Poisonous Plants of the World. Briza, Pretoria.

Index

Note: 'Page numbers followed by "f" indicate figures'.

Printed in the United States
By Bookmasters